Gold Medal Nutrition

FIFTH EDITION

Glenn Cardwell, APD

Nutrition Impact

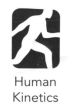

Human
Kinetics

Library of Congress Cataloging-in-Publication Data

Cardwell, Glenn, 1956-
  Gold medal nutrition / Glenn Cardwell. -- 5th ed.
    p. cm.
  Includes bibliographical references and index.
  ISBN 978-1-4504-1120-2 (soft cover) -- ISBN 1-4504-1120-7 (soft cover)
1. Athletes--Nutrition. I. Title.
  TX361.A8C35 2012
  613.2024'796--dc23

                              2012002719

ISBN-10: 1-4504-1120-7 (print)
ISBN-13: 978-1-4504-1120-2 (print)

The web addresses cited in this text were current as of January 2012, unless otherwise noted.

Acquisitions Editor: Peter Murphy; **Developmental Editor:** Anne Hall; **Assistant Editor:** Tyler Wolpert; **Copyeditor:** Patsy Fortney; **Indexer:** Alisha Jeddeloh; **Permissions Manager:** Martha Gullo; **Graphic Designer:** Nancy Rasmus; **Graphic Artist:** Tara Welsch; **Cover Designer:** Keith Blomberg; **Photographer (cover):** Axel Schmidt/Getty Images; **Photographer (interior):** © Human Kinetics; **Photo Asset Manager:** Laura Fitch; **Visual Production Assistant:** Joyce Brumfield; **Photo Production Manager:** Jason Allen; **Art Manager:** Kelly Hendren; **Associate Art Manager:** Alan L. Wilborn; **Illustrations:** © Human Kinetics, unless otherwise noted; **Printer:** Edwards Brothers Malloy

Human Kinetics books are available at special discounts for bulk purchase. Special editions or book excerpts can also be created to specification. For details, contact the Special Sales Manager at Human Kinetics.

Printed in the United States of America   10 9 8 7 6 5 4 3 2 1

The paper in this book is certified under a sustainable forestry program.

Human Kinetics
Website: www.HumanKinetics.com

United States: Human Kinetics
P.O. Box 5076
Champaign, IL 61825-5076
800-747-4457
e-mail: humank@hkusa.com

Canada: Human Kinetics
475 Devonshire Road Unit 100
Windsor, ON N8Y 2L5
800-465-7301 (in Canada only)
e-mail: info@hkcanada.com

Europe: Human Kinetics
107 Bradford Road
Stanningley
Leeds LS28 6AT, United Kingdom
+44 (0) 113 255 5665
e-mail: hk@hkeurope.com

Australia: Human Kinetics
57A Price Avenue
Lower Mitcham, South Australia 5062
08 8372 0999
e-mail: info@hkaustralia.com

New Zealand: Human Kinetics
P.O. Box 80
Torrens Park, South Australia 5062
0800 222 062
e-mail: info@hknewzealand.com

E5471

This edition is dedicated to Sports Dietitians Australia, the dietitians who created the organisation in 1996, and the team that keeps it a leading professional sports nutrition body today.

Contents

Foreword

Glenn and I live on opposite sides of a big country, so we sadly don't get to see each other that often. Recently, however, we got together to celebrate a happy occasion: the 15th anniversary of the creation of Sports Dietitians Australia, the professional body to which this book is dedicated. It can be quite jarring to look back over old photos of yourself. The clothes! The hair! (Except for Glenn, of course.) What were we thinking?

Gold Medal Nutrition is a testament to our changes in thinking about sports nutrition. The various editions track our progress in understanding the ways that nutrition can help an athlete achieve goals in training and competition. Like previous editions, the fifth edition provides the latest evidence-based information on eating for your best outcome in sport. It's all delivered in Glenn's expert style, which means that complicated stuff becomes understandable, even the most mundane stuff becomes memorable, and the factual stuff becomes practical to achieve.

I have always learned new things by reading *Gold Medal Nutrition*. Each successive edition has collated new or updated information, demonstrating the exciting and evolving nature of the science of sports nutrition. Who would have thought at the time of the fourth edition that we would be talking about beetroot juice or worrying about athletes who trained indoors? Yet nitrate supplementation and vitamin D status are now the hottest of topics at conferences and sports institutes.

Of course, data are only as good as the practice they allow or inspire. Here is where *Gold Medal Nutrition* is at its best. Glenn presents facts on sports nutrition with the insight of someone who has worked at the coalface of elite sport, understood the passion of the weekend warrior and been blessed with the skills of an entertainer. The book is filled with information that helps athletes translate concepts into activities and convert present eating patterns into better choices. I particularly enjoy the Final Score element. After you take the journey through the narrative and fascinating sidebars of each chapter, it is good to be able to cut straight to the bottom line and to check off your understanding.

It has been exciting to be part of the journey of sports nutrition and to see it has grown both in sophistication and recognition. *Gold Medal Nutrition* has played a role in this journey, and I hope to see the number of editions continue into double figures!

Louise Burke, OAM, PhD, APD
Fellow of SDA
Head of Sports Nutrition
for Australian Institute of Sport

Preface

Back in the early 1980s, a colleague of mine suggested we run a marathon. Purchasing the only two books we could find on eating and sport, we set about learning about the best nutrition to complete the distance. They told us that sports drinks were of little value, that fit people could safely lose 4 to 5 per cent of their body weight through sweating before their performance is affected and that athletes probably need less protein than sedentary people because they use protein more efficiently. These books were based on the very little research available at the time. Today, we know differently. There is a huge foundation of research on nutrition and hydration for sports performance, so our advice has greatly improved, yet there is so much more to learn. Now, virtually all elite athletes use the services and advice of sports dietitians and adhere to the nutrition guidelines in this book. Guidelines are the best anyone can offer in a book because athletes differ greatly. Some sweat heavily, whereas others seem to lose very little sweat; as a result, fluid intake advice is going to be different for different athletes. Some will respond to a creatine supplement; others won't. Specific monitoring by a sports dietitian will be invaluable, as will personal experimentation within the guidelines at training sessions.

This fifth edition of *Gold Medal Nutrition* is divided into three parts. Part I discusses the fuel systems used in generating muscle power and gives the principles of good nutrition for healthy body function. It then covers the key aspects of sports nutrition, such as how much carbohydrate, protein, fluid and the key minerals are needed for peak performance, whether for endurance, strength or speed. There has been both confusion and great debate about the athlete's needs for protein, carbohydrate and fluid, and this section makes a big effort to clarify the science.

Part II gets into the practical side of sports nutrition: cooking and the food purchasing habits needed to perform at one's best at training and in competition. Starting with the digestive process, it details the best times to eat meals and snacks so they enhance performance, and how to deal with the all-too-common gastrointestinal distress many athletes experience. You will learn the best nutrition to have before, during and after the event. One chapter discusses the best nutritional supplements for your sport and why some supplements are unlikely to improve your performance.

The final part covers a concern of most athletes—how to control their body fat stores and gain muscle, if necessary. This issue is perhaps the hardest for many athletes. The body seems to have a preconceived view of how much body fat to store. This level of body fat may not be what judges, coaches or the athlete deems ideal. Athletes sometimes must accept a compromise, as getting too lean can weaken performance just as can carrying too much body fat. Increasing muscle mass sounds simple in principle, but it is hard work, and there is a limit to what good nutrition can do. Weight training is going to be the main contributor to an increase in muscle mass.

The first edition of this book, written in 1996, was a small publication for fitness leaders and students looking for a simple explanation of the basics of nutrition for sports performance. The book became so popular that second and third editions were produced in 1999 and 2003. Readers said they loved it because, unlike a textbook, it was easy to read and understand, it was fun and it cut straight to the key points. With international interest, the fourth edition was taken over by Human Kinetics and was expanded to cater to all students of the topic. It was so popular that this fifth edition was requested. Although it has an Australasian bent, the principles are universal and are based on research conducted throughout the world.

Thanks must go to Chris Halbert for her continued support of the manual. I am most grateful to Mike Bahrke and Chris Drews for making the fourth edition a wonderful template for the fifth edition, admirably managed by Anne Hall. Their efforts have greatly improved the manual for an international audience. Many of my sports nutrition colleagues from around the globe have given me tips and ideas to place in the manual.

The members of Sports Dietitians Australia, the first exclusively sports nutrition professional organization in the world, have been frequent sources of inspiration.

You are most welcome to send in ideas to include in the next edition. Although many websites and books profess to give information on sports nutrition, sadly, very few provide high-quality, unbiased advice. For those readers who want to go deeper and broader than this book allows, please make use of the resources suggested on page 241.

PART I

Sports Nutrition Principles for Athletes

Nutrition and Fuel Systems for Sport

> He must rise at five in the morning, run half a mile at the top of his speed up hill, and then walk six miles at a moderate pace, coming in about seven to breakfast, which should consist of beef steak or mutton chop, under-done, with stale bread and old beer.
>
> *Captain Robert Barclay Allardice's nutrition advice to long-distance walkers (c. 1810)*

If I asked you to define healthy eating, you would likely give a very acceptable answer: 'Plenty of fruits and vegetables, whole-grain cereals . . . include lean meats and dairy foods . . . go easy on the cakes and take-aways'. Basically, this is correct, but it is easy to become confused by what we hear from the media and friends and what we read in books and magazines. As a result, we often go against our basic instincts. This chapter will help you think about what foods to eat both for health and to get the best out of your body, as well as the nutrients in these foods. We will be going into more detail about the components of food in chapter 2 (protein), chapter 3 (carbohydrate) and chapter 4 (vitamins and minerals).

Good nutrition is quite simple to achieve. Eat lots of minimally processed foods such as vegetables, grains, nuts, fruits, lean meats and reduced-fat dairy foods (except Camembert and premium ice cream because they taste the best with the fat left in!). Figure 1.1 on page 4 shows the Healthy Eating Plate with the major food groups in the proportion needed for good nutrition and to fuel an active body. This Healthy Eating Plate, from the Commonwealth Department of Health and Ageing in Australia, is very similar to the food guidelines of most Western nations and is especially suited to athletes and other active people.

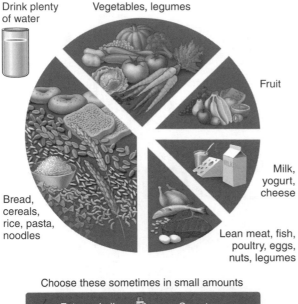

Drink plenty of water

Vegetables, legumes

Fruit

Milk, yogurt, cheese

Lean meat, fish, poultry, eggs, nuts, legumes

Bread, cereals, rice, pasta, noodles

Choose these sometimes in small amounts

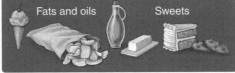

Fats and oils

Sweets

FIGURE 1.1 The Healthy Eating Plate.

Food Groups

Foods are divided into groups, each of which provides essential nutrients. The underlying science is well established and similar across every reputable health source, although health authorities sometimes differ in how they name the food groups (e.g., fruit and vegetables might be in separate groups or the same group). Table 1.1 lists the minimum serves recommended from each food group for good health.

Fruit, Vegetables and Legumes

This group should make up about a third of what you eat because it plays an essential role in protecting the body from disease now and in the future. This group is the major source of antioxidants and fibre in your diet. These foods also provide appreciable amounts of essential

minerals and vitamins. The legumes can be a major protein source for vegetarians (legumes are beans such as kidney beans, lentils and baked beans). This food group is underconsumed by many people in the Western world. Eating more fruit and vegetables can be the single biggest nutritional improvement many people can make. Around the world, 'Eat more fruit and vegetables' campaigns encourage people to eat two serves of fruit (about 300 g [10 oz]) and at least 2 cups of vegetables (about 400 g [14 oz]) each day. Australia has the Go for 2&5 campaign (2 serves of fruit and 5 serves of vegetables; www.gofor2and5.com.au), the USA has the 5 A Day campaign (www.cdc.gov/nccdphp/dnpa/5aday/) and the UK promotes five portions a day (www.eatwell.gov.uk/healthydiet/nutritionessentials/fruitandveg/; www.nhs.uk/Livewell/5ADAY/Pages/Whatcounts.aspx).

▶ **One serve of fruit**
150 g or 5 oz (e.g., 1 medium apple or orange or 2 apricots or 1 cup canned fruit); one serve of vegetables = 1/2 cup cooked vegetables or legumes or 1 cup salad

Bread and Cereals

This group should also comprise around one third of the diet. It includes pasta, rice, bread, breakfast cereals, muesli and porridge. This group is also a major source of fibre for regularity and general bowel health. Breads and cereals provide some antioxidants, especially in the least processed, whole-grain variety. These foods are your best carbohydrate source; they get broken down to glucose, the main fuel source for active muscles, the liver and the brain.

Some people suggest cutting down or cutting out carbohydrate foods to be healthy and lose weight. In reality, if you do so, you are cutting down on fibre and muscle fuel, making you more prone to tiredness and constipation! High-carbohydrate foods are only likely to make you fat if you are inactive or they come with a lot of added fat, such as pastries and cakes. The least processed grain and cereal foods provide

TABLE 1.1 Minimum Serves From Each Food Group for Good Health

Fruit	Vegetables	Bread, cereals	Milk, yogurt, cheese	Meats, legumes	Oil, fat	Treats
2	5	4	2	1	1	1

more nutrients per serve than biscuits, cookies or pastries.

▶ **One serve of breads and cereals**
2 slices of bread; 1 bread roll; 1 cup of cooked pasta, rice or porridge; or 40 g (1.4 oz) breakfast cereal

Milk, Yogurt and Cheese

Dairy foods are your main source of calcium and also provide an appreciable amount of riboflavin and protein. I recommend the lower-fat varieties of milk and cheese because they provide less saturated fat and more protein and calcium. Virtually all reduced-fat milks and yogurts have more protein and calcium than the regular versions. Some milks are specifically calcium fortified, allowing you to get up to 400 milligrams of calcium in a 200-millilitre glass. If you don't fancy dairy foods, then take some calcium-fortified soy drinks as a substitute. (Make sure soy drinks state that they are calcium fortified on the label because there is very little naturally occurring calcium in soy.)

▶ **One serve of dairy**
1 cup milk; 1 cup calcium-fortified soy drink; 40 g (1.4 oz) cheese; or 200 g (7 oz) yogurt

Lean Meat, Fish, Poultry, Eggs, Nuts and Legumes

This group of foods is very important in providing protein and essential minerals. Lean meat is a very good source of easy-to-absorb iron and zinc. Fish have gained prominence because the omega-3 fat found in cold-water fish has been strongly linked to a reduced risk of heart attacks. Eggs, nuts and legumes are very important protein sources for many vegetarians. Both nuts and legumes provide fibre and antioxidants, so it is no surprise that they appear to lessen the risk of heart disease, some cancers and possibly diabetes. You will often see legumes listed with protein foods and also in the vegetable group because they are a very important source of protein in vegetarian diets, while providing fibre and nutrients common to vegetables.

▶ **One serve of meats**
100 g (3.5 oz) cooked meat, chicken; 120 g (4.2 oz) cooked fish; 2 eggs; 1/2 cup legumes; or 1/3 cup nuts

Oil and Fat

Oil and unsaturated margarine provide vitamins D and E and help improve the flavour of many foods. Oil is 100 per cent fat, whereas butter and margarine are around 80 per cent fat. 'Light' margarine may be as low as 40 per cent fat with some of that fat being replaced by water. Most people need to limit oil and fat because they are high in energy (kilojoules/calories), although athletes can afford a higher fat intake because they are likely to burn it up in training. Note: Technically, *calories* is often capitalised when referring to kilocalories, but in keeping with common public usage of the term, in this book we will use *calories* to mean kilocalories, even though it is not capitalised. However, kilojoules are never referred to as joules; hence, we use the term *kilojoules* for countries that use metric.

▶ **One serve of oil and fat**
1 tbsp oil, butter, margarine or 1 1/2 tbsp reduced-fat spread

Treats

OK, this is not really a food group, but many people enjoy treats in small amounts during or between meals. Some treats provide essential nutrients. Ice cream provides calcium and protein and is a nutritious dessert with canned fruit. Chocolate provides essential vitamins and minerals, along with antioxidants (in dark chocolate, in particular), but being 30 per cent fat, it cannot be eaten in large amounts. Biscuits, cookies, cakes, pastries, pies and take-aways are often high in saturated fat, salt or both; these should be enjoyed, but greatly limited.

▶ **One serve of treats**
25 g (0.9 oz) chocolate; 40 g (1.4 oz) cake; 30 g (1 oz) crisps; 1 doughnut; one 375 mL (12.7 oz) can soft drink; 200 mL (7 oz) wine; 400 mL (13.5 oz) regular beer; 12 hot chips or french fries; or 2 cream cookies or biscuits

Water

Yes, water is a nutrient and a most essential one as well. Your body loses fluid each day through exhaled air, urine, sweat and feces. These losses vary depending on the air temperature and how much sweat you lose each day, but a loss of 1,500 to 3,000 millilitres (3 to 6 pints) of water a day is an average range for active people. You can get your fluid needs from water, tea, coffee, fruit juice, cordial, soft drinks, sports drinks and high-water foods such as milk, ice cream, fruits, vegetables and soup. Water requirements are discussed later in the chapter.

Essential Components of Food

Food comprises protein, fat, carbohydrate, fibre, vitamins, minerals and many bioactive compounds such as the antioxidants found mainly in fruits and vegetables. Alcoholic drinks also include alcohol (ethanol), which is technically a nutrient. We will look at each nutrient in turn.

Protein

Protein is composed of long chains of amino acids (see figure 1.2). Amino acids are the building blocks that make up large protein molecules. The digestive process breaks the protein mainly into groups of one, two or three amino acids, which are then absorbed from the intestine and into the blood to be made into body proteins such as haemoglobin, ferritin, antibodies, enzymes, hair and muscle. Some amino acids must come from food (indispensable, or essential, amino acids), whereas the body can make the others (dispensable, or nonessential) even though they still come from food.

Protein has many functions in the body:

- Enzymes are forms of protein that enable chemical reactions to take place in the body; they are involved in the digestive breakdown of food via digestive enzymes.
- Cell membranes, tendons and cartilage are composed of structural protein.

- Blood has important forms of protein, such as haemoglobin, which transports oxygen around the blood; transferrin is a protein that transports iron around the body; and albumin is a protein that controls water balance in the cells.
- Antibodies are a specialised form of protein that helps protect us from disease.
- Muscle strength comes from the contractile proteins actin and myosin, which allow muscles to contract and relax in exercise.
- Skin, nails and hair are made of strong proteins that can cope with the rigours of daily life.

In Western countries, animal foods provide most of the protein. Foods such as meat, chicken, fish, milk, cheese, yogurt and eggs have protein that provides all of the essential amino acids for life (see table 1.2). This is not to discount other valuable sources of protein. About one third of our protein comes from cereal foods (e.g., bread, rice), legumes, fruits and vegetables. Some plant foods will be low in some of the essential amino acids. A combination of plant foods, however, can provide all of the essential amino acids at one meal (complete protein). Some examples are legumes with cereal foods (e.g., beans on toast, lentils with rice) and seeds or nuts with grains (e.g., peanut butter sandwich). In some countries, rice and beans are a major source of complete protein.

If we eat more protein than we require, the excess protein is used as muscle fuel (glucose) during exercise or possibly stored as body fat (but not muscle). Most people, even vegetarians, have no difficulty eating enough protein each day, and protein deficiency is rare in Western

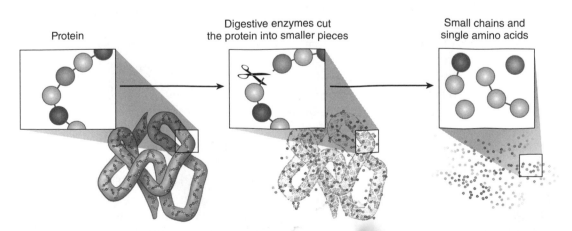

FIGURE 1.2 Through digestion, chains of amino acids in protein are broken down into small chains or single amino acids. They are then absorbed into the blood to be made into body proteins.

TABLE 1.2 Protein in Food

Good sources	Moderate sources
Meat	Bread
Chicken	Breakfast cereal
Fish	Rice
Seafood	Pasta
Cheese	Oats
Milk	Legumes (e.g., baked beans, lentils)
Milk powder	Nuts
Yogurt	Seeds
Eggs	

countries. Those who may be at risk of low protein are those who eat no animal foods (vegans) and those on highly restrictive weight loss diets.

We discuss amino acids and protein needs, as well as protein supplements, in chapter 2.

Fat

Although fat in food has received a bad name over the years, it is actually an essential nutrient. Fat is part of each cell membrane, and in the skin it helps form a barrier against water penetration. Fat is eaten as triglycerides, which consist of a molecule of glycerol bound to three molecules of fatty acids. The two fatty acids essential to life are linoleic acid and linolenic acid. These and other fatty acids can be made into a range of compounds called eicosanoids that control blood clotting, inflammation and immune function.

Fat is found in oils (100 per cent fat), butter and margarine (both about 80 per cent fat); it naturally occurs in oats, whole-grain cereals, nuts, peanut butter, seeds, eggs, avocado, milk, yogurt and cheese. Fat may be added during the manufacture of foods such as cakes, cookies, biscuits and snack foods; or it may be removed, such as in the production of non-fat milk or low-fat yogurt.

For many years there has been a constant message to eat less fat. 'Eat less fat' is an easy take-home message, whereas the more accurate 'Eat less saturated fat' was more difficult to market. Unfortunately, the 'eat less fat' campaigns have given the impression that all fat is bad. More recently we have heard the concept of 'good' and 'bad' fat. The truth has always been that we should be eating less of the 'bad' saturated fat because it causes atherosclerosis (fatty build-up in artery walls) and thrombosis (blood clots). Other types of fat, 'good' unsaturated fat, are unlikely to cause health problems. Table 1.3 shows the types of fat in foods.

Unfortunately, all types of fat eaten in excess are easily converted to body fat. The problem with people in many Western countries, and some athletes, is that they consume too much dietary fat and the excess gets converted to body fat. The more active people are, the less likely this is to happen. Don't see this advice as meaning that you should eat next to no fat because some nutritious foods contain a fair amount of 'healthy' fat, such as nuts and avocados. These foods provide many nutrients and antioxidant chemicals that protect you from disease. It would be crazy to eliminate these from your diet.

TABLE 1.3 Fat in Food

Mainly saturated fat	Mainly unsaturated fat
Cream, lard, copha	Monounsaturated and polyunsaturated margarine
Butter	Monounsaturated and polyunsaturated oil
Cooking margarine	Avocado
Commercial cakes, pastries, cookies and biscuits	Nuts
Fatty take-aways	Peanut butter
French fries, hot chips	Seeds
Hard cheeses, milk, yogurt	Tahini (sesame seed paste)
Fatty meats, salami, sausages	Oily fish
Snack foods, crisps	Lean meats

Types of Fat

Three main types of fat are found in food: saturated, monounsaturated and polyunsaturated. Another type of fat, called trans fat, also occurs naturally, although too much trans fat in processed fatty foods has been linked to a higher risk of heart disease. Fat is named after the dominant fat type. For example, olive oil is termed 'monounsaturated' because three quarters of its fat is monounsaturated. Let's take a look at each type of fat found in food.

- **Saturated.** Saturated fat is generally considered the 'bad' fat because of its link to heart disease and raising unhealthy blood cholesterol levels. The term *saturated* is an organic chemistry term meaning that each fatty acid is 'saturated' with the maximum number of hydrogen atoms. The term *saturated*, however, does not mean that the food is 'saturated with fat'. Foods high in saturated fat are listed in table 1.3 on page 7. Saturated fat is generally solid at room temperature and is often added to commercial cakes, biscuits, cookies, pastries and take-away foods. To be fair, some take-away franchises and food manufacturers are working hard to lower their saturated fat content and replace it with unsaturated fat.

- **Monounsaturated (MU).** This type of fat is viewed quite favourably in health terms and doesn't appear to contribute to future disease. Olive oil, canola oil and the avocado have put MU fat in the spotlight and spawned a range of MU margarines. Nuts, seeds and lean meat also provide some monounsaturated fat. In chemistry terms, *monounsaturated* means that one double bond (hence 'mono') exists between the carbon atoms in the fat, which entails dropping two hydrogen atoms; hence it becomes 'unsaturated' with hydrogen. This is not easy to comprehend unless you have a good knowledge of chemistry, which you will not need to understand the nutrition principles of this book.

- **Polyunsaturated (PU).** This type of fat is considered to be unrelated to poor health. Apart from PU margarines and oils, PU fat also appears in lean meat, nuts and seeds. The fats in oily fish are also PU, and are often referred to as omega-3 fats, fish oils or marine oils. The two most common types are EPA (eicosapentaenoic acid) and DHA (docosahexaenoic acid). You will see them listed in fish oil supplements. Fish and fish oil are associated with a lower risk of heart disease and stroke. Some people worry that heating PU fat converts it to saturated fat. Under normal domestic cooking conditions, no unsaturated fat gets converted to saturated fat. In chemistry terms, *polyunsaturated* means that two or more double bonds (hence 'poly', meaning more than one) exist between the carbon atoms in the fat, which results in some hydrogen atoms being dropped; hence it is 'unsaturated' with hydrogen.

- **Trans fatty acids (TFAs).** TFAs are naturally occurring in ruminant animals, so we find TFAs in beef, lamb, mutton, milk, cheese and yogurt. A TFA is technically an unsaturated fat, but it acts like a saturated fat and is linked to heart disease and heart attacks. Fortunately, the amount of TFAs we get from these foods is not a health problem. The production of margarine results in high TFA levels. Although this remains a problem in some countries such as the USA, other countries like Australia and New Zealand now have virtually eliminated TFAs from table margarine since the late 1990s. Check the margarine label because table margarine without TFAs is available in many countries. Hard margarines used in making pastries, cookies and biscuits (also called stick margarine or cooking margarine in supermarkets) are likely to contain TFAs.

How Much Fat Should You Eat?

You are often told that you should eat only 20 to 30 grams of fat a day. Good luck to you. Given that the average man eats more than 100 grams of fat every day, and the average woman, 70 grams of fat, it will take a monumental change and restriction in eating habits to make it down to 20 grams a day. A more realistic daily goal is 40 to 60 grams of fat for a moderately active adult.

Another common piece of advice given to the public is to avoid any individual food or food product that has more than 10 per cent fat by weight (10 g per 100 g). This means the deletion of avocados, olive oil, nuts, peanut butter, seeds, polyunsaturated margarine and good chocolate, none of which adversely affect the health of your heart or other parts of your body.

Any food that includes oats, chocolate, avocados, nuts or seeds will often have more than 10 per cent fat content; for example, muesli is commonly 10-12 per cent fat because of the oats and nuts present; peanut butter is 55 per cent fat. There is good evidence that these foods all have nutritional qualities that actually improve your health so there is little point in eliminating them.

When choosing food, you should consider more than just the fat content. If left on a deserted island, I would choose peanut butter (55 per cent fat) over jam (0 per cent fat) because it is more nutritious and higher in antioxidant compounds, and the fat is unsaturated. The total fat content of a single food is not the issue; we need to consider the total fat intake of the day, the type of fat and what other nutrients are associated with the fat. If we take a holistic view of fat in the diet, then the basic points are as follows:

- Eat less saturated fat, because it generally increases the risk of atherosclerosis and thrombosis (e.g., most take-aways, cookies, biscuits, pastries). Note: These foods shouldn't be banned, just respected and eaten in sensible amounts.

- Consume most of your fat as unsaturated fat (e.g., lean meats, nuts, seeds, wholegrain cereals, unsaturated oils and margarines).

- Don't eat too much fat, especially during periods of inactivity, such as injury, because it is easy to convert dietary fat to body fat.

Carbohydrate

Without carbohydrate, you just cannot perform at your best. Carbohydrate foods provide the crucial energy for muscle contraction and brain function. Many unrefined carbohydrate foods also provide the fibre necessary for normal bowel function and health, as well as antioxidants that protect the body from heart disease and some cancers. Good sources of carbohydrate are fruits, root vegetables (e.g., potatoes), rice, pasta, bread, breakfast cereal and legumes. Milk and yogurt have a small amount of carbohydrate in the form of lactose.

Forms of carbohydrate include sugar, of which there are six main types, and starch, of which there are two types. Sugar consists of either a single molecule or two molecules joined together, whereas starch consists of hundreds of sugar molecules joined together. Despite the simple difference, there is much fantasy, emotion and misinformation about the two.

First let me offer you the basic chemistry behind sugar and starch. Although sugar is often thought of as only table sugar, there are other types.

Types of Sugar

The main sugars in nature are either a single molecule (monosaccharide) or two molecules joined together (disaccharide) (see figure 1.3). The monosaccharide sugars are as follows:

- Glucose
- Fructose
- Galactose

Galactose is found mainly joined to glucose to form the disaccharide lactose, the sugar found in the milk of almost every mammal. The main disaccharide sugars in nature are as follows:

- Lactose (glucose + galactose)
- Sucrose (glucose + fructose)
- Maltose (glucose + glucose)

The digestive enzymes that break down these disaccharides are called lact*ase*, sucr*ase* and malt*ase*, respectively. (The suffix *–ose* indicates a sugar, and the suffix *–ase* indicates an enzyme; all enzymes are proteins.) About two thirds of the world's adult population lacks the enzyme lactase, meaning that they have a lactose intolerance (*not* an allergy, as some think). A small amount of lactose eaten with a meal usually presents no problem to these people.

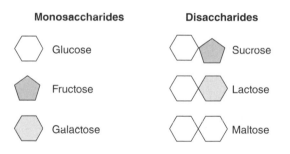

FIGURE 1.3 The main sugars in food are either monosaccharides (single sugars) or disaccharides (double sugars).

Types of Starch

Starchy foods include bread, breakfast cereal, pasta, rice, potatoes and peas. To the amazement of many, starch is made of hundreds of molecules of just one type of sugar. That sugar is glucose. When starch is digested, it ends up just as glucose, which can then be absorbed. This is important for athletes because this glucose is required to fuel muscle contractions and is needed for brain functioning, allowing them to perform well and think well. Too little carbohydrate means too little glucose for the muscles to work efficiently, which can result in the onset of fatigue. Too little glucose will also affect brain function, meaning that you may not make the best decisions during sport.

Starch is broken down by the digestive enzyme amylase, which breaks down the long chains of glucose to maltose, allowing maltase to break it down further to individual glucose molecules for absorption into the bloodstream. Starch comes in two main forms, amylose and amylopectin, with their different structures affecting the rate at which they are digested. This greatly influences the glycemic index (GI). Carbohydrate and the GI are discussed in greater detail in chapter 3.

Fibre

Since the 1970s fibre has been on the nutrition agenda. Fibre is the indigestible carbohydrate found in plant foods such as grains, vegetables and fruit. It started out being called just plain roughage, something to keep you regular. Dr. Denis Burkitt came up with the simple, but unattractive, idea of measuring the weight of human stools (as in waste, not furniture) around the world and linking it to disease. He found that daily stool weight varied from 450 grams in rural Africa to a mere 100 grams in Western societies. His conclusion: More fibre meant more waste and less constipation, hiatus hernia, gallstones, hemorrhoids and bowel cancer. Subsequent studies confirmed that the risk of bowel cancer was less in those who ate their fibre (http://epic.iarc.fr/keyfindings.php). That got everyone adding wheat bran to breakfast cereals. It wasn't tasty, but think of the roughage.

And why all the fuss about fibre? Well, apart from the protection Dr. Burkitt found, it also decreases your risk of high blood cholesterol and helps keep blood sugar levels healthy. That means that eating enough fibre reduces your risk of heart disease and diabetes, so the long-term benefits are substantial. These are all good reasons to enjoy fruits, vegetables, legumes and whole-grain cereals. Fibre is not just one nutrient or component of plant food; rather, it is composed of a range of water-soluble components (pectins, gums and mucilages) and water-insoluble bits (cellulose and hemicellulose). Fibre is a mix of the two types. Wheat bran is a common example of being high in insoluble fibre, the type of fibre most responsible for keeping us 'regular'.

Some foods are high in soluble fibre; good examples are oat bran and psyllium, which is available mainly as a supplement or added to commercial breakfast cereals. Soluble fibre helps control blood cholesterol and keep it in the healthy range. Researchers have found that relatively small amounts of psyllium have a modest cholesterol-lowering effect, which could, in turn, reduce heart disease risk. A tasty and enjoyable way to get your soluble fibre is by eating foods such as fruits, rolled oats (porridge), muesli and legumes (e.g., kidney beans, baked beans).

You may have recently heard of resistant starch, a type of starch that is resistant to digestion and moves through the small intestine and into the large intestine to act a lot like fibre. Resistant starch has a gel-like consistency. When it reaches the large intestine, it is consumed by healthy resident bacteria, just like other fibre that enters the large intestine, producing short-chain fatty acids to protect the large intestine from disease. For that reason, resistant starch is called a prebiotic: compounds eaten by colonic bacteria to help keep harmful bacteria levels low. (Prebiotics are not to be confused with probiotics, which are bacteria often taken as a supplement or added to foods such as yogurt.) Some white breads and breakfast cereals now have added resistant starch. Although not classified as fibre on food labels, resistant starch provides similar benefits to fibre. Resistant starch is common in legumes, bananas and potato salad (when the potato cools, starch gels are formed to become resistant starch).

Alcohol

The alcohol found in alcoholic drinks is called ethanol, a substance that is toxic to the body. When you hear the word *toxic*, you might start to worry. Don't. It just means that ethanol must be metabolised by the liver as soon as possible, or else it might build up to dangerous levels, which it does when you have had a few too many. Alcohol seems to be safe when consumed in sensible quantities, although we don't know if there is a safe level for babies. For this reason, pregnant and breastfeeding women are recommended to avoid alcohol altogether. However, there is good evidence that having around one standard drink a day can reduce heart disease risk. That's a maximum of one or two standard drinks a day, not an average. Exceeding two standard drinks in a single day increases the risk of liver damage, brain damage, high blood pressure and some cancers.

The drinking guidelines provided by the National Health and Medical Research Council in Australia (2009) are as follows:

- For healthy men and women, drinking no more than two standard drinks on any day reduces the lifetime risk of harm from alcohol-related disease or injury.

- For healthy men and women, drinking no more than four standard drinks on a single occasion reduces the risk of alcohol-related injury arising from that occasion.

- For women who are pregnant or planning a pregnancy, not drinking is the safest option. For women who are breastfeeding, not drinking is the safest option.

Research suggests a maximum of two standard drinks a day for long-term health in men and non-pregnant women. Many countries now have similar guidelines on the maximum number of daily alcohol serves. From a sporting perspective, remember that alcohol is a diuretic, meaning that it can make you pass a greater volume of fluid (as urine) than you take in from the alcoholic drinks, possibly contributing to dehydration. For this reason, you will need more non-alcoholic fluids in your diet when drinking alcohol. Smart athletes keep their alcohol intake safe and remain hydrated by alternating an alcoholic drink with a non-alcoholic 'spacer'.

Water

Around 60 per cent of your total body weight is water. That's about 40 litres (10.5 gal) of water in a 70-kilogram (154 lb) person. Water makes up most of your blood, urine and sweat, and it is the main component of each body cell. Water is crucial to the regulation of body temperature to prevent overheating, which will quickly impair sports performance. Too little water in the body is called dehydration and can lead to thermal stress and heatstroke. Fluid replacement is discussed in more detail in chapter 5.

I've heard many times—and no doubt you have too—that you should drink 6 to 8 glasses of water each day. If this statement is based on human physiology, then it is flawed from the start. I originally thought that the claim was based on the physiology textbooks that state that the average human produces 1,500 millilitres (50 oz) of urine each day. If a glass is 200 to 250 millilitres (7 to 8 oz), then that means that you produce

the equivalent of 6 to 8 glasses of urine a day. It makes logical sense that you should drink enough water to replace urine losses, but this may not be as logical as it seems. There are other water losses from the body via the skin (500 mL [17 oz]—more if you sweat through exercise or in hot conditions), exhalation (350 mL [12 oz]) and in feces (150 mL [5 oz]). Does that mean you need more than 8 glasses of water a day?

A lot of the 'solid' foods you eat contain appreciable amounts of water. Vegetables and fruits are around 90 per cent water, as is milk, fruit juice and soft drinks. Cooked meats and fish are over 50 per cent water, and breads are about one-third water (see table 1.4 on page 12). So, a meat and salad sandwich will provide 160 millilitres (5.5 oz) of water. Add a piece of fruit and a glass of milk, and you have around 470 millilitres (16 oz) of water. As you can see, water doesn't have to be your only source of water.

Under most conditions, your thirst response works wonderfully well, as you would expect after years of human evolution, mostly in the warm to hot environment of Africa. When you get thirsty, drink non-alcoholic beverages. The thirst response becomes less reliable as an indicator of fluid needs when exercising and working under hot conditions. Under those conditions it is wise to drink at the rate of 1 litre (1 qt) per hour to minimise your risk of dehydration (more if you sweat heavily). One rider in the 2010 Tour de France was reported as drinking 11 litres of fluid during a hot day on the tour.

You should drink as much fluid as you need to keep hydrated. In most cases, this is the amount of fluid that will produce pale urine about five or six times a day. On a hot day, that might be 3 litres or more; on a rest day in winter, that might be only 4 cups of tea or coffee, with your food providing the rest of your fluid needs. That's right, even tea and coffee are fluid sources to the body (see the section on diuretics in chapter 5).

Vitamins

Vitamins are compounds critical to the normal function of the body, yet required (see table 1.5 on page 13) in very small amounts measured in milligrams (one thousandth of a gram) and micrograms (one millionth of a gram). They do not provide kilojoules like protein, fat, carbohydrate and alcohol, but they do help to release the energy from these nutrients. Just about every action and metabolic function in the body requires vitamins.

TABLE 1.4 Approximate Water Content of Some Foods

Food	Water content
Sports drink, 200 mL (7 oz)	190 mL (6.4 oz)
Soft drink, 200 mL (7 oz)	185 mL (6.2 oz)
Fruit juice, 200 mL (7 oz)	185 mL (6.2 oz)
Milk, 200 mL (7 oz)	180 mL (6.0 oz)
Fruit salad, 200 g (7 oz)	170 mL (5.7 oz)
Yogurt, 200 g (7 oz)	160 mL (5.4 oz)
Apple, 150 g (5.3 oz)	130 mL (4.4 oz)
Tomato, 100 g (3.5 oz)	93 mL (3.1 oz)
Mushrooms, 100 g (3.5 oz)	92 mL (3.1 oz)
Broccoli, 100 g (3.5 oz)	90 mL (3.0 oz)
Potato salad, 100 g (3.5 oz)	75 mL (2.5 oz)
Baked beans, 100 g (3.5 oz)	75 mL (2.5 oz)
Avocado, 100 g (3.5 oz)	73 mL (2.4 oz)
Ham 100 g (3.5 oz)	70 mL (2.3 oz)
Chicken 100 g (3.5 oz)	50 mL (1.7 oz)
Egg, boiled, 50 g (1.8 oz)	35 mL (1.1 oz)
Cheddar cheese, 30 g (1 oz)	10 mL (0.3 oz)
Bread, 1 slice	10 mL (0.3 oz)
Breakfast cereal, 100 g (3.5 oz)	5 mL (0.2 oz)
Peanuts, raw, 100 g (3.5 oz)	5 mL (0.2 oz)
Vegetable oil, 1 tbsp	0 mL

Vitamins are often divided into water-soluble and fat-soluble types. The water-soluble ones are vitamins C and the B group vitamins (thiamin, riboflavin, niacin, pyridoxine, biotin, pantothenic acid, folate and vitamin B_{12}). The fat-soluble ones are vitamins A, D, E and K. Although most people get their daily vitamin needs by eating well, about half of all athletes take a vitamin supplement. The B vitamins and vitamin C can be lost through light exposure and heat in cooking, so foods such as vegetables should be well cared for and cooked quickly (see also the discussion of the role of vitamins in sport in chapter 4).

Minerals

Minerals are less prone to destruction through food preparation. They are inorganic compounds that play significant roles in body functions, such as iron in blood and calcium in bones and teeth. Getting too few minerals is not a common problem for most men because their needs are usually met by food intake (see table 1.6 on page 14). For example, iron deficiency anaemia is not common in men because they can usually get enough iron through eating lean meat and iron-fortified breakfast cereals alone. Inadequate mineral intake, especially of iron, calcium and zinc, is of concern to many women, with over half of women getting less than the recommended intake of these minerals. (See chapter 4 for more on iron and calcium.)

One mineral of concern is sodium, which is most commonly found in high levels in processed foods as sodium chloride (salt). Too much salt is not good for long-term health and may contribute to bone loss and high blood pressure. I recommend that you choose low-salt or reduced-salt versions of processed foods and

TABLE 1.5 Vitamins in Food

Vitamin	Good food sources	Australia and New Zealand recommended daily needs (RDI)	United States and Canada recommended daily needs (DRI)	UK recommended daily needs (RNI)
Thiamin	Whole grains, nuts, legumes, bread, fortified breakfast cereals, meat, yeast extract	1.1 mg women 1.2 mg men	1.1 mg women 1.2 mg men	0.8 mg women 1.0 mg men
Riboflavin	Milk, yogurt, yeast extracts, fortified breakfast cereals, almonds, meat	1.1 mg women 1.3 mg men	1.1 mg women 1.3 mg men	1.1 mg women 1.3 mg men
Niacin	Meat, poultry, fish, yeast extracts, peanuts, legumes, whole-grain bread	14 mg women 16 mg men	14 mg women 16 mg men	13 mg women 17 mg women
Vitamin B_6 Pyridoxine	Meats, whole grains, vegetables, nuts	1.3 mg	1.3 mg	1.2 mg women 1.4 mg men
Biotin	Widely distributed in food	Adequate intake: 25 mcg women 30 mcg men	Adequate intake: 30 mcg women 30 mcg men	N/A
Pantothenic acid	Widely distributed in whole foods	Adequate intake: 4 mg women 6 mg men	Adequate intake: 5 mg women 5 mg men	N/A
Folate	Fruit, avocado, vegetables (especially green leafy), lentils, folate-fortified breakfast cereals, yeast extract	400 mcg	400 mcg	200 mcg
Vitamin B_{12}	Fish, meats, egg, milk, cheese, yogurt	2.4 mcg	2.4 mcg	1.5 mcg
C	Fruit, fruit juice, canned fruit, vegetables	45 mg	75 mg women 90 mg men	40 mg
A	Milk, butter, margarine, cheese, egg, liver; yellow and orange fruits and vegetables for beta-carotene	700 mcg women 900 mcg men	700 mcg women 900 mcg men	700 mcg women 700 mcg men
D	Oily fish, margarine, liver, cheese, mushrooms exposed to sunlight, Aktavite, action of sunlight on skin	Adequate intake: 5 mcg (young adult) 15 mcg (adults over 70 yr)	15 mcg (young adult) 20 mcg (adults over 70 yr)	10 mcg (adults over 50 yr)
E	Wheat germ, nuts, avocado, margarine, meat, poultry, fish	Adequate intake: 7 mg women 10 mg men	15 mg women 15 mg men	N/A
K	Green leafy vegetables, liver, legumes	Adequate intake: 60 mcg women 70 mcg men	Adequate intake: 90 mcg women 120 mcg men	N/A

Note: The figures given represent the amount that will provide the requirements for virtually everyone and are not minimum requirements. RDI = recommended dietary intake; DRI = dietary reference intake; RNI = reference nutrient intake; mg = milligrams; mcg = micrograms. Adequate intake: No recommended daily requirement has been established. The level at which intake should be adequate for normal body function has been determined from the best available data.

TABLE 1.6 Minerals in Food

Mineral	Good food sources	Australia and New Zealand recommended daily needs (RDI)	United States and Canada recommended daily needs (DRI)	UK recommended daily needs (RNI)
Iron	Meats, iron-fortified foods (e.g., breakfast cereals and Milo)	8 mg men 18 mg women <50 yr 8 mg women >50 yr	8 mg men 18 mg women <50 yr 8 mg women >50 yr	8.7 mg men 14.8 mg women <50 yr 8.7 mg women >50 yr
Calcium	Milks, yogurt, cheese, calcium-fortified soy milk and drinks, ice cream, canned fish with soft edible bones, milk chocolate	1,000 mg 1,300 mg women >50 yr 1,300 mg men >70 yr	1,000 mg 1,200 mg women >50 yr 1,200 mg men >70 yr	700 mg 700 mg women >50 yr 700 mg men >50 yr
Zinc	Meats, seafood, nuts, milk, cheese	8 mg women 14 mg men	8 mg women 11 mg men	7 mg women 9.5 mg men
Chromium	Nuts, meat, fruit, vegetables, cheese, egg	Adequate intake: 25 mcg women 35 mcg men	Adequate intake: 25 mcg women 35 mcg men	N/A
Copper	Seafood, nuts, legumes, chocolate	Adequate intake: 1.2 mg women 1.7 mg men	0.9 mg women 0.9 mg men	1.2 mg women 1.2 mg men
Selenium	Fish, meats, cereals, grains	60 mcg women 70 mcg men	55 mcg women 55 mcg men	60 mcg women 75 mcg men
Iodine	Seafood	150 mcg	150 mcg	140 mcg
Magnesium	Green vegetables, nuts, legumes, bread	320 mg women 420 mg men	320 mg women 420 mg men	270 mg women 300 mg men
Sodium	Many processed foods contain added salt or sodium	Adequate intake: 460–920 mg Maximum: 2,300 mg	Maximum: 2,300 mg	Maximum: 1,600 mg
Potassium	Fruit, vegetables	Adequate intake: 2,800 mg women 3,800 mg men	Minimum: 2,000 mg	3,500 mg

Note: The figures given represent the amount that will provide the requirements for virtually everyone and are not minimum requirements. RDI = recommended dietary intake; DRI = dietary reference intake; RNI = reference nutrient intake; mg = milligrams; mcg = micrograms. Adequate intake: No recommended daily requirement has been established. The level at which intake should be adequate for normal body function has been determined from the best available data.

that you wean yourself from the taste of salty foods. Note that some salty foods don't taste salty. Often breakfast cereals, such as cornflakes, don't taste salty, yet they may contain 800 milligrams of sodium per 100 grams. Compare that to salty potato crisps at 600 milligrams per 100 grams. A breakfast cereal with more than 400 milligrams of sodium per 100 grams is considered quite high in salt. A low-salt food has less than 120 milligrams of sodium per 100 grams. Thankfully, many major food companies are now modifying their manufacturing processes to reduce the amount of sodium in foods, especially in breads and breakfast cereals.

Vitamin and Mineral Supplements

Your doctor may recommend that you take a vitamin or mineral supplement based on an established deficiency. Some researchers suggest that you take a multivitamin supplement after the age of 65 because your body may have a reduced ability to absorb certain nutrients, such as vitamin B_6. These supplements can also be very useful on other occasions, such as when you travel overseas and cannot be sure you are eating well. If you are bushwalking or camping for weeks at a time, consider a supplement to make up for the limited range of foods you are eating. Other than that, it is pretty much an individual decision.

Don't expect wonderful results from taking a vitamin supplement. Some people take them in the hope that they will give them vitality and diffuse the general fatigue they suffer, when a change of job or relationship, or improving their diet, would have had a far better outcome. Vitamin supplements will not compensate for poor nutrition choices. The evidence suggests that eating fruits and vegetables and being active provide far more health benefits than taking a supplement does. If you do choose a supplement, make sure it provides only 50 to 100 per cent of your daily needs (refer to tables 1.5 [page 13] and 1.6). More than this is generally excreted in the urine. (Hence the iridescent glow-in-the-dark stream!)

In general, no vitamin and mineral supplements are required if an athlete is consuming adequate energy from a variety of foods to maintain body weight. A multivitamin/mineral supplement may be appropriate if an athlete is dieting, habitually eliminating foods or food groups, is ill or is recovering from injury, or has a specific micronutrient deficiency.

Position of the American Dietetic Association, Dietitians of Canada and the American College of Sports Medicine: Nutrition and Athletic Performance (2009, 510)

Antioxidants

Without oxygen, you would die quickly. Oxygen keeps you alive, but it is also slowly killing you because oxygen is toxic over a lifetime. Inhaling air naturally produces harmful free radicals that cause a slow rusting, or aging, of the body. The rusting is properly termed *oxidation* and is the reason we slowly age. To slow down the oxidation process, antioxidation chemicals are needed—hence the term *antioxidants*.

There is now evidence that the harm caused by oxygen can accumulate and contribute to diseases such as heart disease and cancer and other health problems such as eye cataracts and rheumatoid arthritis. The free radicals may cause damage to DNA molecules so that new body cells mutate and become cancer cells. Free radical damage to blood cholesterol can make the cholesterol far more damaging to your artery lining than previously realised. (Note: Free radicals are not always harmful. Clever blood cells called phagocytes produce free radicals to kill disease-causing microbes.)

Fortunately, through evolution, humans have devised ways to minimise the toxic damage of oxygen. The body produces special antioxidant enzymes to soak up free radicals. They have names such as glutathione, catalase and superoxide dismutase. Certain minerals can help those enzymes do their job efficiently, such as selenium, copper, manganese and zinc. The antioxidants we eat as food are a bonus that helps reduce our chance of developing heart disease and some cancers.

Vitamins can also act as antioxidants, the best known being vitamin C, vitamin E and beta-carotene. More recently, the spotlight has been on non-nutrient antioxidants found in food, such as phenols, flavonoids and carotenoids other than beta-carotene. These antioxidant compounds have been found in red wine, coffee, tea and chocolate and are widely distributed in the plant kingdom (fruit, vegetables, mushrooms, nuts). If you don't like wine, grape juice has similar antioxidants as red wine.

It is estimated that at least 5,000 compounds in foods have antioxidant properties; many of them are in fruits and vegetables. For example, there are over 500 different carotenoids in food. Scientists uniformly agree that the highest consumers of fruits and vegetables are the least likely to get heart disease or cancer.

Manufacturers add antioxidants to foods to stop them from deteriorating and 'going off', hence giving them a longer shelf life. Many foods containing fat and oil have added antioxidants to protect against rancidity as a result of exposure to oxygen. Even a small amount of rancid fat will ruin the flavour and smell of a food. Sulphur dioxide is added to dried apricots to stop the discolouration caused by oxygen. Vacuum sealing of foods also helps keep the food away from oxygen.

Fuel Systems

We have discussed foods and nutrients and the amounts you need for good health. Before we cover specific nutrient needs in fitness and sport, we will explore how the body produces the energy you need for exercise. Many nutrients are involved in energy production during exercise. The two major fuels for energy are fat and carbohydrate. This section will look at how we burn energy.

Your body is perfectly designed to move by a coordinated series of muscle contractions. When your brain tells your body to move, nerve signals trigger a powerful release of muscle energy through a special molecule called adenosine triphosphate (ATP). ATP is a high-energy molecule that, when its phosphate bonds snap apart, provides the energy for muscle contraction and away you go. ATP is generated in mitochondria, the powerhouses of each body cell, from the energy you eat as food. Each muscle cell contains thousands of mitochondria. Three systems in the body create the ATP energy required for physical activity.

ATP-CP System

The ATP-CP system provides enough energy for a five- or six-second sprint or other rapid muscle contraction such as lifting weights. Creatine phosphate (CP) is a high-energy molecule that can deliver its energy to manufacture ATP very quickly. A resting muscle has about four times more CP than ATP. During muscle contraction the CP transfers its energy to ATP production (see figure 1.4), but the CP reserves are drained quite quickly. Stocks of CP in the muscles are remade during the next rest period between sprints.

Many strength and sprint athletes now take creatine supplements to make sure they have maximum creatine phosphate levels in their muscles. (See chapter 9 for more on creatine.)

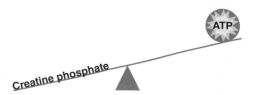

FIGURE 1.4 Creatine phosphate transfers its energy to produce more ATP for quick bursts of muscle contraction, leading to a drop in creatine phosphate and a rapid rise in ATP.

No oxygen is required for this system to work, so you don't need to inhale during a very short sprint. Because no oxygen is required, it is called anaerobic (without oxygen) exercise.

Glycolytic System

The glycolytic system is most important for high-power efforts lasting up to two minutes. When CP levels are low, the muscles turn to glucose for rapid production of ATP, again with little requirement for oxygen. This anaerobic system generates only two ATP molecules from each glucose molecule (see figure 1.5).

Unfortunately, lactic acid is a by-product of the glycolytic system, and too much lactic acid causes muscle fatigue. The muscle avoids acid fatigue by switching to a third system that requires oxygen, the aerobic system. As exercise intensity rises, the body relies more on the glycolytic system fuelled by glucose. When the intensity is lower (e.g., during walking or jogging), the body prefers the aerobic system that uses both fat and glucose for muscle fuel.

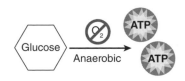

FIGURE 1.5 In the anaerobic glycolytic system, the glucose molecule produces two ATP molecules.

Aerobic System

The word *aerobic* is a combination of the Greek words *aero* (air) and *bios* (life). As the name implies, plenty of oxygen is required for this system to work efficiently. This system is most important in any exercise that lasts longer than two minutes. It is also known as oxidative phosphorylation and uses both glucose and fat as its fuel source. All this action takes place in the mitochondria, which are abundant in muscle cells and in the cardiac cells of the heart.

The inhaled oxygen helps the muscles produce an extra 34 ATP molecules from one glucose molecule, making a total of 36 ATPs compared to only two without oxygen (see figure 1.6). Glucose is the most efficient fuel because it produces more ATP with each breath than does fat or protein. Your major source of glucose is the carbohydrate (sugar and starch) in your diet.

However, body stores of glucose are limited compared to body stores of fat. Endurance train-

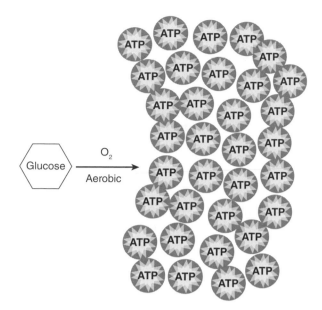

FIGURE 1.6 While you are exercising at low to medium intensity, one glucose molecule is metabolised to produce an extra 34 ATP molecules, for a total of 36.

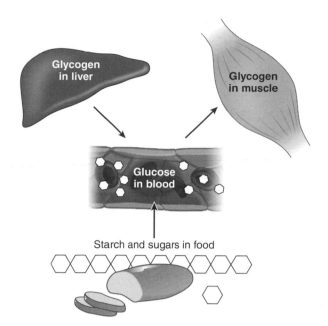

FIGURE 1.7 Starches and sugars in food become glucose in the blood or are stored as glycogen in the muscles and liver. Glycogen then breaks down to glucose as required by the body.

ing helps muscles use fat more efficiently as a fuel, thereby making fewer demands on glucose and improving endurance. Amino acids from protein are sometimes used as a fuel, mainly near the end of endurance sports when glucose stores are low. Note: The three energy systems operate at the same time, but their relative contributions vary with the intensity and duration of the sport.

Maximum Fuel Stores

Glucose is stored in the muscles as long chains that form the giant molecule called glycogen. Hence, we refer to glycogen as the primary muscle fuel. Glycogen is specially structured to break down quickly to glucose as required by muscles.

Carbohydrate in food is digested, absorbed into the blood and transported to muscles to be converted to glycogen (see figure 1.7). Glycogen is stored in both your muscles and your liver. The average fit 70-kilogram (154 lb) person has 165 kilojoules (40 calories) of glucose in the blood and stores around 1,100 kilojoules (262 calories) of glycogen in the liver and 5,900 kilojoules (1,409 calories) of glycogen in the muscles. If you want to train and compete efficiently, you need a full fuel tank of glycogen every time you exercise.

During exercise the body burns a mixture of fat and glycogen, but glycogen is the fuel that runs out the quickest. The glycogen molecule

releases glucose units as they are needed by the muscle. Glucose is the preferred muscle fuel, especially as exercise intensity increases. During high-intensity exercise, glycogen is used at a very fast rate and may become depleted after 30 to 45 minutes, yet it may last for 180 minutes in a brisk walk.

At lower intensities (e.g., walking, recovery sessions) both body fat and glycogen are used

Muscles burn glucose at a faster rate during high-intensity exercise.

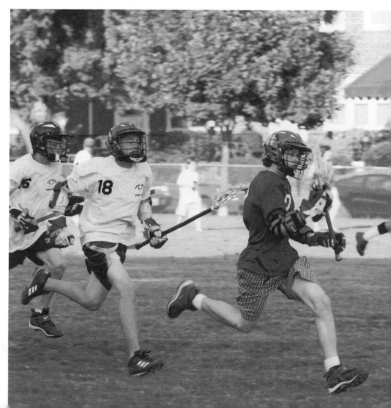

▶ Glycogen Power

Time-and-motion analyses of soccer games have revealed that players travelled 9 to 12 kilometres (5.5 to 7.5 miles) in 90 minutes of play. Players with plenty of glycogen travelled 12 kilometres, with only a quarter (3 km) of that at a walk. Players with low glycogen stores travelled only 9.5 kilometres and about half (4.7 km) of that was at a walk. Researchers concluded that 'the more glycogen, the further and faster the player ran' (Kirkendall 1993, p. 1372).

as fuel. Even a slim person carries 250,000 kilojoules (about 60,000 calories) or more of fat, so fat fuel never runs out. (Theoretically, 250,000 kilojoules is enough energy to run 1,000 kilometres or 620 miles!) Glycogen is the 'limiting' fuel; in other words, there is a limit to how much the body can store. In hot weather glycogen may be burned at a faster rate than in cooler weather.

Carbohydrate in food replenishes the glycogen fuel tank in working muscles.

Maintaining Fuel Levels

Muscle glycogen levels vary among people. A trained athlete has more muscle glycogen than someone doing little activity. Fit people aim to keep muscle glycogen levels as high as possible so they can train effectively for long periods and recover quickly, whether from weight training or endurance training. Adequate glycogen is also important for completing everyday activities such as walking and gardening.

Glycogen is stored mainly in the active muscles; hence, cyclists and runners preferentially store, and then use up, the glycogen in their leg muscles. Swimmers store lots of glycogen in their arm and leg muscles. Unfortunately, if your leg muscles run out of glycogen, you can't bring in more from your arms, or vice versa.

When muscle glycogen levels are low and blood glucose levels start to drop, it is called 'hitting the wall' (cyclists, strangely, call this 'bonking'), an altogether unsavoury feeling of extreme fatigue, dizziness and hunger. This feeling can be partially reversed by consuming some quick-to-absorb carbohydrate, such as a sports drink or soft confectionery (candy). If you ever do hit the wall, evaluate your eating habits in the 24 hours before the event and your nutrition during the event. There is a good chance you didn't consume enough carbohydrate before or during the event.

Liver glycogen is the main source of blood glucose, and overnight your liver glycogen can drop by two thirds. This is a key reason you should eat something before an event, especially after an overnight fast (i.e., sleeping). There should be enough fuel for an early morning training session of 60 minutes, however, provided you ate enough carbohydrate the night before.

When you run out of muscle glycogen, your muscles begin to take up more glucose from your blood (see figure 1.8). At this point your liver comes to the rescue. The hormone glucagon races off to the liver and asks the liver to now convert its glycogen to glucose and pump it into the blood. Taking a sports drink or a carbohydrate gel will also help keep blood glucose levels up during long events.

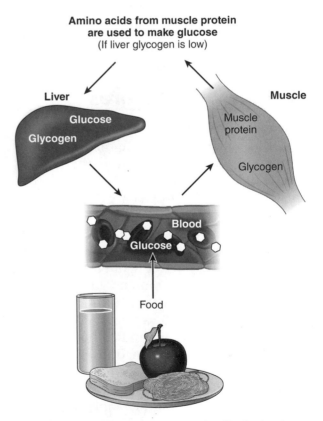

FIGURE 1.8 The glucose cycle. Carbohydrate-containing food and drinks are absorbed as glucose into the blood. From there, glucose is transported to the muscles and liver to be stored as glycogen.

When liver glycogen levels run low, the adrenal gland releases the hormone cortisol. Cortisol tells some of the muscle protein to break down to amino acids, which then go to the liver to be made into glucose and released into the blood. You can see why it's smart to have lots of glycogen in your muscles and liver before you start—it means you won't burn up muscle protein.

FINAL SCORE

- Protein is plentiful in most people's diets. Most people eat more than they need, unless the diet is highly restricted.
- Fat is essential to health. It is mainly saturated fat that should be limited because it can be harmful to overall health.
- If you are active and relatively lean, you don't have to severely limit your unsaturated fat intake.
- Forms of carbohydrate include both sugar, of which there are six common types in nature (glucose, fructose, galactose, sucrose, lactose and maltose), and starch, of which there are two main types (amylose and amylopectin).
- Sugars are a normal part of the diet. They are not harmful, except when you eat so much added-sugar foods that they displace other nutritious foods.
- Some sugar-containing foods are very nutritious, such as fruit, milk, yogurt, soy drinks and chocolate.
- Starches are long chains of glucose molecules. Starchy foods generally also provide essential minerals, vitamins, antioxidants and fibre.
- Fibre is found only in plant foods. If you eat plenty of fruits, vegetables, legumes and whole-grain cereals, you will likely be getting enough fibre for health.
- Plant foods are very protective against future disease because of their high levels of essential nutrients, fibre and antioxidants.
- The first five or six seconds of a sprint activity relies on creatine phosphate to activate the ATP.
- High-intensity exercise relies mainly on glucose for energy.
- Lower-intensity activity relies on the aerobic system, which uses both fat and glucose as fuels.
- Glycogen is the rate-limiting fuel. When glycogen stores are low, fatigue results. For greatest endurance, a high-carbohydrate diet is required.

Protein for Growth and Maintenance

> **Protein recommendations for endurance and strength-trained athletes range from 1.2 to 1.7 g/kg (0.5 to 0.8 g/lb) body weight per day. These recommended protein intakes can generally be met through diet alone, without the use of protein or amino acid supplements. Energy intake sufficient to maintain body weight is necessary for optimal protein use and performance.**
>
> *Position of the American Dietetic Association, Dietitians of Canada and the American College of Sports Medicine (2009, 510)*

In the sixth century BC, the Greek athlete Milo of Crotonia won wrestling gold in six Olympic games and was recognised as one of the world's strongest men. He may have developed the first progressive resistance exercise program by lifting a calf daily. As the calf grew, Milo continued to lift it, and his muscles became stronger. When the calf was four years old, Milo had her for dinner. It was common for him to eat 5 to 8 kilograms (11 to 18 lb) of meat a day, or so the legend goes. Was it Milo who sparked the great protein debate?

The popular view of most athletes today is that muscles, being made of protein, will get bigger the more protein the person eats. Lean steaks, skinless chicken, amino acids and protein powders attract those in search of the larger latissimus, the bigger biceps, and the gargantuan gastrocnemius. Do we know how much protein an athlete needs? Let's take a look at the science.

What Are Proteins and Amino Acids?

Protein is composed of long chains of amino acids. The amino acids that the body can make are called non-essential amino acids. Eight amino acids, called essential amino acids, can't be made by the body and must be provided by foods (see table 2.1). (Scientists now use the terms *indispensable* and *dispensable* for essential and non-essential amino acids, respectively, but because the latter two terms are better known and understood, we will continue using them.)

High-protein foods of animal origin such as meat, chicken, fish, milk, cheese, yogurt and eggs provide all of the essential amino acids. This is not to discount other valuable sources of protein from plant foods. About one third of our protein comes from cereal foods (e.g., bread, rice), legumes, fruits and vegetables. Table 2.2 lists some of protein's most common food sources.

Some plant foods are low in some of the essential amino acids. A combination of plant foods can provide all the essential amino acids at the one meal, with one food compensating for a low level of an essential amino acid in another food. For example, grains can be low in the essential amino acid lysine, whereas legumes may be low in the essential amino acid methionine. By combining legumes with cereal foods (e.g., beans on toast, lentils with rice) and seeds or nuts with grains (e.g., peanut butter sandwich), the body gets adequate amounts of both amino acids from a meal.

Many believe that all the essential amino acids need to be eaten at each meal, but this is not necessary. If a person consumes a range of protein foods throughout the day, enough amino acids will be circulating in the body from which it can select the essential amino acids it needs. As long as the diet provides the minimum essential amino acids over 24 hours, there is no risk of a protein deficiency. This is quite simple for ovo-lacto vegetarians because they eat eggs, milk, cheese and yogurt, all of which contain adequate amounts of essential amino acids. Only the vegan, who eats no animal foods, is at risk of too little protein. Soy milk, tofu, nuts, seeds, legumes, wheat germ and grains can provide sufficient protein for vegans, although I do suggest that vegan athletes consult a sports dietitian to ensure that they are getting adequate nutrition.

Getting enough protein each day is not difficult, and virtually all athletes and active people can get what they need from regular meals and snacks.

TABLE 2.1 Amino Acids

Essential amino acids	Nonessential amino acids
• Isoleucine	• Alanine
• Leucine	• Arginine
• Lysine	• Asparagine
• Methionine	• Aspartic acid
• Phenylalanine	• Cysteine
• Threonine	• Glutamic acid
• Tryptophan	• Glutamine
• Valine	• Glycine
	• Histidine
	• Proline
	• Serine
	• Tyrosine

TABLE 2.2 Common Sources of Protein

Food	Protein (g)
Meat, lean, 100 g average	27.0
Fish, cooked average 100 g	22.0
Poultry, lean meat, 100 g	27.0
Cheese, cheddar, 30 g	7.0
Milk, 200 mL	7.0
Soy milk, 200 mL	7.0
Yogurt, 200 mL, average	10.0
Egg, 1 whole 50 g	7.0
Bread, 1 slice	3.0
Breakfast cereal, 1 serve, average	4.0
Vegetables, ½ cup, average	1.0
Mushrooms, ½ cup	1.5
Potato, baked, 1	3.0
Legumes, ½ cup average	7.0
Fruit, 1 serve, average	1.0
Pasta, cooked, 1 cup	8.0
Rice, cooked, 1 cup	5.0
Muesli & nut bar, 40 g	3.5
Protein sports bars 60 g	18.0
Nuts, 30 g, average	4.0
Peanut butter, 1 tbsp (30 g)	7.0
Milk chocolate, 50 g	4.0
Popcorn, 1 cup	1.0

There are more protein figures in the Nutrient Ready Reckoner on page 215.

Protein Digestion: From Mouth to Blood

A small amount of the protein we eat is digested in the stomach, but the majority is digested in the small intestine. Here the protein is broken down into smaller chains of amino acids (peptides) by digestive enzymes. The results of digestion are single amino acids and small peptides of two or three amino acids joined together (figure 2.1). These are then absorbed from the intestine into the blood to be made into body proteins such as hemoglobin, ferritin, antibodies, enzymes, hair and muscle. Amino acids in the form of small peptides are more rapidly and efficiently absorbed than single amino acids (called 'free form' amino acids) because they are absorbed through different pathways. We have known this since 1962, yet the notion that 'free form' amino acids are the best way to get amino acids is still widely promoted. The most efficient way to take your amino acids is as food protein, preferably a low-fat version such as non-fat milk, lean meat or chicken breast.

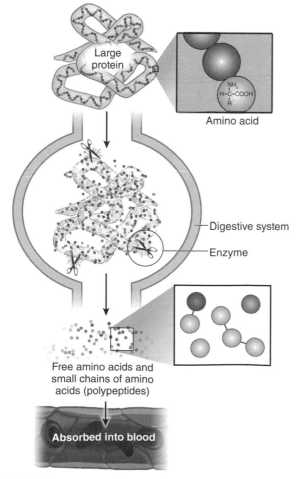

FIGURE 2.1 Long chains of amino acids in protein are broken down by digestive enzymes for absorption into the blood.

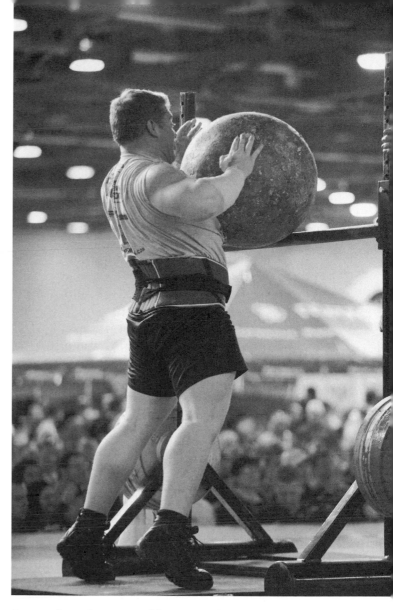

Strength and power athletes need the most protein; however, this extra protein can be obtained through smart eating.

Christophe ate the most enormous steak, and I knew then that we had the man for the job.

David Redvers, horse breeder, after jockey Christophe Lemaire won the 2011 Melbourne Cup on Dunaden

Protein Needs of Athletes

The value of protein to athletes has been debated for over 100 years in scientific literature. In the early 1900s protein was considered essential for muscle strength and the most important fuel for exercise. In the 1970s the scientific opinion was that the protein needs of athletes were the same as those of sedentary people. Now there is universal agreement that active people, especially athletes, require more protein than sedentary people do.

There is still a lot of debate over the protein needs of different athletes under various sporting conditions. I have given a table of protein requirements (see table 2.3), based on the research at the time of writing. This advice will be refined with further research, although don't expect the amount of protein recommended to change dramatically. New research will provide a better idea of the timing of meals, the type of protein mix, protein distribution through the day and what other nutrients to consume with the protein to ensure that the protein is most effectively converted to muscle.

It seems that female athletes don't need as much protein as male athletes do, about 10 to 20 per cent fewer grams of protein for an equivalent body weight. For example, a 65-kilogram (143 lb) female endurance athlete requires about 66 grams of protein daily. This is calculated by multiplying 65 by 1.2 grams per kilogram of body weight (78 g) and then reducing this figure by 15 per cent (78 g × 0.85 = 66 g).

If you are carrying excess body fat, then base your protein requirements on your ideal weight, not your current weight. If you are already well muscled and have normal body fat levels, then calculate your protein needs based on your current weight.

During exercise the body relies mainly on muscle glycogen, liver glycogen and fat stores for fuel. However, athletes doing high-intensity training or endurance training for more than an hour may use some protein for muscle fuel, especially if glycogen stores are low. In other words, when people consume too little carbohydrate, muscle protein and amino acids in the blood are converted to glucose to be used as muscle fuel. Weight training uses mainly carbohydrate as a fuel during intense sets. Protein is also needed for muscle growth and repair after resistance training, intense exercise or endurance training, hence the higher protein needs of athletes.

Protein may account for 5 to 10 per cent of the energy men use in endurance training. This percentage is normally lower in women, who make better use of fat as a fuel and are therefore better fat burners than men are. A greater amount of protein is used as muscle fuel if muscle glycogen stores are low. For this reason, be sure to pump your glycogen stores with plenty of carbohydrate before sport to stop your body from using protein as fuel. Note: High-carbohydrate foods are generally cheaper than protein foods, so fuelling your body right could save you money.

TABLE 2.3 Recommended Daily Intake of Protein (Grams)

Type of person	Grams/kg IBW[a]/day	75 kg man	65 kg woman[b]
Adults, non-athletes	0.8	60	52
Elite endurance athletes	1.6	120	88
Moderate intensity endurance athletes	1.2	90	66
Power sports	1.4–1.7	105–127	77–94
Strength athletes (early training)	1.5–1.7	112–127	83–94
Strength athletes (steady state)	1.0–1.2	75–90	55–66
Recreational athletes	0.8-1.0	60-75	55
ACTUAL DAILY INTAKE OF PROTEIN			
Average adult eats	1.0–1.5		
Average female athlete eats	1.0–2.8		
Average male athlete eats	1.5–4.0		

[a]IBW = ideal body weight.

[b]Female athletes require about 15% less protein than male athletes.

Sources: Nutrient Reference Values for Australia and New Zealand 2006; Tarnopolsky, M. 2010. *Clinical Sports Nutrition*. Sydney: McGraw-Hill.

How Much Protein Do You Need?

Sports nutrition experts agree that the healthy eating ideals covered so far in this book will provide the needs of virtually all athletes. The quote at the beginning of the chapter and the one that follows, both from authoritative voices, suggest that getting your protein needs is quite simple.

A dietary protein intake that represents about 15% of the total energy intake with an energy-sufficient diet should easily cover the requirements for nearly all strength and endurance athletes. Given the increase in energy intake by most athletes, there is no need to use protein supplements to attain these levels.

Professor Mark Tarnopolsky
(2010, 83)

These opinions reflect the protein research since 1990. Most active people use 10,500 to 12,500 kilojoules (about 2,500 to 3,000 cal) per day, and 15 per cent of that is 1,570 to 1,875 kilojoules (375 to 450 cal), which is around 94 to 112 grams of protein. This will cover the protein needs of many athletes, as shown in table 2.2 on page 22. Although athletes need more protein than the unfit, their extra protein needs are covered by their bigger appetites, making protein a perceived, rather than a real, concern for most athletes.

Athletes just beginning a training program might need the higher end of the range, whereas seasoned athletes probably require less protein. There is no benefit in taking more than 2 grams of protein per kilogram of body weight, providing you are consuming enough carbohydrate, yet many strength athletes believe that the more protein they take in, the better.

To put this in perspective, the average sedentary person eats 1.0 to 1.5 grams of protein per kilogram of body weight; the average female athlete eats 1.0 to 2.8 grams per kilogram; and the average male athlete eats 1.5 to 4.0 grams per kilogram—so there is a good chance you are getting enough protein. But don't take my word for it. Use the Nutrient Ready Reckoner on page 215 to see whether you are getting enough protein to cover your training needs.

Can You Eat Too Much Protein?

Almost everyone in Western society eats more protein than necessary. The average athlete often eats twice the recommended amount of protein. If more protein is eaten than is required, the excess protein is used as muscle fuel during exercise or possibly stored as body fat (but not muscle). There is probably no harm in a healthy adult having a relatively high protein intake. Although it is widely agreed that no athlete needs more than 2 grams of protein per kilogram of body weight, there is no evidence of harm when consuming 2.5 to 3.0 grams per kilogram (about 240 g in an 80 kg, or 176 lb, athlete).

Protein is high in nitrogen, and this nitrogen needs to be excreted daily via the kidneys. Therefore, more protein in the diet means more nitrogen that must be excreted, which means that more urine has to be produced, which in turn requires the athlete to drink more water. Anyone with kidney or liver disease, or a family history of kidney disease, should see a specialist for specific protein recommendations.

The sample menu in table 2.4 on page 26 provides around 127 grams of protein and 11,370 kilojoules (2,715 cal), showing that getting plenty of protein in a day is quite easy. A daily intake of 11,370 kilojoules is modest—most active people eat more than this.

Should You Consume Protein Just Before Sport?

The current view is that unless the preexercise meal doubles as a recovery meal from the last exercise session, such as having only a two- to three-hour break between workouts, there is no clear evidence that you will benefit by having protein just before sport. Your presport meal will already provide some protein (e.g., cereal and milk, sandwiches or a banana smoothie). We are really in the early days of research regarding whether protein taken in the hour prior to sport provides an extra benefit to athletes.

Should You Consume Protein During Sport?

Many have wondered whether protein consumed in a beverage during sport will reduce protein breakdown or reduce muscle damage. Although we are not certain of the answer,

TABLE 2.4 Sample High-Carbohydrate, High-Protein Meal Plan

Food	Protein	Fat	Carbohydrate
Weet-Bix, 3	6	1	30
Milk, reduced fat, 200 mL (7 oz)	8	4	12
Bread, 2 slices	5	2	30
Margarine, 2 tsp	0	8	0
Marmalade, jam, 4 tsp	0	0	14
Fruit juice, 150 mL (5 oz)	0	0	15
Banana	2	0	22
Ham and salad sandwich, 2	24	21	60
Flavoured milk, 300 mL (10 oz)	12	6	25
Flavoured yogurt, 200 mL (7 oz)	9	4	25
Sports drink, 500 mL (17 oz)	0	0	30
Steamed rice, 2 cups	10	2	100
Chicken breast, 150 g (5.3 oz)	42	6	0
Vegetables, 1 cup	3	0	10
Fruit salad, 1 cup	1	0	24
Ice cream, 1 scoop	2	5	10
Milo (2 tsp Milo + 40 mL, or 1.4 oz, milk + water)	3	2	8
TOTALS	**127**	**61**	**415**

some early research hints that a little protein in a sports drink could be beneficial in endurance sport. Long-distance cyclists were given either a sports drink or a sports drink with added whey protein (1.8 g per 100 mL). The cyclists who were given sports drinks with added protein were able to ride 29 per cent longer before exhaustion. The researchers also found less muscle damage in the cyclists who were given the sports drink with protein (Saunders, Kane and Todd 2004). More research is needed in this area to clarify whether protein taken during sport will help some athletes. (For a more detailed discussion on protein in sports drinks, see chapter 5.)

Before we can give more precise information on protein requirements during sport, we need more research into the best type or mix of protein and whether protein should be taken in solid or liquid form.

Should You Consume Protein Straight After Sport?

Yes, some protein is needed after exercise to build muscle and help repair any muscle damage, probably in the region of 20 grams of protein. The best current advice is to eat a combination of protein and carbohydrate soon after intense exercise because that provides both amino acids and glucose for muscle repair and growth and helps replenish muscle fuel.

A regular meal including lean protein sources and high-carbohydrate foods does stimulate the uptake of amino acids, mainly through the action of the hormone insulin released after a meal. Any reasonable meal provides around 30 grams of protein and 80 grams of carbohydrate (e.g., one ham and salad roll with one fruit and 240 mL of juice are around 30 g of protein and

85 g of carbohydrate; a Triple G drink described in chapter 12 and two pieces of fruit provides 26 g of protein and 80 g of carbohydrate). This should allow the body to quickly repair any muscle damage caused by a workout and provide amino acids to help increase muscle mass in strength training.

It is wise to spread your protein intake evenly throughout the day. In Western societies we often have an evening meal that is laden with protein, especially animal protein, and skimp on protein through the day.

Protein Supplements

The protein supplement was born mainly in response to the demands of bodybuilders. Although protein is a popular supplement, few athletes or bodybuilders need extra protein in addition to the protein they get from food. One advantage of protein supplements is that they are convenient. If your training venue is a long way from home, then taking a protein supplement soon after training will help muscle repair and growth until you are able to get home and have a meal. If you don't feel like eating in the two hours after a workout or event, then a protein supplement, preferably with carbohydrate to replace muscle fuel, can be handy to help repair muscle damage.

I worked with an elite Rugby Union team that had training in the early morning, followed by stretching, rehabilitation for the injured, and visits to the doctor, physiotherapist or dietitian. We provided a breakfast and a protein supplement after training because it would have been too long before they got home to some food.

Some athletes, such as vegans, other strict vegetarians and those on a restricted energy diet, benefit from a protein supplement because they cannot get enough in their diets. Vegans may prefer to meet their extra protein needs through a soy protein supplement. For athletes who expend a lot of energy each day, the protein supplement is a simple way of getting the nutrients and kilojoules they need.

Whether you are buying a supplement drink or meal replacement for weight loss, muscle gain or improved performance, what appears on the label is usually the scientific terms for each ingredient. That can make it sound more impressive than it is or just plain confuse you. Here are some examples:

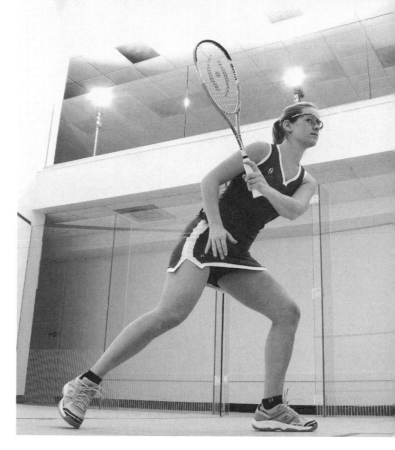

Eating a mix of protein and carbohydrates soon after finishing sport helps replace muscle fuel and repair any muscle damage.

- Calcium caseinate—milk protein (milk protein is about 80 per cent casein)
- Whey protein—another milk protein (left over from cheese manufacturing)
- Lactalbumin—a specific whey protein
- Non-fat milk solids—non-fat, or skim, milk powder
- Soy protein isolate—protein extracted from soybeans
- Egg albumin—egg white
- Dextrose—glucose
- Maltodextrins—small chains of glucose molecules
- Xantham, carrageenan, guar—vegetable gums often used as thickening agents
- Lecithin—an emulsifier that stops any fat from rising to the top of the drink

All of the previous ingredients are inexpensive and do not generally deserve to be sold to consumers at premium prices. Even the vitamins added to such products are inexpensive. Whey protein has become a very popular protein supplement, and there is good evidence that it assists muscle development (Hayes 2008). There may be an advantage in having a mix of casein, whey and soy protein in a protein supplement. Each is

▶ Protein Supplements

Protein powders, protein bars and weight gain powders have virtually the same ingredients as weight loss powders: milk powder, milk protein, soy protein, sugar, vitamins and flavour.

GLENNERGY DIY

If you really believe you need a protein supplement, here's one that will save you a lot of money. You can make it for around 20 per cent of the retail cost of a similar protein powder.

Ingredients

1 kg (2.2 lb) non-fat milk powder

7 tbsp sugar

7 tbsp flavour (e.g., Milo, Nesquik)

Method

Mix together to make a powder in bulk.

To make one drink add 4 tbsp powder to 200 mL (7 oz) of water. Add sugar and flavour to your taste.

Compare the nutrition analysis of Glennergy DIY with the ones on your protein powder.

NUTRITION ANALYSIS

	Per 100 g of powder	4 tbsp (30 g/1 oz)
Protein (g)	27	9
Carbohydrate (g)	62	21
Fat (g)	2	<1
Calcium (mg)	980	325
Energy	1,540 kJ (370 cal)	510 kJ (122 cal)

a complete protein, providing all of the essential amino acids. Whey protein is digested quickly, soy protein is digested at an intermediate speed, and casein is digested slowly. That means that the whey and soy protein assist in muscle synthesis straight after a workout, whereas casein provides an amino acid source a bit later. The mix of the three proteins could be an ideal blend to minimise muscle breakdown while enhancing muscle synthesis in the hours after exercise (Paul 2009).

At the time of this writing, protein supplements range from $42 to $98 per kilogram, or $19 to $44 per pound. A homemade protein and energy supplement that a client named after me (Glennergy DIY) is inexpensive ($8 per kilogram $3.60 per pound) and can be made in the comfort of your own kitchen.

Many protein supplements list their amino acid content. Compare them with the amino acid profile of the common foods listed in table 2.5.

Fill in the blank column with information on the amino acid content of your favourite supplement. It may be cheaper to get your protein from food. Some specific amino acids are promoted as a sport supplement, but there is little scientific evidence to suggest that they are useful to athletes, as explained in more detail in chapter 9.

Remember the following:

- Most recreational athletes can get their protein needs from food. Protein supplements may only benefit the elite athlete doing more than 10 hours of training each week.

- Your body cannot tell the difference between protein in a protein powder and protein from milk powder (a mix of casein and whey protein). If you truly believe you need extra protein, then an affordable drink such as Glennergy is the way to go.

TABLE 2.5 Approximate Amino Acid Content (mg) of Some Foods

Amino acid (mg)	Protein or amino acid supplement	Baked beans, 1 cup	Milk, 250 mL (8.5 oz) glass	Egg, 50 g (1.8 oz)	Skim milk powder, 100 g (3.5 oz)
Isoleucine		565	495	343	2,124
Leucine		1,012	802	534	3,438
Lysine		745	650	452	2,784
Methionine		117	205	196	880
Phenylalanine		667	395	334	1,694
Threonine		373	370	302	1,584
Tryptophan		128	115	76	495
Valine		650	550	384	2,349
Histidine		330	223	149	952
Arginine		572	298	377	1,271
Alanine		507	283	350	1,210
Aspartic acid		1,577	622	632	2,663
Cysteine		92	75	146	325
Glutamic acid		2,000	1,718	822	7,350
Glycine		465	173	212	743
Proline		600	795	250	3,400
Serine		800	445	468	1,909
Tyrosine		302	395	256	1,694

Amino acid (mg)	Protein or amino acid supplement	Lean chicken breast, 100 g (3.5 oz)	Lean beef, 100 g (3.5 oz)	Bread, 1 slice (30 g; 1 oz)	Rice, 1 cup cooked (150 g; 5.3 oz)
Isoleucine		1,638	1,198	105	153
Leucine		2,328	2,095	188	292
Lysine		2,635	2,226	85	127
Methionine		859	686	43	84
Phenylalanine		1,231	1,040	130	189
Threonine		1,310	1,052	83	126
Tryptophan		362	173	39	40
Valine		1,539	1,307	124	216
Histidine		963	840	63	84
Arginine		1,871	1,703	126	295
Alanine		1,692	1,601	75	205
Aspartic acid		2,764	2,399	108	333
Cysteine		397	340	60	72
Glutamic acid		4,645	3,954	825	690
Glycine		1,524	1,604	80	162
Proline		1,275	1,255	315	166
Serine		1,067	1,037	140	186
Tyrosine		1,047	839	81	118

Data from USDA National Nutrient Database for Standard Reference, Release 17 (2004)

www.nal.usda.gov/fnic/foodcomp/Data/SR17/reports/sr17page.htm.

- Your protein powder may have more protein per 100 grams than Glennergy, mainly because the carbohydrate has been extracted. Compare the cost per gram of protein.

- Glennergy also makes an ideal presport meal. You may want to blend in some fruit rather than adding flavouring.

FINAL ANALYSIS

- Active people and athletes need more protein than spectators do.
- The current evidence doesn't suggest that performance can be significantly enhanced by protein or amino acid supplementation, except in the unlikely event that the athlete is getting inadequate protein.
- The protein needs of an athlete can be met adequately with a variety of healthy foods. Use the Nutrient Ready Reckoner in the appendix on page 215 to assess your own protein intake.
- An inexpensive milk-based protein drink such as Glennergy or Triple G (described in chapter 12) can be a useful adjunct to a healthy training diet.
- To assist muscle repair and growth after resistance or endurance training, eat protein foods throughout the day and soon after completing a training session.
- You can boost the protein content of your diet by adding milk powder, wheat germ, powdered food drinks and nut meal to foods and dishes.
- Protein can be converted to glucose to be used as a muscle fuel, but this usually occurs only near the end of endurance sports such as triathlons, marathons and ironman events, or if an excessive amount of protein is consumed.
- Future research may show that taking protein or amino acids before or during endurance exercise reduces muscle protein breakdown to glucose.

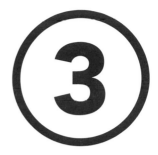

Carbohydrate for Energy

> Animal diet alone is prescribed, and beef and mutton are preferred. Biscuits and stale bread are the only preparations of vegetable matter which are permitted. Vegetables are never given as they are watery and of difficult digestion. Fish must be avoided. Salt, spices, and all kind of seasonings, with the exception of vinegar, are prohibited. Liquors must always be taken cold, and home brewed beer, old but not bottled, is best. Water is never given alone. It is an established rule to avoid liquids as much as possible.
>
> *Captain Robert Barclay Allardice,*
> *long-distance walker, c. 1810*

Our knowledge of sports nutrition has come a long way since Robert Barclay Allardice walked 1,600 kilometres (1,000 miles) in 1,000 hours, about 38 kilometres (24 miles) a day for 42 days. In 1999 long-distance runner Pat Farmer was able to run 70 kilometres (43 miles) a day for 200 days to run around Australia by being on the right fuel. All sport scientists agree that an athlete's diet must be high in carbohydrate to fuel muscles.

Why Carbohydrate?

Carbohydrate is your main source of glucose, the sugar used by the body to produce ATP for muscle contraction (see chapter 1). If you do not stock up on carbohydrate, then your glycogen stores will be low and you will quickly run out of glycogen during exercise. Once you run out of glycogen (i.e., 'hit the wall'), you will need to rely heavily on muscle protein and body fat for energy. Unfortunately, these are less efficient than carbohydrate as muscle fuel.

You may have been told to avoid carbohydrate in an attempt to lose excess body fat. This is misguided because in doing so you are depriving the body of its favourite fuel for exercise. If you are involved in aerobic exercise, then you need carbohydrate and fat for fuel. As the intensity of exercise increases, your muscles need mainly glucose (carbohydrate). If you do mainly weight training, then you rely heavily on carbohydrate for fuel because each muscle contraction uses glucose. Some weight training athletes avoid carbohydrate foods not realising that they must then produce glucose from the protein they eat. That's not necessarily a problem, it's just that high-protein foods are usually more expensive than high-carbohydrate foods.

Blood Glucose and Glycogen

When you eat carbohydrate, your blood glucose level rises, which stimulates the release of the hormone insulin. Blood glucose is commonly called blood sugar, and insulin is needed to lower the blood sugar level after a meal and promote storage of glucose as muscle and liver glycogen. Some people believe that this release of insulin inevitably results in low blood sugar and, therefore, decreased sports performance. But this is misguided because in most cases the insulin brings blood glucose back to normal. Should blood glucose drop too low, another hormone called glucagon steps in to raise it back to normal. This happens naturally in most healthy adults.

Another common misconception is that insulin converts carbohydrate to fat. This is not true. Instead, insulin promotes the storage of glucose as muscle and liver glycogen, not as fat! Insulin also helps the muscles take up amino acids for muscle repair, and fat for fuel during aerobic exercise. So, in summary, the digestive enzymes break down the starch molecules, and the resulting glucose molecules are absorbed into the bloodstream, causing a rise in the blood glucose levels. The hormone insulin then lowers the blood glucose levels and promotes storage of glucose as muscle and liver glycogen.

Athletes generally eat lots of high-carbohydrate foods, so they are able to store more glycogen, allowing them to train and compete for long periods. Glycogen is a long sequence of glucose molecules with many branches, similar to amylopectin in starch. This branching is very useful because it allows glycogen to be quickly broken down to individual glucose molecules that provide muscle energy during exercise.

How Much Carbohydrate Should You Eat?

Plenty, if you are a very active person. Almost all surveys of athletes reveal that they eat too little carbohydrate for their training level. Most adults eat only 150 to 250 grams of carbohydrate a day. That might be OK if you are sedentary. Unfortunately, that amount of carbohydrate daily is not enough to fuel an athlete's body, so it's no wonder so many feel tired. Most recreational athletes need 300 to 400 grams of carbohydrate daily. Elite athletes need 500 to 700 grams every day.

Just how much carbohydrate you need to eat depends on your sport, training level, gender, size, appetite and so on. I'll try to help you find your carbohydrate needs, which will be expressed in grams of carbohydrate for every kilogram of your ideal weight (see table 3.1).

Carbohydrate recommendations for athletes range from 6-10 g/kg (2.7-4.5 g/lb) body weight per day. Carbohydrates maintain blood glucose levels during exercise and replace muscle glycogen. The amount required depends upon the athlete's total daily energy expenditure, type of sport, sex, and environmental conditions.

Position of the American Dietetic Association, Dietitians of Canada and the American College of Sports Medicine: Nutrition and Athletic Performance (2009, 510)

Based on table 3.1 and your body weight, you can get an approximate idea of your carbohydrate needs by using this simple formula:

Your weight (in kg) × grams of carbohydrate per kg of body weight = your carbohydrate needs each day

For example, from table 3.1 we can see that a serious amateur athlete might need 6 grams of carbohydrate per kilogram of body weight per day. If the athlete weighs 70 kilograms (154 lb), the equation would look like this:

70 kg × 6 g carbohydrate per kg per day = 420 g carbohydrate per day

Be warned: When you do your calculations, you will see that you need a lot of carbohydrate,

TABLE 3.1 Your Carbohydrate Needs

Carbohydrate (g per kg of body weight per day)	Activity level sustained
1	• The amount of carbohydrate you get with some weight loss programs • Very little aerobic activity possible
2	• Sleeping, watching TV, sitting
3	• Daily chores (The amount most adults eat)
4–5	• A good intake for active people. • Walking, moderate exercise, recreational sports, fitness programs (3–5 hr/wk)
5–7	• Serious amateur sports, football, rugby, netball, bodybuilding, weight training • Medium level of exercise (6–10 hr/wk)
7–9	• Serious professional sports • Endurance sports, marathons • Training 10+ hours a week
10+	• Full-time athletes • Ultra-endurance, ironman events • Olympic athlete • Training 15+ hours a week

Note: This is a guide only. Women generally can sustain activity at the lower end of the range of carbohydrate intake for each activity level.

and you're going to think, 'How will I ever eat that much?' If your carbohydrate needs are high, then you will likely need to eat frequent snacks or meals throughout the day just to get enough food. I'll show you later in this chapter how it's done in food terms. Make your first goal to eat a little more carbohydrate (say, an extra 50 g a day). Just make sure you choose good-quality carbohydrate foods such as bananas, baked beans and whole-grain bread, not doughnuts and biscuits. One trick is to cut back on the fatty foods to make more room for high-carbohydrate foods. You will certainly feel and perform better if you do. Less fat in your meals may take a little getting used to. Remember, it's less fat, not zero fat.

Certainly, men find it easier than women to eat enough carbohydrate because women, generally, eat less food than men do. Part of the reason could be that women seem to be better fat burners than men are and therefore need less carbohydrate during endurance events. Women should choose the lower-carbohydrate figure for their activity level in table 3.1, eating more if that amount is clearly not enough.

Carbohydrate Loading

The classic carbohydrate-loading regimen was first described in 1966 by Scandinavian researchers (Bergström and Hultman 1966). To boost muscle glycogen stores, their athletes endured three days of low-carbohydrate eating, followed by three days of high-carbohydrate eating just before the big event. This regimen does increase the amount of glycogen stored in muscle, but in the three days without carbohydrate, the athlete suffers severe fatigue and irritability and feels like an invalid with a sack of potatoes under each arm. This manner of increasing glycogen stores is no longer considered necessary, although some athletes still swear by it.

Now we realise that a moderate- to high-carbohydrate diet throughout the pre-event week, especially the two days before, has the same effect of raising muscle glycogen to high levels as the Scandinavian regimen. For this reason sports dietitians recommend moderate- to high-carbohydrate eating all the time for serious athletes. Enjoyable carbohydrate loading now consists of a week of tapered training, working down to light training during the two or three days before the event, while at the same time consuming high-carbohydrate meals. This pattern is illustrated in figure 3.1 on page 34. Be aware that as training tapers, you are likely to feel less hungry than you usually do. Just make sure that the foods you choose are relatively high in carbohydrate, especially in the two days before the event.

This message can get confused. Some see carbohydrate loading as cake overloading, or as

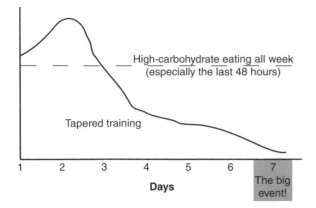

FIGURE 3.1 Carbohydrate loading combined with tapered training in the week before a big endurance event.

just including some rice, potatoes or pasta in a meal. Certainly, carbohydrate loading is not an excuse to eat until you are bloated! The idea is to eat plenty of carbohydrate, not lots of any food that tastes sweet. Cake may taste sweet, but a lot of its kilojoules (40 per cent) comes from fat.

Pasta is a favourite pre-event meal for most athletes. Unfortunately, many think that just because they have pasta on their plate, they're carbohydrate loading. It's not the case, however, if the pasta is suffocating under a mountain of meat sauce and cheese. Pasta should be the mountain; and the sauce and cheese, the snow-cap.

An athlete might eat more bread for extra carbohydrate, yet be totally unaware that a 290 kilojoule (70 cal) slice of bread has been smeared with 420 kilojoules (100 cal) or more of margarine or butter. This is fat loading, not carbohydrate loading. It's smarter to have only a scrape of butter or margarine to allow enough room for two slices of bread. Likewise, potatoes should not be served with lots of sour cream, and rice shouldn't be fried with lots of oil. In both cases more energy is coming from fat than from carbohydrate.

Sugar and Your Health

You will note that some of my suggestions to boost carbohydrate include foods that have sugar such as sorbet, confectionery (candy) and ice cream. Fortunately, active people have a great deal of flexibility with their diet and can include some sugar-containing food without compromising their health. Some foods with sugar such as flavoured yogurt, ice cream and chocolate also provide essential nutrients. Sugar confectionery is used by many athletes as a carbohydrate source during, or just after, sport. Let's take a brief look at two issues that usually arise when sugar is discussed.

Sugar in Food

Part of the emotion of the debate of sugar versus starch is that most people don't understand the real difference between the two. It is not rational

▶ Boosting the Carbohydrate (But Not the Fat)

- Eat at least two pieces of fruit a day.
- Eat plenty of starchy vegetables, such as peas, corn, potatoes, baked beans.
- If you like chips, choose low-fat oven fries (frozen food section).
- Eat all kinds of pasta (go easy on cheese and oil).
- Choose low-fat milk and yogurt (flavoured versions OK).
- Eat steamed rice instead of fried rice.
- Eat fruit instead of biscuits, cookies or cakes.
- Eat a bread roll instead of pies, pastries or sausage rolls.
- Breakfast cereals and mueslis are high in carbohydrate (avoid toasted varieties).
- Eat more bread, but use less butter or margarine.
- Try a banana sandwich for a carbohydrate-packed snack.
- Halve the oil, margarine or butter in standard recipes—doing so usually doesn't affect the end result and makes more room for carbohydrate.
- Have lots of canned fruit and one scoop of ice cream for dessert.
- Sorbet and gelato make great desserts.

to state that sugar-containing foods are implicitly bad given that foods such as fruit, milk, yogurt and soy drinks provide their carbohydrate only as sugars (e.g., fruit provides glucose, fructose and sucrose; milk provides lactose). Some of the sweeter vegetables also contain sugar. Because fruits provide a handsome dividend in antioxidants (chemicals that slow the aging of the body), it would be ridiculous to malign them based on their sugar content.

The real problem is not sugar per se, but foods with a lot of sugar that provide little else in nutrition. Often this sugar is in the form of 'added sugar' (sugar not naturally present in a food). High-sugar foods can displace more nutritious foods from the diet. A can of soft drink will easily fit into an active person's diet, but 2 litres (68 oz) a day is not wise nutrition for anyone. Naturally, if you become inactive or need to lose excess body fat, then you need to limit high-sugar foods because they contribute energy (kilojoules, or calories) you need to burn.

There is no scientific link between sugar and diabetes, heart disease, arthritis or any other disease you care to name. The reason many adults get adult-onset diabetes is that their bodies have a reduced sensitivity to insulin and their blood sugar levels rise to unhealthy levels. This is commonly due to being overweight, itself caused by overeating and underexercising. Remember that table sugar is merely fructose and glucose, two molecules we have been consuming for millennia. Although sugar does not cause life-threatening disease, it may be involved in dental disease.

Sugar and Your Teeth

If you don't take care of your teeth, excess sugar in your diet can cause tooth decay. Any carbohydrate (both sugar and starch) that remains in the mouth after meals can be converted to lactic acid by bacteria in the mouth. The lactic acid can then eat away at the enamel of the tooth and, over time, cause decay. It is not scientific, however, to blame solely sugar for tooth decay. All forms of carbohydrate, including dried fruit and bread, have the potential to cause tooth decay.

There are a number of ways to stop tooth decay. Naturally, saliva has tooth-protective elements, and regular brushing and flossing of teeth also help maintain dental hygiene. Saliva also helps raise the pH to buffer the acids produced by oral bacteria or taken in the diet. For example, sports drinks, soft drinks and fruit juices are quite acidic and shouldn't stay in the mouth in contact with teeth for too long. It is wise to take these drinks via a straw so the fluid has minimal contact with the teeth, or at least use a drink bottle to squirt the liquid to the back of the tongue and drink them quickly.

Looking after your teeth is more a case of dental hygiene than of avoiding sugar. Dentists recommend that you allow at least two hours between eating times to give your saliva time to raise the pH and repair any damage caused to tooth enamel.

Artificial Sweeteners

For hundreds of years we have sweetened foods with sugar and honey. As a result of an occasional shortage of sugar, people became interested in using other sweeteners as tabletop sweeteners or in food manufacturing. Saccharin and cyclamate were two early examples. Common artificial sweeteners include:

- aspartame—found in Equal and Nutrasweet
- sucralose—Splenda
- saccharin—tends to have a bitter or metallic aftertaste
- cyclamate—often mixed with saccharin to reduce its aftertaste
- sugar polyols such as sorbitol and mannitol—often found in chewing gum, these are based on carbohydrate, so still contain some kilojoules; can cause gastrointestinal upset when eaten in large amounts
- stevia—derived from the sweet leaves of the stevia plant; one example is the brand called Truvia
- acesulfame potassium
- neotame—related to aspartame but much sweeter so it can be used at much lower levels

Despite widespread campaigns against them, there has never been a convincing argument to stop the use of artificial sweeteners on health grounds.

Agencies such as the U.S. Food and Drug Administration and the National Health and Medical Research Council in Australia rigorously check all of the research on sweetening agents before they are permitted on the market. Sweeteners can be added only to specific foods, and there is a limit to how much sweetener

▶ Smart Carbohydrate Eating

The idea of getting 400 grams of carbohydrate or more each day may sound like a lot of eating. Well, it isn't, if you choose wisely. Following are three sample menus that provide over 400 grams of carbohydrate.

HIGH-CARBOHYDRATE MENU 1

Food, Carbohydrate (g)			
BREAKFAST		**SNACK**	
4 Weet-Bix, Vita Brits	40	1 apple	14
200 mL (7 oz) reduced-fat milk	12	300 mL (10 oz) flavoured milk	25
2 tsp sugar	10	**TRAINING**	
2 slices toast	30	1,000 mL (34 oz) sports drink	60
1 tbsp jam/marmalade	14	**DINNER**	
SNACK		Meat	0
1 bread muffin	28	2 medium potatoes	32
1 banana	22	1 cup peas	9
LUNCH		1 cup carrots	5
4 slices bread + lean meat + salad	60	2 scoops ice cream	20
(sandwich)		1 cup canned fruit	21
250 mL (8.5 oz) fruit juice	25	250 mL (8.5 oz) fruit juice	25
1 chocolate bar, 50 g (1.8 oz)	30		
		TOTAL CARBOHYDRATE	**482**

HIGH-CARBOHYDRATE MENU 2

Food, Carbohydrate (g)			
BREAKFAST		**SNACK**	
1 cup canned spaghetti	30	300 mL (10 oz) flavoured milk	25
4 slices toast	60	**DINNER**	
250 mL (8.5 oz) fruit juice	25	2 cups steamed rice	100
SNACK		Meat/chicken/fish	0
Food bar	25	Stir-fried vegetables	15
LUNCH		1 cup fruit salad	24
2 bread rolls + avocado + salad	60	Yogurt, flavoured nonfat	25
1 banana	22		
1 iced fruit bun	40		
		TOTAL CARBOHYDRATE	**451**

HIGH-CARBOHYDRATE MENU 3

Food, Carbohydrate (g)			
BREAKFAST		**SNACK**	
2 cups breakfast cereal	50	2 mandarins	12
200 mL (7 oz) reduced-fat milk	12	**DINNER**	
2 tsp sugar	10	1 cup meat or seafood sauce	0
1/2 cup canned fruit	11	2 cups pasta	100
SNACK		Side salad	5
1 breakfast bar	28	2 scoops ice cream	20
1 medium apple	14	1 cup canned fruit	21
LUNCH		250 mL (8.5 oz) fruit juice	25
2 bread rolls with chicken and salad	60		
Triple G (see chapter 11)	47		
		TOTAL CARBOHYDRATE	**415**

Carbohydrate Confusion

Following are two menu examples of an athlete who has eaten enough calories but hasn't reached his carbohydrate goals. As a result, he faded badly during training. This person thought he was getting enough carbohydrate because he ate carbohydrate foods at each meal. Unfortunately, his choices were not ideal (e.g., french fries provide 40 per cent of their energy as fat), or they were inadequate (one cup of pasta is not likely to be enough for an active person).

CARBOHYDRATE FADEOUT 1

Food, Carbohydrate (g)			
BREAKFAST		**SNACK**	
2 slices toast with margarine	30	Doughnut	20
1 cup white tea	2	**DINNER**	
1 tsp sugar	5	1 cup pasta	50
LUNCH		Meat sauce	0
Bacon and cheese hamburger	50	Parmesan cheese	0
French fries	50		
375 mL (12 oz) diet soft drink	0		

TOTAL CARBOHYDRATE 207

CARBOHYDRATE FADEOUT 2

Food, Carbohydrate (g)			
BREAKFAST		**SNACK**	
2 slices toast	30	300 mL (10 oz) Flavoured milk	25
2 eggs	0	**DINNER**	
2 rashers bacon	0	3 pieces fried chicken	0
200 mL (7 oz) fruit juice	20	1 cup mashed potato	30
SNACK		Vegetables	10
2 biscuits	14		
LUNCH			
1 bread roll with filling	30		
1 slice of cake	36		

TOTAL CARBOHYDRATE 195

can be added to each food. Despite a common belief that artificial sweeteners cause cancer, the National Cancer Institute in the USA states that there is no evidence of any link of human cancer to sweetener use (www.cancer.gov/cancertopics/factsheet/Risk/artificial-sweeteners). A hoax e-mail that has done the rounds for many years claims that sweeteners cause a range of medical conditions such as multiple sclerosis. These claims have all been refuted by scientific testing. Sweetening agents do not interfere with sports performance.

Meeting Your Carbohydrate Needs

Although your regular meals will provide the majority of your carbohydrate needs, sometimes other products can supplement your carbohydrate intake. We will take a look at three of these.

Food Bars

There is a great range of food bars to choose from. Some are marketed as sports bars and energy bars, but these are nowhere near as magical as they might imply. Although they are generally a good-quality product and low in fat, you can usually get better value for your money with a wisely chosen muesli bar, fruit bar or other food bar. Many specialty food bars claim to encourage body fat loss or increase endurance or strength. They are unlikely to have a singular benefit based solely on the protein, fat and carbohydrate content and added nutrients. I know there is a wonderful attraction to bars promising the result you seek, but they are probably

▶ Guinness Book of Records

Although I do recommend that you eat an adequate amount of carbohydrate and enjoy your meals, some people have taken carbohydrate eating to the extreme. Years ago, the Guinness Book of Records documented individual cases of gluttony before they stopped those kinds of records. The 27th edition of the GBR (McWhirter 1980) contained a few records for eating carbohydrate foods. How's this for carbohydrate loading?

- Martin Moore ate 2,380 baked beans one by one with a cocktail stick in half an hour.
- Dr. Ronald Alkana ate 17 bananas (2.2 kg [4.8 lb]) in two minutes way back in 1973.
- It took only 82 seconds for Peter Dowdeswell of England to chug down 1.4 kilograms (3 lb) of potatoes. Peter also has an earlier record for eating 40 jam butties (jam sandwiches) in just under 18 minutes.
- Finally, 91.5 metres (300 ft) of spaghetti slid down the throat of Steve Weldon in 29 seconds.

no substitute for good, wholesome eating and hard training. Beware of food bars claiming to 'mobilise' body fat or increase the amount of fat used ('metabolised') as muscle fuel. There is no evidence to support their claims.

Use the 4 and 20 rule of food bars: As a general rule, any food bar providing less than 4 grams of fat and more than 20 grams of carbohydrate is a good choice. Check the ingredient list as well because food bars that include nuts, oats and seeds may naturally be higher in fat. Nutritious food bars also provide 1 to 3 grams of fibre and 2 to 5 grams of protein. See the snack section in the Nutrient Ready Reckoner in the appendix at the end of the book for some examples.

Food bars are convenient for pre- and postevent snacks because they don't need refrigeration and can be sat on and don't spoil so they can be stashed in a gym bag for days. Remember, bars are not a substitute for meals, just a quick and handy snack to have in your sport bag or car to tide you over to your next meal.

Carbohydrate Supplements

During high-level training, many athletes have difficulty eating enough food to match the calorie and carbohydrate needs of their bodies. This is particularly common in elite athletes and endurance athletes training many hours a day. They have less rest time for eating and don't want too much food in their stomachs when exercising. If this sounds like you, then you may benefit from carbohydrate supplements and liquid meal supplements.

Some carbohydrate supplements are available in the form of gels or powdered sugars. Generally these are glucose based (e.g., Glucodin, Carboshotz) because glucose is one of the least sweet sugars and is well tolerated during exercise. Equally important is that glucose is the sugar that muscles can use instantly. Carbohydrate gels are very popular with cyclists and other endurance athletes. Glucose powder can be added to fruit juices, drinks and canned fruit. Like sports bars, carbohydrate supplements are convenient and easy to carry, but use them wisely. It may be cheaper to get your extra carbohydrate as fruit juices, food bars, breakfast cereals, sports drinks, cordials or soft drinks (soda).

Because liquids are generally easier to consume than solids, liquid meals and snacks can be very helpful in meeting your high-energy needs. Commercial varieties are available, or you can make your own (see chapter 12, page 173).

Snacks

Snacking is another way to meet your carbohydrate needs. When you are so hungry that food dominates your thoughts, think smart and snack smart. Sure, a piece of fruit is still the quickest nutritious snack around, but sometimes it doesn't fill the spot, nor is it convenient. Food bars are a favourite with athletes—fruit bars, breakfast bars, muesli bars, sports bars and even chocolate bars.

Snacks of all types can offer good nutrition—fruit muffins, toast, fruit bread, half a sandwich or roll, cracker or crisp breads, yogurt, baked potato, dried fruit, flavoured milk, doner kebab, popcorn or baked beans. Even cereal and milk is a quick snack any time of the day. A low-fat treat could include sorbet, confectionery, soft drinks or fruit juice. Your imagination will provide more ideas.

The more active you are, the more likely you are to need a snack and the more freedom you have with your food choices. For example, a soft drink may provide only sugar and water, but if it is only a small part of a 12,000+ kilojoule (3,000+ cal) diet, there's still plenty of room for more nutritious food choices. You are smart enough to get the balance right. It's not whether you snack, it's what you snack on that will affect your performance and your health.

Glycemic Index

Back in the old days we used to divide carbohydrate into simple and complex forms. It was generally agreed that simple forms of carbohydrate were honey, syrups, soft drinks, confectionery and sugars (glucose, fructose, sucrose, maltose, dextrose); and complex forms were breads, rice, pasta, cereals, fruits and starchy vegetables. It was assumed that all simple forms of carbohydrate were digested quickly and that complex forms were digested slowly. As scientists discover more amazing things about food, nature and human beings, it should be no surprise that our understanding becomes more refined. And so it is with carbohydrate.

Some of the 'simple' forms of carbohydrate aren't so simple, and some of the 'complex' forms aren't as complex as we thought. A carbohydrate food is now classified by how quickly it is digested and absorbed into the blood as glucose; this classification is known as its glycemic index (GI). The GI is essentially the measurement of the blood glucose response to eating foods with carbohydrate. There is no GI for a food without carbohydrate such as meat or oil, or very little carbohydrate such as lettuce or mushrooms.

Determining GI

The GI of a food is determined from eating the amount of that food that provides 50 grams of carbohydrate, and then measuring its effect on blood glucose levels (see figure 3.2). For example, three large apples provide a total of 50 grams of carbohydrate. All foods have been compared to 50 grams of glucose, which has

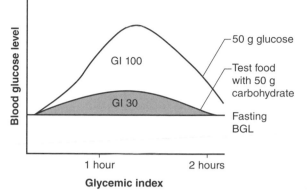

FIGURE 3.2 The blood glucose response to 50 grams of glucose is given a GI of 100. The blood glucose response to other foods with carbohydrate are compared to glucose.

been given an arbitrary GI figure of 100. A food with a GI of 70 raises blood glucose to 70 per cent of the level achieved with pure glucose. The basis of the glycemic index is the rate of digestion of all carbohydrates. High GI foods are quickly

Carbohydrate supplements such as gels are popular with cyclists and triathletes as they are convenient to consume during events.

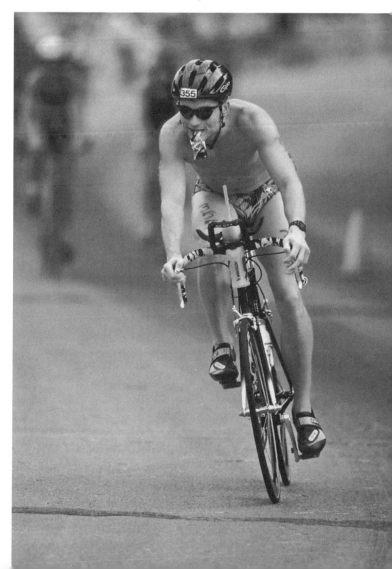

converted to blood glucose, and low GI foods are slowly converted to blood glucose. Some of the results of testing for GI have been surprising: Sugar has a lower GI than bread and potatoes! That finding has resulted in relaxing the restrictions on people with diabetes; they can now include some sugar in their diets.

Slow Starch and Quick Starch

Starch comes in two main forms, amylose and amylopectin. All starchy foods are a mixture of the two forms of starch (see figure 3.3).

- Amylose is a straight chain of glucose molecules and takes longer to digest.
- Amylopectin has a number of branches of smaller glucose chains and is quicker to digest.

The enzyme that breaks down starch can work only on the end glucose molecules, breaking them off in chunks of one or two molecules. Amylose, being a long, straight chain of glucose molecules, has two end molecules. It takes longer to digest than amylopectin, which has a number of branches of glucose chains, and therefore many end molecules. For this reason starchy foods have different rates of digestion. Starches high in amylopectin digest more quickly and have a greater effect on blood glucose than starches high in amylose do. For example, bread is made from wheat, which is high in amylopectin. Pasta, on the other hand, is made

from durum wheat, which is high in amylose. Therefore, bread has a higher GI than pasta because it is digested more quickly.

Note that the GI of maltose, glucose and honey are high because of their high glucose content and rapid absorption into the blood, whereas another sugar, fructose, has a low GI because it has little effect on blood sugar levels. Table sugar (sucrose) is a molecule made of glucose and fructose joined together; hence, its GI (68) is halfway between those of glucose and fructose (see table 3.2). The least processed starchy foods are generally slower to digest and have a lower GI. This can be very relevant to people with diabetes because the lower the rise in blood glucose levels, the easier it is to control diabetes. The processing of starchy foods can break the amylose into smaller pieces, providing more end glucose molecules and enabling quicker digestion. Other factors that influence the GI of a food are discussed later in the chapter.

GI and Nutritional Value

If you are thinking that the GI of a food is some kind of league table of nutritional value and that those with the lowest GIs are better for you than those with the highest GIs, then hold up a moment. First, be aware that a food does not have a set GI, but a range of GIs. The GI for rice can be as low as 54 (e.g., Doongara rice, which is higher in amylose) or as high as 90 for those that are low in amylose, such as jasmine rice. The variation is due to the different botanical types having different proportions of the two types of starch. Underripe bananas have a GI of 40, whereas ripe bananas are around 50 or 55 because the ripening process breaks down starch to produce a higher level of glucose. So don't get hung up on the absolute GI number. The GI allows you to compare foods within the same food grouping such as breakfast cereals.

Second, remember that the GI is a comparison of carbohydrate foods based on 50 grams of carbohydrate. Only a few common serves of food provide 50 grams of carbohydrate, such as a cup of cooked spaghetti. Many foods you generally won't eat in amounts that provide 50 grams of carbohydrate; for example, most serves of fruit provide only 15 grams of carbohydrate. You sometimes hear of people avoiding watermelon because it has a high GI of 76. Yet, a slice of watermelon provides only 6 g of carbohydrate, so a slice has only a modest effect on blood glucose. This brings us to the concept of the glycemic load.

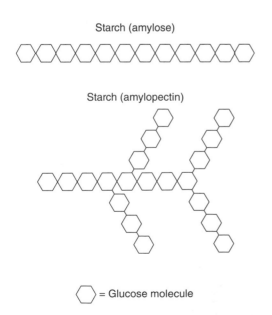

Starch (amylose)

Starch (amylopectin)

◯ = Glucose molecule

FIGURE 3.3 Amylose starch is a long, straight chain of glucose molecules. Amylopectin starch is composed of branched chains of glucose molecules.

Glycemic Load

Because we don't eat carbohydrate foods in an amount that always provides 50 grams of carbohydrate, the concept of the glycemic load (GL) was established.

$$GL = \text{Grams of carbohydrate per serve} \times GI\ 100$$

I have mentioned the watermelon has an average GI of 76 and is therefore classified as high GI, but you would eat only one or two 120-gram slices providing only 6 to 12 grams of carbohydrate (not the 50 grams on which the GI is based). Therefore, the glycemic load (GL) for one slice is $6 \times 76 / 100 = 4.56$, or 4 rounded to the nearest whole number. Compare that to a bagel, which has an average GI of 72, but a single bagel provides 35 grams of carbohydrate. The GL of a bagel is $35 \times 72 / 100 = 25.20$. That's two foods with a similar GI, but one has potentially six times the effect on blood glucose levels of the other when eaten in normal serves. The point I am trying to make is that you should not judge a food solely on its GI. A high GI food such as watermelon is natural and nutritious, so you wouldn't avoid it based on its GI. For health and sport you should ask two important questions: (1) Is it minimally processed, and (2) does it meet my carbohydrate goals?

Don't get the impression that you should check only the GL; if you do, you could end up eating very little carbohydrate and find yourself tiring very quickly in sport and exercise. Take a look at table 3.2. Although the foods have been listed in order of descending GI, the GL per serve varies greatly. Also note that the GI can vary greatly between batches, brand names and countries of origin; therefore, the GI given is often an average and should be used only as a guide. For example, Special K breakfast cereal has a GI of 54 in the Australian version and 69 in the U.S. version, and Coca-Cola has a GI of 53 in Australia and a GI of 63 in the USA because the two versions use different sugar blends. For more specific GIs based on brand names and regions, visit www.glycemicindex.com.

Another issue in determining GIs is that many of the foods are not eaten on their own. The bagel is likely to have a filling, which will affect the GI of the meal. The GI of a meal is approximately the average of the GI of the individual foods based on their carbohydrate content. So, if half of the carbohydrate in a meal came from rice (GI 83) and the other half came from kidney beans (GI 27), then the GI of the meal would be around 55 ($83 + 27 = 110$; divide 110 by 2 and you get 55).

What Can Influence GI?

Many other aspects of a meal can affect its GI and GL. Other components of the meal, such as fat, soluble fibre and protein, usually lower the GI, whereas cooking and processing usually raise the GI. Fat, fibre and protein lower the GI of the meal because they get in the way of the enzymes that break down the carbohydrate in the intestine. Imagine that you are in a large room and you see a friend on the other side. It would take no time for you to walk over and greet your friend. Imagine now that same room full of people. It will take you longer to get over to the other side of the room to talk to your friend. Similarly, in the gut, fat molecules, fibre and chains of amino acids can get in the way of carbohydrate enzymes, slow down the rate of carbohydrate digestion and therefore slow down glucose absorption into the blood.

Highly processed foods generally have a high GI because processing breaks up the starch molecules into smaller chains. If, for example, you have one long amylose molecule, you have only two ends for the digestive enzymes to work on. If that chain gets broken in half, you now have four ends to digest. If they, in turn, are broken in half, there are now eight ends and potentially it could be digested four times as quickly, giving rise to a higher blood glucose level.

Use the GI to compare GI foods within the same group (see tables 3.3 and 3.4). Use the GL to compare different foods with varying carbohydrate content. As an example, pumpkin has a high GI, but a low GL; just because it has a high GI doesn't mean that it will significantly raise your blood glucose levels.

GI and Your Health

The GI and the GL can be somewhat confusing. Many people believe that high GI foods are bad for their long-term health, yet the GI is not the best way to determine the health benefits of a food. This is the main thing to remember: The GI hasn't really changed our nutrition advice to healthy, fit people. If you eat plenty of wholesome food that has been minimally processed, such as fruits, vegetables and whole-grain cereals, and have the occasional treat, your overall diet is likely to have a low GI.

Scientists generally agree that low GI foods such as legumes, vegetables and whole-grain breads may help to prevent diseases such as type 2 diabetes and heart disease. Low GI foods are generally more filling and better able to control your appetite such that you don't overeat and put on body fat. Low GI foods are also less energy dense than high GI foods are, another factor in helping you not to overeat. Evidence also suggests that eating lots of high GI foods puts a strain on insulin production, to the extent that it can cause insulin resistance and type 2 diabetes. So, eat well and your future will likely be a healthy one.

Applying GI to Training and Competition

Now that we've explored the glycemic index of food in general, let's look at how you can use this information in training and competition. Choosing carbohydrate food and drinks based on their GI may provide a performance edge in some sport situations, especially when you are considering what to eat just before, during and just after exercise.

Before Exercise

You may have heard that athletes should eat low GI foods a couple of hours before exercise for a long and sustained release of glucose into the blood during exercise. This advice was based mainly on research conducted in the early 1990s. Studies in which athletes exercised until exhaustion (e.g., in long tennis matches, ultra-marathons and ironman events) often showed that low GI foods improved endurance. Because most of us don't exercise to the point of collapse, however, some scientists argue that the GI is not relevant to normal exercise, especially exercise that lasts less than 90 minutes. Research shows that the GI of the food or meal eaten before sport won't make a big difference to regular performance. The most important thing is that you eat enough carbohydrate before exercise so you will have enough glycogen for sport, and that you choose nutritious foods you enjoy. On the other hand, the GI of what you consume during and after sport could make a difference.

During Exercise

Experts recommend that athletes consume only food and drink with a high GI during exercise to access the glucose quickly. Taking carbohydrate such as sports drinks or sports gels during pro-longed exercise makes more glucose available to the muscles so athletes can exercise for longer. Because sugars generally have a moderate to high GI, they will be easily digested and absorbed. The only exception is fructose, which is easily absorbed but takes some time to be converted to glucose for muscle contraction. For this reason, it is used sparingly in sports drinks (high fructose sports drinks are not recommended for this reason).

Sports drinks such as Gatorade have a GI of around 74 because they need to be quickly absorbed into the blood to replace the glucose burned during exercise. Avoid sports drinks that claim to have a low GI (you want the sugars now, not when you have finished exercise!). Low GI foods are not usually taken during sport, except in ultra-endurance events. In this case you need to experiment with foods to make sure they don't cause gut discomfort. Jelly beans and other jelly confectionery such as jelly snakes and gummy worms, with their high GI, are very popular blood glucose replacers in sports such as cycling, rugby, football, basketball and netball.

After Exercise

There is good evidence that moderate to high GI foods eaten after exercise are converted into muscle glycogen more readily than are low GI foods. Eating high GI foods such as rice and potatoes, along with sports drinks, can be especially useful if you have two or more training sessions or events in a day or you are involved in round-robin competitions that require you to play each day. However, if you have 24 hours or more between training sessions or events, the GI seems less important for glycogen replacement over that time. It is more important that you eat enough great-tasting foods rich in carbohydrate rather than being unduly concerned about the GI of your meals.

The GI of foods is an area of active research, so we may have to refine the advice once further studies are done. If you feel that your choice of food affects your performance based on their GI, then listen to your body and choose low to moderate GI foods before sport, and higher GI foods and drinks during and after sport in your recovery meal.

Because the role of GI in sport is inconclusive, it appears that eating nutritious carbohydrate foods and fluids is all that is required to keep the muscles well fuelled (Donaldson 2010).

For more information on GI and GL, get the book *The New Glucose Revolution* (Brand-Miller et al., 2007), or visit the website www.glycemicindex.com.

TABLE 3.2 Average Glycemic Index (GI) and Glycemic Load (GL) of Carbohydrate (CHO) Foods

Food	GI	CHO per serve	GL per serve
HIGH GLYCEMIC INDEX (70 OR MORE)			
Maltose, 10 g (0.4 oz)	105	10	11
Glucodin tablets (glucose), 50 g (1.8 oz)	102	50	50
Glucose, 50 g (1.8 oz)	100	50	50
Roll-Ups fruit snack, 30 g (1 oz)	99	25	25
Lucozade, 250 mL (8.5 oz)	95	42	40
Jasmine rice, 1 cup cooked	89	40	36
Rice Bubbles (Kellogg's), 30 g (1 oz)	88	26	23
Potato, instant, 150 g (5.3 oz)	87	20	17
Turkish bread, white, 30 g (1 oz)	87	17	15
Lamington, 50 g (1.8 oz)	87	29	25
Potato, baked, av., 1 medium, 150 g (5.3 oz)	86	26	22
Lebanese bread, white, 120 g (4.2 oz)	86	45	39
Rice (Calrose), 1 cup, cooked	83	43	36
Rice cakes, 25 g (0.9 oz)	82	21	17
Potato, 1 boiled, av., 150 g (5.3 oz)	82	25	21
Crispbread, puffed, 25 g (0.9 oz)	81	19	15
Rice (Sunbrown quick), 1 cup	80	38	31
Puffed wheat (Sanitarium), 30 g (1 oz)	80	21	17
Morning coffee biscuits, 2	79	19	15
Rice milk, 250 mL (8.5 oz)	79	22	17
Jelly beans, av., 30 g (1 oz)	78	28	22
Water crackers, 25 g (0.9 oz)	78	18	14
Cereal bar, av., 30 g (1 oz)	78	23	18
Gatorade, 250 mL (8.5 oz)	78	15	12
Licorice (soft), 60 g (2 oz)	78	42	33
Coco Pops (Kellogg's), 30 g (1 oz)	77	26	20
Cornflakes, 30 g (1 oz)	77	25	19
English muffin, 30 g (1 oz)	77	14	11
Waffles, 35 g (1.2 oz)	76	13	10
Watermelon, 120 g (4.2 oz)	76	6	5
Mashed potato, av., 150 g (5.3 oz)	76	20	15
Bread, wholemeal, av., 1 slice 30 g (1 oz)	74	12	9
Sports drink, av., 250 mL (8.5 oz)	74	16	13

▶ *continued*

▶ Table 3.2 (continued)

Food	GI	CHO per serve	GL per serve
HIGH GLYCEMIC INDEX (70 OR MORE) (CONTINUED)			
Bread, fibre-enriched, 1 slice	73	14	10
Bread, white, av., 1 slice	73	14	10
Miniwheats (filled), 30 g (1 oz)	72	21	15
Swede, 150 g (5.3 oz)	72	10	7
Kavli crispbreads, 25 g (0.9 oz)	71	16	12
Life Savers, 30 g (1 oz)	70	30	21
Sao biscuits, 25 g (0.9 oz)	70	17	12
MEDIUM GLYCEMIC INDEX (56–69)			
Bagel, 1 white, 70 g (2.5 oz)	69	35	24
Weet-Bix (Sanitarium), 30 g (1 oz)	69	17	12
Special K (Kellogg's USA), 30 g (1 oz)	69	21	14
Crumpets, 2	69	19	13
Milk arrowroot biscuits, 2	69	18	12
Fanta soft drink, 250 mL (8.5 oz)	68	34	23
Gnocchi, 1 cup cooked	68	48	33
Hot dog roll, white, 60 g (2 oz)	68	33	22
Sucrose (table sugar), 10 g (0.4 oz)	68	10	7
Weet-Bix Multi-grain (Sanitarium), 48 g (1.7 oz)	68	34	23
Taco shells, 2 shells, 20 g (0.7 oz)	68	12	8
Croissant, 65 g (2.3 oz)	67	26	17
Rockmelon/cantaloupe, 120 g (4.2 oz)	67	6	4
Shredded wheat, av., 30 g (1 oz)	83	20	17
One minute oats, av., 1 cup	66	26	17
Cordial, diluted, 250 mL (8.5 oz)	66	20	13
Pineapple, 120 g (4.2 oz)	66	10	6
Nutrigrain (Kellogg's), 30 g (1 oz)	66	15	10
Popcorn, plain, av., 20 g (0.7 oz)	65	11	7
Couscous, cooked 150 g (5.3 oz)	65	14	9
Pumpkin, 80 g (2.8 oz)	64	9	6
Vita Brits (Uncle Tobys), 30 g (1 oz)	64	20	13
Sultana bran (Kellogg's), 30 g (1 oz)	64	19	12
Beetroot, canned, 80 g (2.8 oz)	64	7	5
Raisins, 30 g (1 oz)	64	22	14
Shortbread biscuit, 25 g (.9 oz)	64	16	10
Cherries, 120 g (4.2 oz)	63	14	9

Food	GI	CHO per serve	GL per serve
Golden syrup, 1 tbsp	63	17	11
Mars bar, 60 g (2 oz)	62	40	25
Honey, av., 25 g (0.9 oz)	61	19	12
Sweet potato, av., 1 medium 150 g (5.3 oz)	61	18	11
Figs, dried, 30 g (1 oz)	61	13	8
Muesli bar, with dried fruit, 30 g (1 oz)	61	21	13
Just Right cereal, 30 g (1 oz)	60	22	13
Digestive biscuit, av., 2	59	16	9
Vege Burger (McDonalds)	59	55	32
Mini Wheats, plain, 30 g (1 oz)	58	21	12
Bread, rye, av., 1 slice	58	12	6
Kiwi fruit, 2 medium	58	12	7
Potato crisps, plain, 50 g (1.8 oz)	57	18	10
Bread, pita, 30 g (1 oz)	57	17	10
Sultanas, 30 g (1 oz)	57	22	12
Rice, basmati, av., 1 cup	57	38	22
Clif bar, 65 g (2.3 oz)	57	38	22
Wild rice, boiled 1 cup	57	32	18
Muesli, Swiss, 30 g (1 oz)	56	16	9
Paw paw, 120 g (4.2 oz)	56	8	5
Oat bran, 10 g (0.4 oz)	56	5	3

LOW GLYCEMIC INDEX (55 OR LESS)

Food	GI	CHO per serve	GL per serve
Jatz, 25 g (0.9 oz)	55	17	10
Semolina, dry, 65 g (2.3 oz) cooked	55	50	28
Marmalade, orange, 30 g (1 oz)	55	20	11
Porridge, rolled oats, av., 1 cup	55	24	13
Sustain (Kellogg's), 30 g (1 oz)	55	22	12
Bread, multigrain, 1 slice	54	15	8
Special K (Kellogg's Australia), 30 g (1 oz)	54	21	11
Buckwheat, av., 150 g (5.3 oz)	54	30	16
Rice (Doongara), 1 cup	54	39	21
Yam, av., 150 g (5.3 oz)	54	37	20
Coca-Cola, 250 mL (8.5 oz)	53	26	14
Power bar, av., 65 g (2.3 oz)	53	42	22
Sweet corn, av., 150 g (5.3 oz)	52	32	17

▶ continued

Food	GI	CHO per serve	GL per serve
LOW GLYCEMIC INDEX (55 OR LESS) *(CONTINUED)*			
Parsnip, 80 g (2.8 oz)	52	8	4
Ribena fruit syrup reconstituted, 250 mL (8.5 oz)	52	32	17
Peas, green, average, 1/2 cup	51	7	4
Mango, 120 g (4.2 oz)	51	15	8
Fruit bread, av., 1 slice	50	15	8
Orange juice, 250 mL (8.5 oz)	50	24	12
Two-minute noodles, av., 180 g (6.3 oz)	50	24	12
Sushi, salmon, 100 g (3.5 oz)	48	36	11
Cape seed loaf (Bakers Delight), 2 slices	48	13	6
Banana (ripe), 1 medium	47	24	11
Ice cream, regular, average, 1 scoop	47	13	6
Ryvita, 25 g (0.9 oz)	47	14	7
Grapes, av., 120 g (4.2 oz)	46	18	8
Pineapple juice, unswtnd, 250 mL (8.5 oz)	46	34	15
Tomato soup, canned, 1 cup	45	17	8
Chocolate, white, 50 g (1.8 oz)	44	29	13
Sustagen Sport, 250 mL (8.5 oz)	43	49	21
Nectarine, 120 g (4 oz)	43	9	4
Lactose, 10 g (0.4 oz)	43	10	4
Custard, homemade, 100 mL (3.4 oz)	43	17	7
Muesli, toasted, 30 g (1 oz)	43	17	7
Milk chocolate, 50 g (1.8 oz)	43	28	12
Carrot juice, homemade, 250 mL (8.5 oz)	43	23	10
Peach, fresh, av., 1 large	42	11	5
Orange, av., 1 medium	42	11	5
Spaghetti, whole-meal, 1 cup	42	40	17
Choc Nesquik with milk, 250 mL (8.5 oz)	41	11	5
Snickers bar, 60 g (2 oz)	41	36	15
Apple juice, av., 250 mL (8.5 oz)	40	28	11
Fettuccine, boiled, 1 cup	40	46	18
Soy drink, 250 mL (8.5 oz)	40	17	7
Baked beans, canned, av., 150 g (5.3 oz)	40	15	6
Peaches, canned, natural juice, 120 g (4.2 oz)	40	12	5
Ice cream, low fat, av. 1 scoop	40	13	3

Food	GI	CHO per serve	GL per serve
Ravioli, boiled, meat filled, 1 cup	39	38	15
Carrots, boiled, 80 g (2.8 oz)	39	6	2
Plums, 120 g (4.2 oz)	39	12	5
Apple, av., 1 medium	38	15	6
Pear, av., 1 medium	38	11	4
Spaghetti, white, boiled, av. 1 cup	38	48	18
Tomato juice, no added sugar, 250 mL (8.5 oz)	38	9	3
Ice cream, premium, 1 scoop	37	9	4
Chick peas, canned, 150 g (5.3 oz)	38	23	9
Chocolate flavoured milk, 250 mL (8.5 oz)	37	24	9
Kidney beans, canned, 150 g (5.3 oz)	36	17	6
Milo dissolved in milk, 250 mL (8.5 oz)	36	26	9
Super Supreme pizza (Pizza Hut), 2 slices	36	24	9
Vermicelli, boiled, 1 cup	35	44	16
M&Ms, peanut, 30 g (1 oz)	33	17	6
Yogurt, flavoured, low fat, av. 200 g (7 oz)	33	31	10
Butter beans, cooked, 150 g (5.3 oz)	32	21	7
Milk, nonfat, 250 mL (8.5 oz)	31	14	4
Milk, full cream, 250 mL (8.5 oz)	31	12	4
Banana smoothie, 250 mL (8.5 oz)	30	26	8
All-Bran (Kellogg's), 30 g (1 oz)	30	15	4
Lentils, av., cooked, 1 cup	30	17	5
Apricot, dried, 60 g (2 oz)	31	24	7
Split peas, dry, soaked overnight, 1 cup	25	32	8
Nutella, 20 g (0.7 oz)	25	11	3
Grapefruit, av., 120 g (4.2 oz)	25	11	3
Nuts, mixed, roasted and salted, 50 g (1.8 oz)	24	17	4
Peanuts, roasted, salted, 50 g (1.8 oz)	23	6	1
Hummus, av., 30 g (1 oz)	22	5	1
Cashews, salted, 30 g (1 oz)	22	9	2
Milk, 2% fat, 250 mL (8.5 oz)	20	14	3
Fructose, 10 g (0.4 oz)	19	10	2
Rice bran, 30 g (1 oz)	19	14	3
Soy beans, canned, 1 cup	14	6	1
Pecans, raw, 50 g (1.8 oz)	10	3	0

Data from F.S. Atkinson, K. Foster-Powell, and J.C. Brend-Miller, 2008, "International table of glycemic index and glycemic load values: 2008," *Diabetes Care* 31(12) and J.C. Brend-Miller, T.M.S. Wolever, K. Foster-Powell, and S. Colagiuri, 2007, *The new glucose revolution*, 3rd ed. (New York: Marlowe & Co.).

TABLE 3.3 Average Glycemic Index: Sample Foods by Food Group

Food	Low GI (55 or less)	Medium GI (56–69)	High GI (70 or more)
Breads, crispbreads, taco shells	• Multigrain bread • Fruit bread • Ryvita, Jatz	• Rye bread • Croissant, bagel • Pita bread • Crumpet • Taco shells	• Kavli biscuits, Sao Lebanese and Turkish bread; bread white and wholemeal • English muffins • Crispbread • Water crackers
Breakfast cereals	• All-Bran • Toasted muesli • Special K (Australia) • Porridge • Sustain	• Just Right, Sultana Bran • Shredded wheat • Special K (USA) • Nutrigrain • Vita Brits, Weet-Bix • Weet-Bix Multigrain • Miniwheats, plain • Oat bran • Swiss muesli	• Rice Bubbles • Puffed wheat • Coco Pops • Cornflakes • Shredded Wheat • Miniwheats, flavoured
Pasta, rice etc	• Pasta, spaghetti • Vermicelli, fettuccine • Ravioli • Two-minute noodles • Rice bran • Buckwheat, semolina	• Doongara rice • Basmati rice • Gnocchi • Couscous • Wild rice	• White rice • Rice cakes • Brown rice • Jasmine rice
Vegetables, legumes	• Baked beans • Legumes, chick peas • Carrots, carrot juice • Peas, parsnip • Yam, sweet corn • Tomato soup, tomato juice • Hummus	• Sweet potato • Pumpkin • Beetroot	• Potato—boiled, mashed, baked, instant • Swede
Fruit	• Dried apricot • Orange, banana • Grapes, cherries • Apple, pear • Peach, fresh and canned • Grapefruit, mango • Plums, nectarine	• Pineapple • Rockmelon/cantaloupe • Raisins, sultanas • Paw paw • Kiwi fruit • Cherries • Figs	• Watermelon
Dairy foods and soy	• Milk—all types • Milk—flavoured • Smoothies • Yogurt—all types • Ice cream (regular) • Ice cream (low fat) • Ice cream (premium) • Custard • Soy beverages		• Rice milk

Food	Low GI (55 or less)	Medium GI (56–69)	High GI (70 or more)
Snacks, nuts and confectionery	• White chocolate • Milk chocolate • Snickers bar • M&Ms • Peanuts, pecans, cashews • Power bar	• Sweet muffins • Mars bar • Muesli bars • Potato crisps, pop-corn • Clif bar • Shortbread biscuits, digestives	• Lifesavers • Jelly beans • Some biscuits • Lamington • Water crackers • Cereal bars • Licorice • Roll-Ups fruit snack
Sports drinks, soft drinks, fruit juice	• Fruit juice • Coca-Cola • Sustagen Sport • Ribena • Nesquik or Milo (with milk)	• Fanta • Cordial	• Lucozade • Isostar • Gatorade • Sports drinks
Sugars, spreads	• Fructose • Lactose • Nutella • Marmalade	• Sucrose • Honey • Golden syrup	• Glucose • Maltose • Glucodin (glucose powder)

Data from F.S. Atkinson, K. Foster-Powell, and J.C. Brend-Miller, 2008, "International table of glycemic index and glycemic load values: 2008," *Diabetes Care* 31(12).

TABLE 3.4 Average Glycemic Load Per Serve: Sample Foods by Food Group

Food	Low GL (10 or less)	Medium GL (11–19)	High GL (20 or more)
Breads, crispbread, taco shells	• Whole-meal, white or multi-grain bread, 1 slice • Rye bread, 1 slice • Fruit bread, 1 slice • Pita bread, 1 • Taco shells, 2	• Crispbread, 2 • Kavli, 3 • Sao, Ryvita, 2 • Crumpets, 2 • Turkish bread, 30 g • Croissant, 1 • English muffin, 1 • Rice cakes, 25 g • Water crackers, 25 g	• Bagel, 1 • Lebanese bread, 1
Breakfast cereals	• All-Bran, 30 g (1 oz) • Oat bran, 10 g • Swiss muesli, 30 g • Muesli, toasted, 30 g • Nutrigrain, 30 g	• Puffed Wheat • Shredded Wheat, 30 g • Mini Wheats, 30 g • Sustain, Just Right • Weet-Bix, Vita Brits 30 g • Porridge, 1 cup • One minute oats, 1 cup • Special K (Australia and USA), Corn-flakes • Sultana Bran, 30 g	• Rice Bubbles, 1 cup • Coco pops, 30 g • Weet-Bix Multi-grain, 2
Pasta, rice etc	• Couscous, 150 g • Rice bran, 30 g	• Spaghetti, Fettuccine • Ravioli • Rice cakes, 2 • Vermicelli, 1 cup	• Rice, all types, 1 cup • Buckwheat, 150 g • Gnocchi, 1 cup • Semolina, 65 g • Wild rice, 1 cup

▶ *continued*

Food	Low GI (55 or less)	Medium GI (56–69)	High GI (70 or more)
Vegetables, legumes	• Swede, parsnip • Carrots, pumpkin • Baked beans, legumes • Beetroot • Peas • Tomato soup, tomato juice	• Mashed potato, 1 cup • Instant potato, 1 cup • Sweet potato • Sweet corn	• Baked and boiled potato, 1 medium • Yam • Gnocchi, 1 cup
Fruit	• Watermelon • Rockmelon/canta-loupe • Pineapple, paw paw • Mango, grapes, plums • Orange, apple, pear • Figs, cherry, kiwi fruit • Nectarine, peach • Grapefruit	• Banana • Raisins, sultanas 30 g	
Dairy foods and soy	• Ice cream, regular, premium and low fat, 1 scoop • Milo on milk • Flavoured milk, smoothies, 250 mL (8.5 oz) • Flavoured yogurt • Milk—nonfat, full cream • Soy beverage • Custard	• Rice milk, 250 mL (8.5 oz)	
Snacks, nuts and confectionery	• M&Ms, 30 g (1 oz) • Nuts • Potato crisps, 50 g • Shortbread biscuits, 2 • Popcorn, 20 g • Jatz biscuits, 25 g	• Plain biscuits, 2 • Muesli bar • Milk chocolate, 50 g (1.8 oz) • Snickers bar	• Jelly beans, 30 g (1 oz) • Mars bar, 60 g (2 oz) • Lifesavers, 30 g • Clif bar, Power Bar • Lamington, 50 g • Licorice, 60 g • Roll Ups fruit snack
Sports drinks, soft drinks, fruit juice		• Sports drinks, 250 mL (8 oz) • Fruit juice, 250 mL (8 oz) • Cordial, 250 mL (8.5 oz)	• Lucozade, 250 mL (8.5 oz) • Fanta, 250 mL (8.5 oz) • Coca-Cola, 250 mL (8.5 oz) • Sustagen Sport, 250 mL (8.5 oz) • Ribena, 250 mL (8.5 oz)
Sugars and spreads	• Table sugar, 2 tsp • Nutella, 20 g	• Golden Syrup, 1 tbsp • Honey, 25 g • Marmalade, 30 g	• Glucose, 50 g • Glucodin, 50 g

Data from F.S. Atkinson, K. Foster-Powell, and J.C. Brend-Miller, 2008, "International table of glycemic index and glycemic load values: 2008," *Diabetes Care* 31(12).

FINAL SCORE

- Your muscles, your brain and your liver require carbohydrate (in the form of glucose) to function normally. Your body is a glucose-burning machine.

- If you eat too little carbohydrate, you are likely to tire quickly and not be able to sustain aerobic activity. A low-carbohydrate diet is by default a low-kilojoule diet, so you may also lose weight. A low-carbohydrate diet is likely to be low in fibre, antioxidants and other essential nutrients.

- Carbohydrate supplements in the form of sports drinks, food bars or gels can provide useful additional carbohydrate for the very active endurance athlete. Snack foods and commercial liquid meals can help athletes reach their carbohydrate and nutrition goals in heavy training.

- Sugars are a normal part of the diet. They are not harmful, except when so much added-sugar foods are eaten that they displace other nutritious foods.

- Some sugar-containing foods are very nutritious, such as fruit, milk, yogurt, soy drinks and, believe it or not, good chocolate.

- The GI of a food may be of little advantage in meals before sport. It is probably more important that athletes eat enough great-tasting foods rich in carbohydrate, rather than focusing solely on the GI of foods and meals.

- Moderate to high GI foods are quicker to digest, absorb and convert to glycogen than equal amounts of low GI foods. High GI foods could accelerate the replacement of muscle glucose in athletes training or competing more than once a day.

- Low GI foods generally are the least processed foods and are therefore more likely than high GI foods to have reasonable levels of nutrition and fibre.

Calcium, Iron and Vitamins for Health and Performance

> **The primary minerals low in the diets of athletes, especially female athletes, are calcium, iron, zinc, and magnesium. Low intakes of these minerals are often due to energy restriction or avoidance of animal products.**
>
> *Position of the American Dietetic Association, Dietitians of Canada and the American College of Sports Medicine: Nutrition and Athletic Performance (2009, 516)*

This chapter focuses on some key vitamins and minerals that are of particular importance to active people. Of course, all vitamins and minerals are important, but several have particular benefits for athletes. Because iron deficiency impedes sports performance and poor bone strength has long-term consequences, athletes should eat adequate iron and calcium. The vitamins that often get mentioned in sports performance are the B group vitamins because they are involved in energy production, and vitamins E and C because they are proposed to enhance performance.

Vitamin D has generated a lot of interest because low blood levels have been associated with a higher risk of heart disease, diabetes and some cancers. Although athletes exercise outside, they often do so early in the morning or late in the evening when the sun has lost much of its ability to generate vitamin D through the action of sunlight on

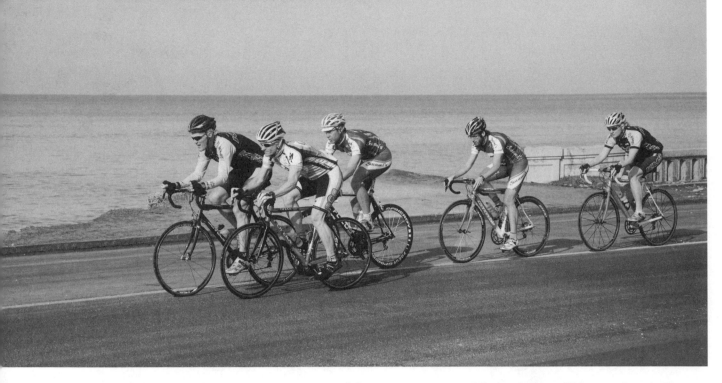

Many athletes are low in vitamin D. Sensible sun exposure while training will keep vitamin D at a healthy level.

the skin, especially during the winter months. One study in a sunny country found that 80 per cent of young indoor athletes and nearly half of outdoor athletes had insufficient levels of vitamin D (Constantini 2010). Athletes training outside during the day in summer should use sunscreen to stop sunburn. Although sunscreen does block the UV rays from sunlight, usually enough sneaks through where sunscreen has not been applied thickly enough, or has rubbed off, to generate some vitamin D during the middle of the day. Be aware that reddened or burnt skin is damaged skin and cannot produce vitamin D.

Let's take a look at calcium and iron in particular.

Calcium

Calcium is an essential mineral that is part of the structure of teeth and bones. The body needs a daily supply of calcium for maximum bone strength throughout life. Our best sources of calcium are dairy foods (yogurt, milk and cheese—but not butter), calcium-fortified foods (e.g., some soy drinks) and the soft bones of canned sardines and salmon. There are lesser amounts in vegetables such as broccoli and nuts such as almonds.

Osteoporosis and Physical Activity

Every day your bones are in a constant state of flux; some bone is manufactured and some is broken down as your bones are modelled and remodelled. Early in life, more bone is made than is broken down; hence, bones get bigger and stronger. Bone mass increases rapidly from puberty and peaks when people reach their 30s. Later in life the trend tends to be the opposite—more bone gets broken down than is formed, so bones become weaker. The aim is to minimise the rate of loss so you have the maximum possible bone strength throughout your life.

If bones break down more quickly than they can be rebuilt, osteoporosis (brittle and weak bones) occurs, making them more likely to break as a result of minor injury. Postmenopausal women experience a more rapid breakdown of bone as a result of the drop in the female hormones estrogen and progesterone. (Estrogen prevents bone loss, whereas progesterone promotes bone formation.) Osteoporosis can occur in men, too, although usually at a slower rate and at a later age than in women. The best way to measure bone strength is by assessing bone mineral density (BMD): the lower the density, the greater the risk of bone fractures.

Bones just love their exercise. Fitter people tend to have stronger bones, which is great for avoiding osteoporosis later in life. Weight-bearing exercise (e.g., running) is a wonderful stimulus to bone growth and strength because the skeleton adapts to the forces applied during running. Strength training also applies greater loads to the skeleton and can reduce bone loss, especially in the later years of life.

Weight-supported sports, such as cycling and swimming, are less effective at increasing bone mass because less force is applied to the skeleton. Most athletes, male and female, have above-average bone mass and are less likely to get osteoporosis compared to those who do not get enough exercise.

Bone-Tired Women

If a female athlete has long and arduous training sessions, her menstrual pattern can become irregular and may even cease altogether (this is called amenorrhea). For some women this comes as a great relief—no more premenstrual tension. Unfortunately, having no periods means that the body is producing less estrogen, which stops bones from reaching their highest mass and strength. This less-than-normal amount of bone is called osteopenia, which may lead to osteoporosis. Runners, especially distance runners, are more likely to stop having periods than are swimmers or team sport players. Non-menstruating athletes tend to have a lower bone mass compared to the rest of the female population, even if they do have enough calcium in their diet.

Young amenorrheic females could be losing bone rather than building it, making them likely to suffer from stress fractures in the short term and premature osteoporosis in the long term. They may have to consume 1,500 milligrams of calcium daily to stop significant bone loss. Because bone loss appears to be most rapid soon after periods stop, experts advise any athlete who stops menstruating for more than three months, or has very irregular periods, to see her doctor.

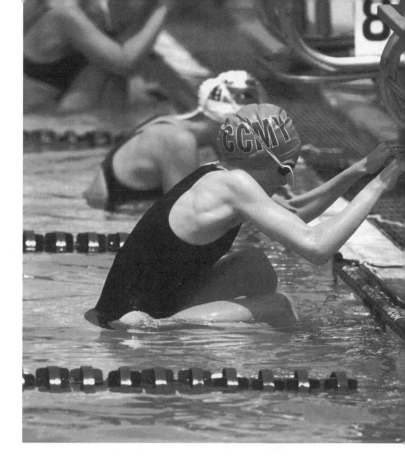

Female athletes especially need to make sure they get enough vitamin D and calcium for maximum bone strength.

Remember that amenorrhea has other causes, too, including not eating enough food (very strict diets), the eating disorder anorexia nervosa, very low body weight and psychological stress. Amenorrheic athletes should check with a sports dietitian to ensure they are getting enough food to fuel performance and normal menstruation and see their doctor for advice. Amenorrhea is also more likely to occur in

⏵ Factors That Increase the Risk of Osteoporosis in Men and Women

- Family history of osteoporosis
- Caucasian or Asian background
- Certain medications (e.g., corticosteroids)
- Inadequate calcium in the diet
- Lack of sunlight exposure leading to low vitamin D levels
- Excessive amounts of sodium (salt) in the diet
- Excessive consumption of alcohol
- A combination of excessive caffeine and low calcium
- Inactivity over many years
- Cigarette smoking
- Early menopause or ovary removal (women only)
- Amenorrhea (women only)

women who had irregular periods before they started heavy training.

As training becomes lighter, amenorrhea is reversible and regular periods can return. Although more research needs to be done, it is heartening to note that bone loss can be reversed if periods recommence, although it may not return to ideal levels for a person's age. Those involved in weight-bearing exercise seem to have greater protection against bone loss during amenorrhea than those in non-weight-bearing sports.

Calcium in Food

Too little dietary calcium has also been implicated as a cause of osteopenia and osteoporosis. More than 99 per cent of the body's calcium is found in bones and teeth. About 70 per cent of our dietary calcium comes from the dairy foods milk, cheese and yogurt. Low-fat yogurt and milk are usually higher in calcium than the regular versions because when the fat is removed, manufacturers add back more milk solids, which includes calcium and protein. Around 20 per cent of all the calcium in our diet is absorbed from our digestive system (mainly the duodenum, the first part of the small intestine). It is often said that we cannot absorb the calcium from milk, but in fact, we absorb around 30 per cent of the calcium from milk.

Table 4.1 shows how much calcium you need each day, and table 4.2 lists the calcium content of some foods. With judicious food choices, you can reach your daily calcium needs.

Calcium Supplements

For various reasons, some people choose not to eat dairy foods or calcium-fortified foods. If you believe you are not getting enough calcium from food, then taking a calcium supplement may be wise. Your doctor or dietitian can give you advice. If you take a supplement, check the label to see how much pure calcium you get, not the total amount of the calcium supplement. For example, 600 milligrams of calcium gluconate gives you only 55 milligrams of calcium, whereas 600 milligrams of calcium carbonate gives you about 250 milligrams of calcium, about five times as much. Calcium carbonate and calcium citrate are considered the better calcium supplements.

Although absorption of calcium from supplements is slightly lower than that from dairy foods, absorption is highest when calcium supplements are taken between meals or at bedtime in doses of 500 milligrams or less. Sometimes

TABLE 4.1 Daily Calcium Recommendations

Female	Age	Australia/New Zealand	United States/Canada	UK
Girls	9–11 yr	1,000 mg	1,300 mg	800 mg
Girls	12–13 yr	1,300 mg	1,300 mg	800 mg
Teenagers	14–18 yr	1,300 mg	1,300 mg	800 mg
Women	19–50 yr	1,000 mg	1,000 mg	700 mg
Women	Pregnant	1,000 mg	1,000 mg	700 mg
Women	Nursing	1,000 mg	1,000 mg	1,250 mg
Women	51+ yr	1,300 mg	1,200 mg	700 mg
Male	**Age**	**Australia/New Zealand**	**United States/Canada**	**UK**
Boys	9–11 yr	1,000 mg	1,300 mg	1,000 mg
Boys	12–13 yr	1,300 mg	1,300 mg	1,000 mg
Teenagers	14–18 yr	1,300 mg	1,300 mg	1,000 mg
Men	19–50 yr	1,000 mg	1,000 mg	700 mg
Men	51–70 yr	1,000 mg	1,200 mg	700 mg
Men	71+ yr	1,300 mg	1,200 mg	700 mg

TABLE 4.2   Calcium Content of Some Common Foods

Food	Calcium (mg)
MILK AND SOY FOODS	
Calcium-fortified milk, 240 mL (8 oz)	500
Sustagen Sport, 200 mL (7 oz), with water	400
Non-fat milk, 240 mL (8 oz)	375
Reduced-fat (2% fat) milk, 240 mL (8 oz)	310
Low-fat (1% fat) milk, 240 mL (8 oz)	310
Flavoured milk, 240 mL (8 oz)	300
Calcium-fortified soy drink, 240 mL (8 oz)	300
Whole milk, 240 mL (8 oz)	275
Tofu, firm (calcium coagulant), 100 g (3.5 oz)	300
Tofu, soft (calcium coagulant), 100 g (3.5 oz)	80
Tempeh (fermented soy), 100 g (3.5 oz)	75
YOGURT, PER 200 G (7 OZ)	
Low-fat, natural	360
Low-fat, fruit flavour	320
Plain, natural	290
Whole, fruit flavour	260
CHEESE, PER 30 G (1 OZ)	
Edam	260
Cheddar	240
Processed	200
Camembert, brie	150
Ricotta	100
Cottage cheese	30
DAIRY DESSERTS, PER SERVE	
Dairy dessert, 100 mL (3.4 oz)	120
Custard, commercial, 100 mL (3.4 oz)	120
Ice cream, regular and low fat, 1 scoop	65
FAT AND OIL, PER SERVE	
Cream, 1 tbsp	15
Butter, 1 tbsp	5
Vegetable oils	0

▶ continued

▶ Table 4.2 (continued)

Food	Calcium (mg)
OTHER FOODS, PER SERVE	
Breakfast cereal, calcium fortified, 40 g (1.4 oz)	200
Sardines with bones, 50 g (1.8 oz)	180
Salmon with bones, 50 g (1.8 oz)	170
Molasses, blackstrap, 1 tbsp	40
Collard, 1/2 cup cooked	70
Prawns, 100 g (3.5 oz)	80
Spinach, 1/2 cup cooked	65
Milk chocolate, 50 g (1.8 oz)	125
Tahini, 1 tbsp	65
Baked beans, 1 cup	80
Soybeans, 1/2 cup	65
Pak choi (bok choy), 1/2 cup cooked	80
Clams, 100 g (3.5 oz)	40
Almonds, 30 g (1 oz)	70
Kidney beans, chick peas, 1/2 cup	50
Brazil nuts, 30 g (1 oz)	45
Sesame seeds, 3 tbsp, 30 g (1 oz)	20
Egg, 1 50 g (1.8 oz)	20
Broccoli, 1 cup cooked	30
Dark chocolate, 50 g (1.8 oz)	25
Fruit juice, 240 mL (8 oz)	25
Fresh fruit, average	20
Bread, 1 slice	20
Peanuts, 30 g (1 oz)	15
Meat, chicken, 100 g (3.5 oz)	20
Peanut butter, 1 tbsp	10
Pasta, 1 cup	10
Rice, 1 cup	5

Data from nutrition information panels on food labels; NUTTAB 2010 Online Version, Food Standards Australian New Zealand (http://www.foodstandards.gov.au/consumerinformation/nuttab2010/nuttab2010onlinesearchabledatabase/onlineversion.cfm); USDA National Nutrient Database for Standard Reference, Release 23 (www.ars.usda.gov/SP2UserFiles/Place/12354500/Data/SR23/nutrlist/sr23a421.pdf); USDA Nutrient Data Laboratory (www.ars.usda.gov/main/site_main.htm?modecode=12-35-45-00).

▶ Tips for Getting More Calcium Into Your Diet

- Change to non-fat (skim) or reduced-fat milk and low-fat yogurt; they generally have more calcium (check the nutrition information panel).
- Use low-fat milk in baking.
- Add yogurt or milk to soup, or a dab of yogurt to tacos, burritos and curries.
- Mix low-fat milk with mashed potatoes.
- Melt cheese on toast, baked potatoes or pasta dishes.
- If you don't like plain milk, blend it with fruit for a smoothie, or add some flavouring such as Milo, Nesquik, AktaVite, Ovaltine or Horlicks.
- Use commercial flavoured milks for a convenient snack. Most are made from reduced-fat milk.
- Eat green leafy vegetables such as broccoli, bok choy or Brussels sprouts because they have easy-to-absorb calcium. The exceptions are spinach and rhubarb, which have calcium in a form that is very difficult to absorb.
- If you don't eat dairy foods, choose a calcium-fortified soy beverage.
- Go easy on salt and salty foods. Too much salt in the diet may cause extra calcium to be lost in the urine. Choose reduced-salt varieties of food.

you will hear that calcium supplements interfere with iron absorption from the intestines. Studies of people taking calcium supplements for long periods show no effect on iron levels. If there is interference, then it appears to be only short term with the body quickly compensating (Lönnerdal 2010).

Iron

If you are very active, then you have an increased chance of becoming low in iron; your chance is further increased if you are a young female. This section addresses iron and explains how to avoid iron deficiency and its symptoms.

Most of the iron in the body is incorporated into haemoglobin, a protein in blood that takes oxygen from the lungs to all parts of the body and retrieves carbon dioxide from body cells to return to the lungs to be exhaled. Iron is also found in myoglobin in muscles, which does a similar job to haemoglobin in that it stores oxygen. Iron is a part of ferritin molecules throughout the body. Some iron is lost from the body each day; ideally, lost iron is replaced by eating iron-containing food.

Iron Depletion in Athletes

If the amount of iron lost exceeds the amount absorbed by the digestive system, then body iron stores are gradually depleted. The first stage is called iron deficiency; at this stage sports performance can drop, yet the athlete may not feel the more obvious symptoms of fatigue. Iron deficiency anaemia occurs when all the body's iron stores have been used up; at this stage the athlete experiences constant fatigue. Iron depletion can occur in athletes when high-level exercise causes an increase in iron losses. Fortunately, anaemia doesn't have to follow if athletes compensate for the extra iron losses by eating more iron-rich food.

Most athletes suspect low iron levels when their training performance deteriorates despite putting in a good effort. If fatigue or poor performance persists and you suspect anaemia, get a confirmation via a blood test from your doctor. Symptoms of low iron include the following:

- Fatigue (for other causes of tiredness, see table 4.3 on page 60)
- Listlessness
- Paler-than-normal skin
- Being more susceptible to infection (iron is needed for a healthy immune system)
- Decline in sports performance

Remember that many conditions can lead to fatigue. Note the serious warning on page 61, and see table 4.3, which lists possible causes of fatigue and their solutions.

TABLE 4.3 Fatigue Guide

Possible causes of fatigue	Solutions
Low iron levels	• Have a blood test to confirm iron levels. • Eat more iron-containing foods. • Take iron supplements, if prescribed by your doctor.
Too little carbohydrate	• Eat more carbohydrate foods and drinks, especially during heavy training programs. • Eat carbohydrate foods five or six times a day.
Overtraining or lack of fitness	• Reduce training. • Increase your training load more slowly. • Check with your coach for a modified training schedule. • Lack of fitness can make people feel tired, especially those who do very little exercise. Increasing fitness makes you more energetic and helps you to sleep better. • Eat more carbohydrate-rich foods if you are training a lot.
Gastric upset	• Don't eat too close to training; allow two hours or more between eating and exercise. • Drink plenty of fluids; avoid dehydration. • Eat familiar foods.
Too much caffeine	• Don't consume caffeinated food and drink close to bedtime. • Cut back on caffeine supplements and caffeine drinks such as high-caffeine energy drinks.
Stress, worry	• Avoid the cause of stress. This may involve changing your job, your work hours, where you live or your relationships. • Learn relaxation techniques.
Dehydration	• Minimise your risk of dehydration during training and events. • Drink until you pass copious amounts of pale urine, especially after training.
Too much alcohol	• Reduce alcohol. • Explore why you need to drink unhealthy amounts.
Shiftwork	• This problem has no simple answer. It is best to get into a routine so that you sleep at the same time each day. • Enjoy light meals at work; don't overeat. • Have your vitamin D levels checked because a lack of sunlight can cause low vitamin D levels.
Premenstrual syndrome	• Reduce salt and salty foods; this can help reduce the bloated feeling.
Skipping meals	• Always eat regularly throughout the day, even if only a light snack. Don't skip breakfast because that will make you tired and reduce your physical and mental performance. • Eat three to six times daily.
Study	• Fitting in study hours can be tough, especially if you work as well. Try to reshape the day by watching less TV and exercising every day.
Smoking	• The answer is obvious: Don't.

Possible causes of fatigue	Solutions
Hay fever, allergies	• See your doctor for the best advice to minimise symptoms. • Attend an allergy clinic at a major teaching hospital.
Timing of meals or snacks	• Leave two hours or more between eating and training. • Leave two hours or more between eating and going to bed. • Don't miss meals.
Overweight	• Lose excess body fat, especially abdominal fat.
Hypoglycemia	• Eat for health over five or six meals or snacks a day. • Note: Very few people have true hypoglycemia. Most tiredness is not due to hypoglycemia.
Weather	• Hot or humid weather can wipe you out until you acclimatise. Train in the cooler part of the day if it is more comfortable. • Seek medical help if hay fever is a problem.

Increased losses of iron from the body may occur in the following ways:

• **Via urine and feces.** Athletes tend to lose more iron this way than do other people. Small amounts of blood loss from the stomach or the intestines can occur in endurance runners. It may be due to some minor damage caused by reduced blood flow to the intestinal lining as much of the blood is redirected to the muscles in sport. Blood loss can also be due to the effects of some drugs such as aspirin. Blood in the urine may be caused by minor damage to the lining of the bladder. It will usually clear up within 48 hours of strenuous exercise. Good hydration can reduce damage because having some urine in the bladder may lessen damage to the bladder lining. For most athletes, blood is not lost in this manner. See your doctor if you see blood in your urine or stools.

• **From running.** Every time the foot hits the ground during running, some red blood cells are destroyed, a process called haemolysis; hence it's called foot-strike haemolysis. This is not a problem for most athletes, but it can become an issue in endurance runners. Some of the haemoglobin released from the broken red blood cells may end up in the urine. Check your running shoes and make sure they are well cushioned and that your running style is efficient. A sports podiatrist can help you here. If you are overweight, reduce your body fat stores to reduce the pressure on your feet.

• **From normal blood loss.** A good deal of iron can be lost during menstruation, which is the main reason young women need twice the iron as men. Blood can also be lost through injury and regular blood donations. I'm not suggesting that you stop being a blood donor, but you will have to consider when in your training schedule it is best to donate blood. One option is to be a plasma donor because you can keep your red blood cells. For most active people, regular blood donations are not a problem, although

▶ Serious Warning

Please do not take iron supplements if you haven't had a blood test to confirm low iron levels or just because you feel a bit tired. About 1 in 250 people has an iron overload condition called hemochromatosis, whereby the body absorbs more iron than needed. It occurs in both men and women, although it is more common in men. Iron builds up in the liver, pancreas and heart, slowly destroying these organs. One of the symptoms is chronic tiredness. If you take an iron supplement in this situation, you will make things worse. See your doctor for a blood test if you are always tired. I know that 1 in 250 doesn't sound like many, but the consequences are dire as the liver, pancreas and heart are organs that are very difficult to repair or replace. Again, do not ever take iron supplements unless recommended by your doctor after a blood test.

you may want to take it easy on the day of the donation. Having noted all of the potential ways an athlete might lose more iron than normal, be aware that the most likely cause of iron deficiency anemia in athletes is menstrual loss in women and insufficient iron in the diet in both men and women.

- **Via sweat.** Because athletes sweat more than sedentary people do, it has been suggested that iron losses can add up over months of heavy sweat loss such as during endurance training. This is unlikely to be a major cause of anaemia in athletes, unless they are heavy sweaters. Estimates of iron loss have been as high as 0.3 milligram per litre of sweat, so an athlete who loses 3 to 4 litres of sweat in a training session may have lost 1 milligram of iron. Because we absorb only about 10 per cent of the iron in food, people who sweat heavily may require an additional 10 milligrams of iron in their daily diet.

Sport Anaemia

In sport anaemia, ferritin and haemoglobin levels in the blood appear low, but this is due to the extra 10 to 20 per cent of plasma (the liquid part of blood) produced by athletes in heavy training. In other words, because there is more plasma, not less haemoglobin, haemoglobin levels only appear to be low. Sport anaemia is not a case of too little iron in the diet and therefore does not require an iron supplement.

Although the concentration of haemoglobin is lower in cases of sport anaemia, the oxygen-carrying capacity of the blood is not affected. Sport anaemia is sometimes impressively called dilutional pseudoanaemia. The dilution makes the blood less viscous (less gluggy) so that blood can travel the blood vessel highways much more quickly, which is ideal for oxygen delivery to the muscles. The extra plasma may also reduce the risk of dehydration. The dilution effect usually occurs early in a bout of increased training and generally doesn't affect sports performance. The dilution reverses quickly over a few days if training ceases.

Some elite athletes make extra red blood cells in response to training, which is also very useful in getting more oxygen to the muscles. Although there may be more red blood cells, there's an even larger increase in plasma, so dilutional pseudoanaemia still occurs.

Blood Tests for Iron Deficiency and Anaemia

A blood test is the best way to see whether you have a true anaemia. Blood should be taken on a rest day or before any strenuous exercise because dehydration will give falsely high readings as a result of the blood having become more concentrated. Table 4.4 lists the range of bloods tests for iron deficiency. Your doctor will advise you on the interpretation of your blood test. You will probably have the some of the following tested:

- Serum ferritin (lower in iron deficiency) is a very good marker for iron stores in the body.
- Serum transferrin, the main transport protein for iron in the blood, is lower in iron deficiency.
- Iron saturation of serum transferrin (the transferrin saturation level falls in iron deficiency).
- Total iron-binding capacity (TIBC) of the blood (higher in iron deficiency).
- Haemoglobin level. Levels under 120 g/L for women and under 130 g/L for men indicate iron deficiency anaemia.

When iron stores become depleted, the body can't make enough haemoglobin. This will lead to anemia and less oxygen being transported to muscles, which causes a deterioration in performance.

The measurement most widely used in sports medicine is that of serum ferritin, a protein in which iron is stored. Iron is toxic to the body so

TABLE 4.4 Blood Tests for Iron Deficiency

Blood test	Iron deficiency
Serum iron	<500 mcg/L
TIBC	>400 mcg/100 mL
Transferrin saturation	<16%
Serum ferritin	<20 mcg/L
Haemoglobin*	<120 g/L female; <130 g/L male

*A low haemoglobin level indicates that iron deficiency has now become clinical anaemia.

it needs to be wrapped in the protective ferritin molecule. Ferritin is found mainly in the bone marrow, but a small amount is found in the blood in proportion to the amount in the bone marrow. The range usually found in athletes is 30 to 200 micrograms per litre. A ferritin value below 20 micrograms per litre is considered to represent depleted bone marrow iron stores and is usually associated with fatigue and a decline in performance. Many sports physicians prescribe iron supplementation when the value is lower than 35 micrograms per litre.

The interpretation of ferritin levels is not straightforward. For example, smaller people, especially those with low muscle mass, have normally lower concentrations of ferritin and haemoglobin. Females have, on average, lower values than males have. A small female distance runner with a haemoglobin of 11 grams per 100 millilitres, or a ferritin of 20 micrograms per litre, may have near optimal levels. However, if a male weightlifter or footballer presented these values, iron deficiency would be suspected. Athletes with iron issues should consult a sports physician. A sports physician is best placed to make a judgment on blood iron studies.

Who Is at Risk of Low Iron Stores?

The following types of people are at highest risk of having low iron stores:

- Male and female endurance runners as a result of foot-strike hemolysis, greater iron loss in feces and urine, and extra iron losses from heavy sweating.

- Females with heavy periods. More blood loss means higher iron needs.

- Females on strict weight loss diets. Strict weight loss diets are generally low in many essential nutrients. It's very difficult to get all your iron needs when food is very restricted. When attempting body fat loss, choose low-fat foods high in iron, such as lean meat and iron-fortified breakfast cereals.

- Athletes avoiding iron-rich foods such as red meat, paté and iron-fortified foods such as breakfast cereals, or avoiding foods high in vitamin C such as fruits and vegetables.

- Vegetarian and vegan athletes because iron is less bioavailable from plant food sources. It is thought that vegetarians may need one and a half to two times more iron in their diets than is recommended to most of the population ('Executive summary' 2005, 189).

Women are generally at greater risk of low iron as a result of menstrual blood losses and consuming less food than men. Very few men eat a low-iron diet.

Iron in Food

The iron in food is found in two forms, heme and non-heme. Heme iron is well absorbed by the body (about 20 per cent is absorbed) and is found in animal flesh foods such as red meat, poultry and seafood. It is abundant in liver and kidney if you fancy that kind of fare. Non-heme iron is found in plant foods, but only around 5 per cent is absorbed from the intestines; the remaining 95 per cent passes through the gut.

The iron in some plant foods such as spinach is poorly absorbed. (Popeye eating spinach for its iron content is a myth!) It is estimated that less than 5 per cent of both the iron and calcium in spinach is absorbed because the minerals are tightly bound to natural compounds called oxalates and can't be absorbed by the intestines. Iron is better absorbed from broccoli because it is low in oxalates.

Cereal foods, vegetables and meat provide three quarters of the iron in a Western diet. There are around 6 to 7 milligrams of iron in every 4,200 kilojoules (1,000 cal) of food, which shows why women who have a restricted food intake have a greater risk of anaemia. Use table 4.5 on page 64 to check that your meals contain enough iron.

There are ways to improve both the amount of iron in your meals and the amount you absorb from your intestines. Follow these tips to pump iron into your meals:

- **Include fruits or vegetables with each meal.** Vitamin C and other natural acids in fruits and vegetables enhances iron absorption, especially from other plant foods. A glass of orange juice with your breakfast cereal can nearly double your iron absorption.

TABLE 4.5 Daily Iron Recommendations

Female	Age	Australia, New Zealand, United States, Canada	UK
Girls	9–13 yr	8 mg	14.8 mg
Teenagers	14–18 yr	15 mg	14.8 mg
Women	19–50 yr	18 mg	14.8 mg
Women	Pregnant	27 mg	14.8 mg
Women	Nursing	9 mg	14.8 mg
Women	51+ yr	8 mg	8.7 mg
Male	Age	Australia, New Zealand, United States, Canada	UK
Boys	9–13 yr	8 mg	11.3 mg
Teenagers	14–18 yr	11 mg	11.3 mg
Men	19+ yr	8 mg	8.7 mg

- **Eat lean red meat three or four times a week.** Red meat is your best source of easy-to-absorb iron. Poultry and fish also provide iron, although less than red meat.

- **Avoid drinking tea and coffee with meals.** The tannin in these drinks reduces iron absorption, by up to half. Drink tea between meals. Coffee contains less tannin than tea, but still needs to be considered because it has other compounds that reduce iron absorption.

- **Eat breakfast cereals.** Most breakfast cereals are fortified with iron. Check the label to see how much iron you get per serve. There will be around 3 to 5 milligrams of iron in the amount you are likely to eat. Because this is non-heme iron, a vitamin C source with your cereal will help with iron absorption, such as slicing a banana onto your cereal. Porridge and muesli are very nutritious, but they are not high in iron.

- **Avoid too much unprocessed bran.** Eat a maximum of 2 level tablespoons of bran daily. Avoid foods highly fortified with bran, as the bran can reduce iron absorption.

Iron Supplements

If you think you suffer from low iron, ask your doctor to do a blood test to check. If iron deficiency is diagnosed, you will probably be prescribed an iron supplement for six weeks or longer to quickly get your iron levels back to normal. Most will provide about 5 milligrams of iron per tablet. Naturally, you will be advised to eat high-iron foods as well (see table 4.6). Iron supplements may cause constipation, so make sure you eat plenty of fibre-containing foods as well.

Vitamins

Thirteen components are considered vitamins. These are conveniently divided into two groups, water soluble (B group vitamins and vitamin C) and fat soluble (vitamins A, D, E and K). Vitamins were one of the earliest supplements to be given to athletes. Because vitamins are involved in the production of muscle energy, healthy immune function and the manufacture of haemoglobin and bone, it was assumed that additional vitamins as a supplement would improve sports performance. Despite much research, there is little evidence that taking a vitamin supplement will make you stronger, faster or more agile, except in the rare athlete who has a clear vitamin deficiency.

Although athletes do need more vitamins than non-athletes do, they generally get them from the extra food they need to fuel their training. An athlete making wise food choices is very unlikely to find a benefit in a vitamin supplement.

B Group Vitamins

The B vitamins thiamin (B_1), riboflavin (B_2), niacin (B_3) and pantothenic acid (B_5) are involved in the metabolism of carbohydrate and fat to provide muscle energy. Pyridoxine (B_6), folate and cyanocobalamin (B_{12}) are involved in

TABLE 4.6 Iron Content of Some Common Foods

Food	Iron (mg)
MEATS, SEAFOOD, EGG	
Liver, 100 g (3.5 oz)	10.0
Lean beef, grilled, 100 g (3.5 oz)	3.0
Lean lamb, grilled, 100 g (3.5 oz)	3.0
Paté, 1 tbsp	1.8
Salmon, 100 g (3.5 oz)	1.2
Lean pork, 100 g (3.5 oz)	1.0
Chicken leg, no skin, 100 g (3.5 oz)	1.0
Tuna, 100 g (3.5 oz)	1.0
Shellfish, average serve	1.0
Egg, 1 whole	1.5
Chicken breast, no skin, 100 g (3.5 oz)	0.5
Fish, grilled, average, 100 g (3.5 oz)	0.6
Prawns, cooked, 100 g (3.5 oz)	0.5
DRINKS	
Sustagen, 240 mL (8 oz)	4.0
Soy beverage, 240 mL (8 oz)	1.0
Milo, Ovaltine, 2 rounded tsp	1.0
Fruit juice, 240 mL (8 oz)	0.4
Milk	0.0
BREAKFAST CEREALS	
Weet-Bix Multigrain, 2 biscuits	3.0
SportsPlus, FibrePlus 45 g (1.6 oz)	3.0
Corn flakes, 30 g (1 oz)	3.0
Just Right, Sustain 30 g (1 oz)	3.0
Iron-fortified cereals, 45 g (1.6 oz)	2.5–5.0
Weet-Bix, 2 biscuits	2.5
Weetabix, 2 biscuits	1.8
Muesli bars, average, 30 g (1 oz)	0.6
Sultana Bran, 30 g (1 oz)	2.0
Muesli, 1/2 cup	2.5
Vita Brits, 2 biscuits	1.0
Porridge, 3/4 cup	1.0
Wheat germ, 1 tbsp	1.0

▶ *continued*

▶ Table 4.6 (*continued*)

Food	Iron (mg)
BREADS, RICE AND PASTA	
Ravioli, beef, 1/2 cup	0.8
Wholemeal bread, 1 slice	0.6
Fruit loaf, 1 slice	0.6
Pasta, 1/2 cup	0.5
Rice, brown, 1/2 cup	0.5
White bread, 1 slice	0.4
Rice, white, 1/2 cup	0.3
VEGETABLES, FRUITS, NUTS, SEEDS	
Spinach, cooked, 100 g (3.5 oz)	3.0
Lentils, kidney beans, 1/2 cup	2.0
Cashews, 30 g (1 oz)	1.5
Baked beans, 1/2 cup	1.3
Peas, 1/2 cup	1.3
Dried apricots, 5 pieces	1.3
Almonds, hazelnuts, 30 g (1 oz)	1.0
Potato, 1 medium	0.8
Sunflower seeds, 1 tbsp	0.8
Raisins, 2 tbsp	0.6
Vegetables, average serve	0.5
Fresh fruit, 1 serve	0.5
Peanuts, 30 g (1 oz)	0.3
Peanut butter, 1 tbsp	0.3
CONFECTIONERY, MUESLI BARS	
Licorice, 50 g (1.8 oz)	4.0
Dark chocolate, 50 g (1.8 oz)	2.2
Milk chocolate, 50 g (1.8 oz)	0.7
White chocolate	0.0

making red blood cells. Although an increased need for these vitamins could be expected in athletes, the vitamin requirements of athletes have not been determined. Because training generally increases appetite, more food is eaten, providing extra B vitamins to meet those increased needs. Table 4.7 lists food sources for the B vitamins.

Vitamin B_{12} is necessary for making DNA (the genetic director in body cells), so it has been hypothesised that it may stimulate muscle growth. However, there is no evidence that B_{12} increases muscle growth or strength. Athletes at greatest risk of getting insufficient B_{12} in their diet are vegetarians and vegans because the main sources of B_{12} are foods of animal origin. Some foods are fortified with B_{12}, such as some soy drinks. See chapter 10 on vegetarian athletes for more information.

TABLE 4.7 Good Sources of B Vitamins

Food	Amount
FOODS WITH THIAMIN (B₁)	
Pork, grilled, 100 g (3.5 oz)	1.3 mg
Fortified breakfast cereal, 50 g (1.8 oz)	0.3–0.6 mg
Hazelnuts, 50 g (1.8 oz)	0.2 mg
Wheat germ, 1 tbsp	0.15 mg
Peas, cooked, 1/2 cup	0.2 mg
Bread, wholemeal, 1 slice	0.1 mg
FOODS WITH RIBOFLAVIN (B₂)	
Milk, low-fat, 240 mL (8 oz)	0.5 mg
Almonds, 30 g (1 oz)	0.4 mg
Yogurt, low-fat, 200 g (7 oz)	0.4 mg
Fortified breakfast cereals, 50 g (1.8 oz)	0.4 mg
Mushrooms, 100 g (3.5 oz)	0.4 mg
Chicken, roasted, 100 g (3.5 oz)	0.3 mg
Egg, 1 whole	0.2 mg
FOODS WITH NIACIN (B₃)	
Ham, lean, 100 g (3.5 oz)	8.0 mg
Beef, grilled, 100 g (3.5 oz)	7.5 mg
Peanuts, 30 g (1 oz)	7.0 mg
Mushrooms, 100 g (3.5 oz)	4.0 mg
Baked beans, 1/2 cup	2.0 mg
Banana, 1 medium	1.0 mg
Bread, wholemeal, 1 slice	0.7 mg
FOODS WITH PANTOTHENIC ACID (B₅)	
Pork roast, 120 g (4.2 oz)	1.2 mg
Mushrooms, 100 g (3.5 oz)	1.1 mg
Avocado, 100 g (3.5 oz)	1.0 mg
Milk, 240 mL (8 oz)	1.0 mg
Egg, boiled, 60 g (2 oz)	1.0 mg
Camembert cheese, 30 g (1 oz)	0.7 mg
Brown rice, boiled, 1/2 cup	0.3 mg

▶ continued

▶ Table 4.7 (continued)

Food	Amount
FOODS WITH PYRIDOXINE (B$_6$)	
Eggplant, grilled, 50 g (1.8 oz)	1.2 mg
Banana, 1 medium	0.4 mg
Pistachios, 30 g (1 oz)	0.4 mg
Tuna, canned, 120 g (4.2 oz)	0.3 mg
Beef, cooked, 120 g (4.2 oz)	0.3 mg
Peanuts, raw, 50 g (1.8 oz)	0.25 mg
FOODS WITH FOLATE	
Folate-fortified breakfast cereals, average serve	100 mcg
Legumes such as kidney beans, cooked, 1/2 cup	100 mcg
Avocado, 100 g (3.5 oz)	59 mcg
Asparagus, 2 spears	43 mcg
Cabbage, cooked, 1/2 cup	40 mcg
Broccoli, 1/2 cup	40 mcg
Peanuts, 30 g (1 oz)	30 mcg
FOODS WITH CYANOCOBALAMIN (B$_{12}$)	
Liver, cooked, 100 g (3.5 oz)	70 mcg
Sardines, canned, 60 g (2 oz)	14 mcg
Salmon, red, 100 g (3.5 oz)	3 mcg
Beef, cooked, 120 g (4.2 oz)	2 mcg
Egg, boiled, 60 g (2 oz)	1 mcg
Pork, grilled, 100 g (3.5 oz)	0.5 mcg

Vitamin D

There are now many reports that around half of the general population in Western countries have low levels of vitamin D in the blood. The main reason is insufficient exposure to sunlight, especially in those who work indoors during the day, or always remain covered up when outside. The few studies on athletes suggest that many are also low in vitamin D, especially if they do most of their training indoors, such as gymnasts. As you remember from high school biology, you need vitamin D to absorb enough calcium from the food you eat, so having a low vitamin D level will compromise your calcium status even if you are consuming adequate amounts of calcium.

Vitamin D is also important for general health. Every organ in the body has vitamin D receptors, and over 2,000 genes are influenced by vitamin D. People getting the least amount of sun seem to have the greatest risk of disease and conditions such as multiple sclerosis, Parkinson's disease, heart disease, diabetes, colon cancer and depression. The foods with greatest amount of vitamin D are oily fish, margarine, eggs, cheese and mushrooms exposed to sunlight. Some vitamin D- and calcium-fortified milks, drink powders and soy beverages are also available. (See table 4.8).

A blood test will show you whether your vitamin D levels are low or healthy. Most adults get less than half of their vitamin D needs through

TABLE 4.8 Good Sources of Vitamin D

Food	Amount
Margarine, 2 tsp (10 g)	1 mcg
Tuna, canned, 100 g	2 mcg
Salmon, canned, 10 g	1 mcg
Egg, 1 whole, 50 g	0.5 mcg
Vitamin D–fortified milk/soy drink, 100 mL	0.5–2 mcg
Cheese, cheddar, 30 g	0.3 mcg
Mushrooms, wild, 100 g	10–40 mcg
Mushrooms, commercial, light exposed, 100 g	20–40 mcg

Data from nutrition information panels on food labels; NUTTAB 2010 Online Version, Food Standards Australian New Zealand (http://www.foodstandards.gov.au/consumerinformation/nuttab2010/nuttab2010onlinesearchabledatabase/onlineversion.cfm); USDA National Nutrient Database for Standard Reference, Release 23 (www.ars.usda.gov/SP2UserFiles/Place/12354500/Data/SR23/nutrlist/sr23a421.pdf); USDA Nutrient Data Laboratory (www.ars.usda.gov/main/site_main.htm?modecode=12-35-45-00).

food and don't make up the remainder with enough sunlight exposure. Too little vitamin D results in an overall health risk as well as weaker bones that are more prone to fractures. Dietary needs of vitamin D are 5 micrograms per day for those under 50 year old, 10 micrograms per day for those 50 to 70 years old and 15 micrograms per day for people older than 70. A 2010 report from the Institute of Medicine in the USA stated that adults should be getting 15 micrograms of vitamin D daily, and those over 70 should be getting as much as 20 micrograms per day. If your doctor, judging from a blood test, says that you have low levels of vitamin D in your blood, then you may be advised to get a bit more sun and take a 25- to 50-microgram (1,000 to 2,000 International Units [IU]) daily supplement of vitamin D.

Following are the types of people who are likely to benefit from a calcium or vitamin D supplement (or both):

- Athletes who eat too little calcium (usually not eating enough dairy or calcium-fortified soy drinks).

- Female athletes with amenorrhea (no periods) or who are postmenopausal.

- Athletes who train mainly indoors or only in the early morning or in the evening and therefore don't get enough sun exposure to generate adequate vitamin D.

Vitamin E

Vitamin E is the common name for eight related compounds comprising four tocopherols and four tocotrienols. Of these, alpha-tocopherol is the most biologically active and the most widely distributed in food. The vast majority of studies since 1955 have reported no useful effect of vitamin E on sports performance. It also appears that the practice of vitamin E supplementation is not harmful, although an upper intake limit has been set at 300 milligrams daily. Table 4.9 lists food sources of vitamin E.

Vitamin C

Vitamin C assists the absorption of iron and has antioxidant activity. Early reports of vitamin C improving sports performance in Eastern European athletes was probably due to correcting a vitamin C deficiency caused by a lack of fruits and vegetables in the diet. Around 100 to 200 milligrams of vitamin C per day will saturate the body's cells, and extra amounts are unlikely to assist the athlete given that this amount is easily obtained by eating fresh fruits and vegetables. For example, as you can see from table 4.10, one

TABLE 4.9 Good Sources of Vitamin E

Food	Amount
Almonds, 30 g (1 oz)	7.3 mg
Mixed nuts, 30 g (1 oz)	3.1 mg
Safflower oil, 1 tbsp	3.6 mg
Margarine, polyunsaturated, 2 tsp	2.4 mg
Avocado, 1/2	2.1 mg
Egg, 1 whole	1.3 mg

TABLE 4.10 Good Sources of Vitamin C

Food	Amount
Red capsicum/red pepper, 1/2 cup	140 mg
Orange juice, 150 mL (5 oz)	75 mg
Orange, 1 medium	70 mg
Mandarin, 1 medium	50 mg
Broccoli, cooked, 1/2 cup	35 mg
Pineapple, 1/2 cup	30 mg
Snow peas, 50 g (1.8 oz)	20 mg

medium orange provides about 70 milligrams of vitamin C. Despite the frequent claim, there is no evidence that taking extra vitamin C prevents the common cold or reduces its duration.

Although vitamin C does act as an antioxidant, the body responds to training by producing more of its own antioxidants. For this reason, taking extra vitamin C as a supplement doesn't seem to offer performance benefits. Indeed, oversupplementation can diminish the body's natural immune system.

Vitamin A

This vitamin is found in liver, oily fish, cheese and eggs (see table 4.11). Common precursors of vitamin A are alpha-carotene and beta-carotene, which are eventually converted to vitamin A in the body. These precursors to vitamin A are found in yellow and orange fruits and vegetables like papayas, mangos, red sweet potato and, of course, the carrot. For vegetarians, plant sources of the carotenes are an important way to get enough vitamin A in the diet. The body is able to extract more carotenes from cooked and well-chewed food than raw versions. Cooking and chewing help release carotenes from the cellulose structures in plant cells. Vitamin A is famous for good vision and a healthy reproductive capability, yet it has broader functions within the body, such as normal gene expression, iron absorption and immune function.

TABLE 4.11 Good Sources of Vitamin A

Food	Amount
Liver, beef, raw, 50 g	7,000 mcg
Carrot juice, 100 mL	1,700 mcg
Carrot, 100 g	1,300 mcg
Vegetable juice, average, 100 mL	1,000 mcg
Sweet potato, cooked, 100 g	1,000 mcg
Pumpkin, cooked, 100 g	500 mcg
Mango, 100 g	350 mcg
Powdered food drink, 1 tbsp	200 mcg
Butter, margarine, 1 tbsp	180 mcg
Apricot, dried, 25 g	100 mcg
Egg, 1 whole, 50 g	90 mcg
Red salmon, 50 g	50 mcg

Vitamin Supplements

Use of vitamin and mineral supplements does not improve performance in individuals consuming nutritionally adequate diets.

Position of the American Dietetic Association, Dietitians of Canada and the American College of Sports Medicine: Nutrition and Athletic Performance (2009, 515).

Any athlete greatly restricting food intake or fasting to lose weight is probably getting too few vitamins. Athletes at most risk would be gymnasts, ballet dancers and anyone in a weight-restricted sport. If you are travelling to a country with a reputation for low-quality food (e.g., poor food safety or variety) or to an area with little access to fresh fruits, vegetables and cereals, then a vitamin supplement may be useful. In these situations, you may benefit from a low-dose multivitamin supplement with no more that the daily needs in a dose. Taking megadoses of single nutrients has no value. If you have low levels of vitamin D, then prudent sun exposure and a vitamin D supplement can be helpful in boosting blood levels.

Clearly, the relationship between vitamins and sports performance needs further investigation. Most research will not be able to pick up a 0.5 or 1.0 per cent improvement in performance. Very little has been done to study the effect of vitamin supplements on recovery or injury prevention in elite athletes. Some vitamins in some athletes in certain conditions could make a small, but useful, difference in performance.

If you truly believe you need a vitamin supplement, then get an inexpensive, low-dose supplement and avoid the popular high-dose, high-priced supplements. Check your vitamin supplement against the recommended amounts needed each day as detailed in chapter 1. Supplements providing more nutrients than twice your daily needs are probably wasteful. Your diet should be providing the recommended amounts or more.

▶ Taking a vitamin supplement is unlikely to cause any harm, but as any sports dietitian will remind you, a vitamin supplement should never be a substitute for good eating habits.

Vitamin O

Some non-vitamin products are promoted as vitamins to athletes and the general public. One example is vitamin O, a supplement of stabilised oxygen molecules in a solution of sodium chloride and distilled water. This supplement is supposed to treat everything from mild fatigue to cancer, heart problems and lung disease. Another variation is 'oxygenated water'. Both have been promoted to athletes as tonics and performance boosters. This is a big hoax.

Although it is called vitamin O, oxygen is not a vitamin, nor is it something deficient in your diet. This is the world's most expensive salty water. Even if the water were as high in oxygen as claimed, it would help only if you were a fish breathing through gills.

The oxygen content of your glass of tap water is around 8 milligrams per litre. If you pressurise the water with oxygen gas, that level might increase to 40 milligrams per litre or more. When you open the bottle of 'vitamin O', most of this extra oxygen is released. In comparison, 1 litre of air contains 146 milligrams of oxygen, and when that runs out, golly, take another breath. Humans take oxygen from their lungs, not their intestines. As one scientist said: 'Ergogenic claims for oxygenated water therefore cannot be taken seriously' (Piantadosi 2006). Give vitamin O and oxygenated water a big miss.

The fact sheet on vitamins and minerals from the Australian Institute of Sport says simply and clearly: 'There is no evidence that supplementation with vitamins and minerals enhances performance except in cases where a pre-existing deficiency exists'(AIS Sports Supplement Program Website Fact Sheet August 2011).

FINAL SCORE

- Exercise in general improves the strength and density of bones. Weight-bearing exercise, such as walking, aerobics, running, netball, football and strength training, offers the greatest protection against osteoporosis.
- Eating a diet rich in calcium reduces the risk of osteoporosis. Avoid excessive amounts of salt because it may trigger calcium loss from the body.
- Adequate vitamin D from prudent sunlight exposure and consumption of vitamin D–containing foods is important for calcium absorption, strong bones and general health.
- Low levels of iron are common in athletes and young women.
- Female athletes with amenorrhea for more than three months should see a doctor and a sports dietitian.
- An inadequate amount of iron in the diet is common in young women, vegans, vegetarians and those on restricted weight loss diets.
- Iron supplements should never be taken unless a doctor has diagnosed an iron deficiency.
- To minimise the risk of low iron intake, eat foods high in heme iron; otherwise, if vegetarian, consume foods containing vitamin C with each meal to enhance iron absorption
- Most athletes can get all their vitamin needs from food. A low-dose vitamin supplement will probably do no harm, but it should not be a substitute for good eating habits.
- Athletes who eat very little food or have a restricted range of foods may be low in certain vitamins and could benefit from a vitamin supplement and professional advice on food choices.

Liquids for Hydration, Cooling and Energy

> **Dehydration (water deficit in excess of 2% to 3% body mass) decreases exercise performance; thus adequate fluid intake before, during and after exercise is important for health and optimal performance.**
>
> *Position of the American Dietetic Association, Dietitians of Canada and the American College of Sports Medicine: Nutrition and Athletic Performance (2009, 510)*

Dehydration and heat stress continue to be major causes of poor sports performance, especially in warm weather. Athletes consider dehydration to be like pregnancy—either you are or you aren't. In fact, performance can decline very early in sport, well before you start to feel thirsty and tired. Dehydration will reduce muscle endurance, aerobic capacity and mental function.

Public interest in dehydration was spurred when Gabriela Andersen-Schiess showed the classic signs of dehydration and heatstroke as she finished the first women's Olympic marathon in 1984. Her legs had lost all coordination. At times she was on all fours, with the crowd shouting encouragement to make sure she made the finish line. The 75,000 spectators created a heroine, and the TV producer loved every rating minute. Those who saw the image of the staggering athlete will likely never forget it, although it happened nearly 30 years ago. Neither did sports physicians and sports dietitians. Since then they have worked actively to prevent dehydration and heat stress in athletes.

Heat Stress

This chapter explains how to avoid heat stress, which includes the heat-related problems of heat exhaustion and heatstroke. Heat exhaustion is a condition in which the body starts to have difficulty maintaining a healthy core temperature. As the ability of the body to lose heat becomes lower than the amount of heat produced by exercise, the body's core temperature begins to rise and performance begins to drop. The symptoms of heat exhaustion during exercise are as follows:

- Nausea and vomiting
- Headache
- Faintness
- Profuse sweating

If you ever experience these symptoms, sit in the shade, drink lots of fluid and stop exercising for the rest of the day. If you were to continue exercising, you would likely go to the next stage, the extremely dangerous heatstroke. Heatstroke is a life-threatening condition in which the body temperature rises dangerously high, with sports performance dropping rapidly.

The symptoms of heatstroke include the following:

- Dizziness
- Nausea
- Cramps
- Headache
- Reduced sweating (due to lack of body fluids)
- Hot, dry skin

Although you may not be aware of it as it is happening, if you have these symptoms, you may be in urgent need of medical attention. People suffering from the flu or fever, and those who are overweight, not acclimatised to hot conditions or drink alcohol during the day before the event are more susceptible to heat stress.

Temperature Regulation

To perform at your best, you need to keep your body from overheating. The three main ways the body can lose the heat generated by muscle contraction during sport are illustrated in figure 5.1 and explained in more detail in this section.

- **Conduction.** When two objects at different temperatures come into contact with each other, heat transfers from the hotter object to the cooler object. For example, when an athlete runs on a hot road, heat is transferred from the road to the athlete's shoes and feet. Being sprayed with cold water can bring relief to the hot athlete because heat is transferred from the body to the water. The loss of too much heat (hypothermia) is common in long-distance open-water swimmers because the water is cooler than the body.
- **Convection.** Convection occurs when heat is transferred from the body to air when the air is much cooler than the body. As air moves across the skin, the warm air on the surface of the skin is replaced by cool air. The process of convection as a cooling mechanism is especially effective in windy conditions. Convection is well known to the snow skier or cyclist coming down a hill. When a cold wind is blowing (i.e., there is a wind chill factor), you may need to put on warmer clothing to prevent hypothermia.
- **Evaporation.** Evaporative cooling is the most important cooling method available to most athletes. About 70 per cent of body heat

▶ City to Surf

The annual City to Surf fun run in Sydney, Australia, attracts over 40,000 participants. Although it is usually held in cool August conditions, runners still suffer from dehydration and heat exhaustion. After two runners died of heatstroke in 1990, the medical directors of the City to Surf surveyed the runners. The survey revealed that the four major risk factors for heat exhaustion were as follows (Lyle et al. 1994):

- Being highly motivated to do a personal best
- Not including at least one training session a week at the same time as the run is scheduled, to help acclimatise for the run
- Failing to drink fluids during the run
- Having a previous history of heat exhaustion

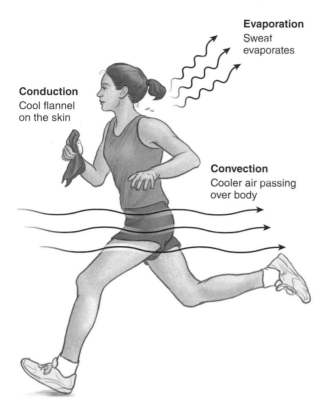

Evaporation
Sweat evaporates

Conduction
Cool flannel on the skin

Convection
Cooler air passing over body

FIGURE 5.1 Heat transfer during sport.

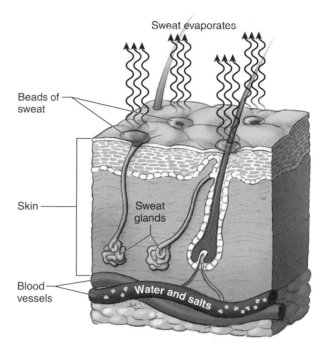

Sweat evaporates

Beads of sweat

Skin

Sweat glands

Blood vessels

Water and salts

FIGURE 5.2 Sweat comes from the blood. More water than salt is lost from the blood during sweating.

is lost when sweat evaporates and the liquid water is converted to water vapour. If the day is humid, this method is less effective because the increased moisture in the air decreases the ability of sweat to evaporate from the skin. Sweat that rolls off the skin is not evaporating and thus has very little cooling effect.

Sweat It Out

During exercise, muscles use the energy from ATP to contract. Only 25 per cent of energy is actually used for muscle contraction. The other 75 per cent is released as heat. So that our muscles don't overheat and 'melt', the heat is transferred to our blood. Our clever bodies then increase the blood flow to the skin so this heat can be released from the warmed blood by evaporative cooling (sweating), convection (breeze) and conduction (cooler ambient temperature).

Sweating from your many sweat glands is a very effective way of keeping your body cool. In fact, it's so good that as you get fitter, you sweat more. As shown in figure 5.2, sweat originates from the water in your blood. Your heart was pumping around every bead of sweat on your brow at one time. Sweat fills your sweat glands, to be released once things get warm. The sweat on the surface of your skin then evaporates to

cool you down. One litre of sweat fully evaporated from the skin dissipates 2,400 kilojoules (573 cal) of heat.

As you sweat, the water level in your blood begins to drop. As your blood volume drops, less blood flows to the skin, which further hinders heat loss. When dehydration is extreme and too much blood volume is lost, the body stops sweating to preserve its remaining blood volume. Unfortunately, the body temperature then quickly rises, and the person suffers heatstroke.

Sweat Glands

There are two types of sweat glands: eccrine (also known as merocrine) and apocrine glands. The estimated 2 to 5 million eccrine sweat glands are all over your body, although the main concentration of them is on the palms of your hands and the soles of your feet. They produce an odour-free mix of water, sodium, potassium and chloride, with a single purpose—cooling the body. The presence of sodium gives sweat its salty flavour.

Apocrine sweat glands are situated in the armpits and groin region. These glands produce fat, protein and various steroids and secrete them into the base of hair follicles. The yellowish fluid has no smell, but bacteria on your skin consume the secretions, producing a range of malodorous compounds. The smell of sweat is actually bacteria excrement. Uh!

▶ Keeping Cool During Exercise

- Avoid sunburn. Apart from the discomfort, sunburned skin sweats less efficiently and stops producing vitamin D.
- Wear loose, light-coloured clothing (it reflects heat better than bare skin does).
- Avoid exercise in the heat of the day.
- Avoid dehydration—drink fluids to closely match sweat losses.
- Apply cool water to your neck and head regions for cooling in warm weather.
- Don't use oil-based sunscreens as they interfere with evaporative cooling.
- Be fit. Unfit people are at greater risk of heatstroke.

How Much Does an Athlete Sweat?

Most athletes produce 500 to 1,000 millilitres (17 to 34 oz) of sweat per hour. This number is higher in hot conditions, when an athlete can easily lose 1 to 2 litres each hour. Replacing that amount during an event is difficult. Swimmers also sweat, although their losses are much lower, around 300 to 350 millilitres per hour.

The stomach empties at around 1,000 to 1,200 millilitres (34 to 40 oz) an hour, but athletes tend to drink much less than that. Research on runners shows that they drink 500 millilitres of liquid (17 oz) or less each hour, while sweating at a rate of 1,000 to 1,500 millilitres (34 to 51 oz) per hour. The volume that most athletes drink voluntarily during exercise is less than half of their fluid losses. Swimmers find it much easier to meet their sweat losses during training. With training and encouragement, land-based athletes can drink 1,000 millilitres (34 oz) each hour (see figure 5.3). Fluids taken during sport are absorbed back into the blood to return the blood volume to normal, keeping proper blood flow to the skin, which in turn promotes sweating and prevents excessive heat build-up in the body.

Sometimes you won't notice yourself sweating. If you exercise in warm, dry conditions, the sweat can evaporate so quickly that you don't appear to be sweating. A good example is bike riding. As your body moves through the air, sweat evaporates almost as quickly as it's produced.

In a sport such as swimming, in which you are constantly wet, it is very difficult to work out how much you have sweated. Yes, you still sweat when you swim. A study of elite swimmers at the Australian Institute of Sport in warm conditions found that 100 to 150 millilitres (3 to 5 oz) of

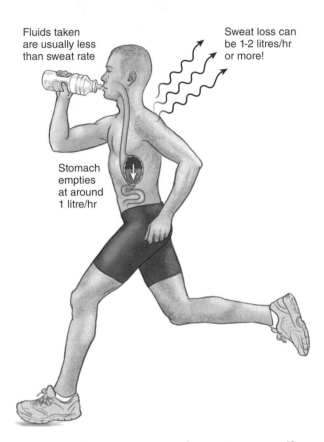

Fluids taken are usually less than sweat rate

Sweat loss can be 1-2 litres/hr or more!

Stomach empties at around 1 litre/hr

FIGURE 5.3 In warm weather, train yourself to drink at least 1 litre of fluid every hour.

fluid was lost for every kilometre swum (Cox et al. 2002). Less fit swimmers may sweat more. Being immersed in water will also suppress the thirst sensation; hence, dehydration may go unnoticed in activities such as swimming and water polo.

Men, Women and Children

Generally, women lose less sweat than men do. It's probably because they are more economical in their sweating and, because of their lower body weight, produce less sweat for the same

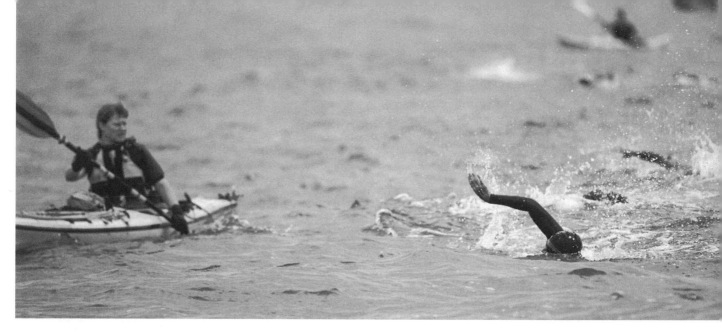

Yes, swimmers do sweat, although at a lower rate than runners. Elite swimmers lose around 100-150 millilitres of sweat per kilometre.

workload. However, women appear to be as effective as men in 'keeping their cool' during exercise in the heat.

Children are at greater risk of overheating than adults are for the following reasons:

- Their sweating is less efficient so they depend more on convection for heat loss.
- Their ability to transfer heat from the centre of the body to the surface of the body (skin) by blood is less than that of adults.
- They produce more heat per kilogram at a given running speed.
- They have a larger surface area to body mass ratio than adults so they can gain heat faster on hot days.

Therefore, even when topped up with fluids, children are at much greater risk of heatstroke than adults. Unfortunately, children, like adults, don't drink enough fluids during exercise in the heat; parents and coaching staff should encourage children to drink by providing frequent drink breaks.

The Thirst Response

In most circumstances, when your body water levels drop, your body triggers a feeling of thirst and you replace the lost water by drinking. Thirst is a very good indicator of your fluid needs during the day around the home or office, while doing daily chores, going for a walk or during light exercise. During higher-intensity sport and when working in hot conditions, however, you can be dehydrated without feeling thirsty. There is no doubt that athletes should start drinking long before they become thirsty. Athletes can

▶ Do You Need Extra Salt?

Sweat does contain sodium (salt), so as you sweat, you lose sodium. This is of little concern to most athletes training or competing for 90 minutes or less. They can replace the sodium they lose by taking a sports drink or in their next snack or meal.

If sweat losses are heavy over a day of physical activity or working in hot conditions, then it is possible that too much sodium can be lost, leading to muscle cramps. Sports drinks with extra sodium can be very useful in replacing sodium losses during activity. Don't take salt tablets, as these are a very concentrated source of sodium and tend to suck fluid from the blood and into the small intestine, possibly causing abdominal pain. (See also the section on cramps later in the chapter on page 93.) As you become fitter, you tend to sweat more to aid cooling and lower the salt concentration in sweat, making you less likely to dehydrate or become low in sodium. Recreational athletes generally won't need extra salt as they are likely to already be taking in enough salt in their regular diets (about 80% of salt in a person's diet comes from that added by food manufacturers). Too much salt can raise blood pressure and increase calcium losses from the bones.

lose 2 per cent of their body weight as fluid (1.4 kg, or 1.4 L, in a 70 kg or 154 lb person) before experiencing the thirst sensation. This delay is called *voluntary dehydration* even though it is not a result of conscious behaviour. If you feel thirsty during training or sport, you are definitely getting too little fluid and will have difficulty catching up on fluid losses during exercise.

You can be dehydrated without feeling thirsty. Athletes should start drinking long before they become thirsty. Don't wait until you feel thirsty before taking a drink during exercise. Try to drink to match your sweat losses, which means drinking every 15 minutes during long workouts.

It was once thought that drinking during an event was a sign of weakness, especially in male sports. Even marathoners weren't allowed to drink before the 11-kilometre (6.8-mile) mark up until 1977. You cannot train your body to cope with dehydration. Coaches who suggest training on little fluid to toughen the body are handing out very old-fashioned advice that could be dangerous. We now appreciate that chronic dehydration can occur in athletes who train frequently without topping up their fluid losses every day.

Remember: Weight loss during exercise is mainly sweat loss and needs to be replaced. Although some fat is used during exercise, it's not likely to amount to more than 50 grams (1.8 oz) in a 90-minute session. That's not to imply that exercise doesn't help you lose body fat. Evidence suggests that exercise is valuable in weight control by helping to 'normalise' your appetite (see chapter 13).

Acclimatisation

If you are going from a cool environment to a warm environment, it is smart to acclimatise to the local conditions for 10 to 14 days before competition (providing you have the time, of course). Remember that the risk of heat exhaustion is higher in those who don't train in local conditions where it is likely to be warm or hot. Exercising in local conditions hastens acclimatisation. If you travel across multiple time zones, you will need around a week just to acclimatise to the new time zone.

When you acclimatise to warmer weather, several things happen:

- Extra blood is produced (up to 12 per cent more) so there is sufficient blood to supply both the exercising muscles and direct blood to the skin for cooling.
- You start sweating earlier and at a lower body temperature.
- You produce more sweat to maximise evaporative cooling (therefore, you will need more fluids).
- You lose less salt (sodium) in your sweat, reducing your risk of sodium-depletion cramps in long events.

Hyponatremia: Can You Drink Too Much Water?

Yes, it is possible to drink too much water. There have been recorded cases of ultra-endurance athletes drinking more fluid than they lost as sweat so they actually gained weight during the event. Overhydrating tends to dilute the amount of sodium in the blood, with plasma sodium dropping below 135 millimole/litre. The low blood sodium (hyponatremia) results in confused thinking, incoordination and weakness. This most commonly occurs in exercise that lasts longer than four hours. In severe cases, people have died.

As athletes sweat, they lose both electrolytes (e.g., sodium and potassium) and water. If, over a few hours, they replace just the water through drinking and not the sodium, the level of sodium drops in the blood. The body thinks there is too much water in the blood and transfers some water out of the blood and into other parts of the body, such as the brain. The brain begins to swell, hence the confused thinking and incoordination. This situation is compounded when the kidneys produce less urine than they should to rid the body of excess fluid, which happens in many cases of hyponatremia.

The common characteristics of those at risk of hyponatremia are as follows:

- Excessive drinking (i.e., drinking more fluid than is lost as sweat)
- Weight gain during exercise due to excess fluid consumption
- Low body weight before starting to exercise
- Female
- Slow running or performance times

- Using non-steroidal anti-inflammatory agents

Adapted from Hew-Butler et al. 2008

The main cause of hyponatremia during sport is the drinking of fluid in excess of fluid lost as sweat or urine (American College of Sports Medicine 2007). Sure, drinking too little fluid is more of a problem with most athletes, but you need to know that overzealous replacement of fluid, either water or sports drinks, is unhealthy. You can see that when advising on fluid needs, we can only provide guidelines and not drinking volume laws that suit everyone.

Those at greatest risk of hyponatremia are ultra-endurance athletes in mild weather conditions who take a long time to complete the course, while drinking plenty of water, such as someone who takes over four hours to finish a 42-kilometre (26-mile) marathon. If you are involved in ultra-endurance events, take a sports drink because they have added sodium, and make sure your snacks and meals have sodium. Sports drinks contain sodium at 20 to 50 milligrams per 100 millilitres to assist in the replacement of sodium lost in sweat. If you replace only water and not sodium during long periods of sweating, the concentration of plasma sodium can become dangerously low. Consult a sports dietitian for food and fluid advice if you are into ultra-endurance sports.

You often hear that you need to drink 6 to 8 glasses of water per day. There have been cases of water intoxication, but only after drinking far more than 8 glasses. In 1999, a 19-year-old U.S. Air Force recruit collapsed during a 10-kilometre (6.2-mile) walk. Doctors say it was the result of hyponatremia and heatstroke. In 2000, a 20-year-old U.S. Army recruit drank over 12 litres of water in an estimated three-hour period. She lost consciousness and died from swelling in the brain and lungs from hyponatremia. Then in 2002, a 19-year-old U.S. marine died from drinking too much water during a 42-kilometre (26-mile) march (Gardner 2002). It is thought that overzealous instructors, not wanting a heatstroke or dehydration victim under their command, pushed the drinking of water to the limit.

To minimise the chance of hyponatremia, the message to endurance athletes is as follows:

- Drink fluids frequently to try to match sweat losses.
- Do not drink more than you sweat. In other words, don't gain weight during an event. A small amount of weight loss, around 1 per cent, is quite OK.
- Choose sports drinks as your main fluid, although the same advice applies—don't overdrink to the point of gaining weight during an event.

▶ Cricketers Caught Behind on Fluids

Australian researchers studied 20 male first-grade cricket players (8 batsmen, 12 bowlers; average age 19 years) under both real match and simulated match conditions and at different temperatures (Gore et al. 1993). Under cool conditions (22 °C or 72 °F) the players sweated at an average of 540 millilitres per hour; in warm conditions (30 °C or 86 °F), at 700 millilitres per hour; and in hot conditions (38 °C or 100 °F), at 1,370 millilitres per hour. Three bowlers on the hot day peaked at a sweat loss of 1,670 millilitres per hour.

During the cool day and the warm day, dehydration was 0.3 per cent and 1.2 per cent, respectively, which suggests that the current drink break schedule (one break each hour) was adequate under these conditions.

But after two sessions of play (each session is two hours long) on the hot day, the average dehydration of the three fast bowlers was a loss of 4.3 per cent (3 kg in a 70 kg person, or 6.6 lb in a 154 lb person) of their starting body weight despite drinking over 2.5 litres of fluid in that time. There is no doubt that this fluid loss compromised their performance.

The researchers stated, 'The implication for cricket is that skill levels, and therefore performance, will diminish as dehydration increases beyond 2% of initial body weight' (Gore et al. 1993, 387).

Now, in international test matches and one-day matches, it is possible for cricketers to get a sports drink or water from a drink bucket on the boundary or from an underground receptacle behind the wickets.

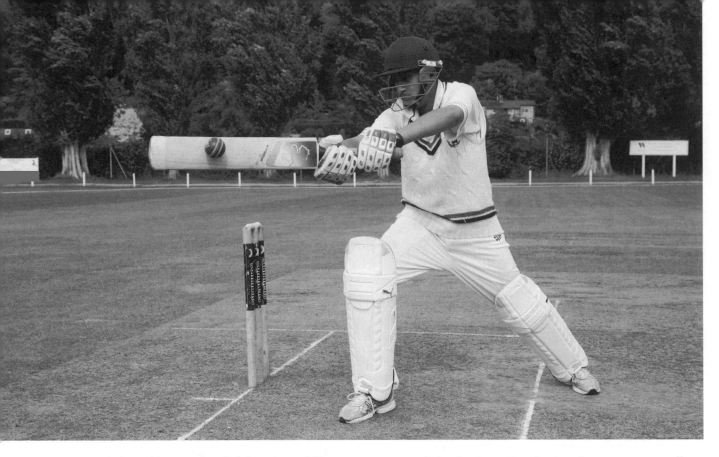

Long, hot days in the field make cricketers prone to dehydration. Breaks in play are an excellent opportunity to replace fluids lost as sweat.

Dehydration, if sufficiently severe, can impair performance in most events, particularly in warm and high-altitude environments. Athletes should be well-hydrated before exercise and drink sufficient fluid during exercise to limit dehydration to less than about 2% of body mass.

International Olympic Committee Consensus Statement on Sports Nutrition (2010)

Dehydration and Sports Performance

Dr. Lawrence Armstrong, Ball State University in the USA, assessed the effect of dehydration on running (Armstrong, Costill and Fink 1985). Running speed was reduced by 6 to 7 per cent with just a 2 per cent decrease in body weight from fluid loss. Even a 1 per cent reduction in body weight added an extra 17 seconds to a 1,500-metre run time. For the serious athlete, that could mean the difference between first place and a huge disappointment. In the 1996 Olympic men's marathon, only eight seconds separated the gold medal winner and the bronze medallist, a mere 0.1 per cent difference in performance!

Another study by Dr. R.M. Walsh (Walsh et al. 1994) at the University of Cape Town Medical School found that a 1.8 per cent drop in body weight during exercise affected sprint performance after 60 minutes of exercise. In practical terms this means that even low levels of dehydration can affect performance near the end of most team games and endurance events. As a general rule, there is a 5 per cent drop in sports performance for every 1 per cent drop in body weight (see figure 5.4). The drop in performance may not be much with a 1 per cent drop in weight, but thereafter the drop in performance is likely to accelerate.

▶ **That's Hot!**

In December 1987, cricket batsman Allan Border lost 5 kilograms (11 lb) during a mammoth innings in a cricket Test match against New Zealand at the Adelaide Oval. He scored 205 (599 minutes) in official temperatures of 40.7 °C (105 °F).

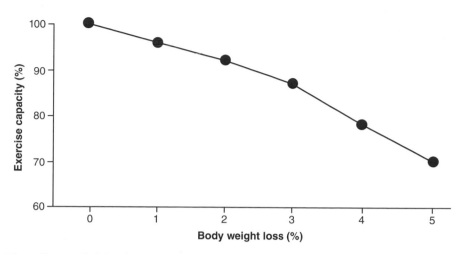

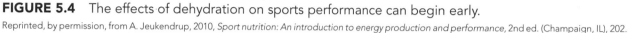

FIGURE 5.4 The effects of dehydration on sports performance can begin early.

Reprinted, by permission, from A. Jeukendrup, 2010, *Sport nutrition: An introduction to energy production and performance*, 2nd ed. (Champaign, IL), 202.

Body weight changes can reflect sweat losses during exercise and can be used to calculate individual fluid replacement needs for specific exercise and environmental conditions.

American College of Sports Medicine 2007

Check Your Water Level

There's a simple way to check your fluid loss during training sessions and events. Weigh yourself before and after training or competition. If possible, weigh yourself nude; if this is not possible, wear minimal clothing (so you are not weighing the sweat lost into your clothing). If you need to pee, do so before you weigh yourself; otherwise you will record a falsely high weight. The other option is to measure any pee you have after you do your weight and factor that into your 'fluid loss'. Although they are not usually accurate in displaying your body weight, bathroom scales will give you a good idea of total weight loss. Ideally, you should be drinking enough fluids to replace most of what you sweat during the event. In my experience it is common for footballers,

basketballers and other athletes to lose 2 to 4 per cent of their body weight during competition.

To determine your percentage of weight loss, use the following formula:

$$\frac{(\text{Presport weight}) - (\text{postsport weight}) \times 100}{\text{Presport weight}}$$

For example, if you are a 70-kilogram person who lost 1.4 kilograms (i.e., 1.4-litre overall fluid loss) in a training session,

$$\frac{(70 \text{ kg} - 68.6 \text{ kg}) \times 100}{70 \text{ kg}} = 2\% \text{ body weight loss}$$

Whatever weight you have lost during sport needs to be immediately replaced by fluids even if you don't feel thirsty. You need to actually drink more than your fluid losses because you will not retain all the fluid you drink after sport. Some will end up as urine. The person in the above example would need to drink more than 2,000 millilitres of fluid to replace the fluid lost.

Athletes who do a lot of training may be dehydrated before they start exercise, so their pretraining weight could be lower than ideal. If you are training a lot, I recommend that you take your nude weight every morning. If you see

▶ Dehydration

Several studies have demonstrated a decreased stomach emptying rate with dehydration and hyperthermia. That means that when you are dehydrated, less fluid is being absorbed to replace fluid losses. This is a reminder to start drinking early in sport. Anxiety associated with sport (e.g., finals) can also greatly reduce the gastric emptying rate.

▶ Drinking Schedule

Here is an approximate fluid replacement schedule for sport. It will vary depending on the temperature of the venue, your sweat rate and your level of fitness. Use it as a guide only.

BEFORE SPORT

Drink 300 to 500 millilitres (two to three glasses) in the 15 minutes before exercise. This is your 'reserve' fluid. Although you will not feel thirsty at the time of drinking, this fluid is being absorbed into your blood at the same time you begin to sweat at the start of your sport. (Remember that there is a delay between drinking and the fluid getting into your blood stream.) For many athletes, especially endurance athletes, this is the most important drink break. I also suggest that you empty your bladder in the 15 to 30 minutes before sport. Water in your bladder cannot be used by the body, so it becomes 'baggage'.

DURING SPORT

Drink 150 to 250 millilitres every 15 minutes, or at suitable breaks in sport. The stomach can empty at a rate of 1,000 to 1,200 millilitres per hour, and in warm weather it is ideal to drink at a similar rate. Even in cool weather, athletes can sweat 1 litre or more per hour.

AFTER SPORT

Drink to replace all lost fluids during sport, plus another 25 to 50 per cent because some of that fluid will be lost as urine. This means that you will need to drink at least 500 millilitres and probably a lot more if you have lost a lot of sweat. For example, if you have lost 1 kg (1 litre) of weight due to sweat loss during sport, then you will need to drink 1.25 to 1.5 litres of fluid after you have finished. To determine how much fluid you have lost, you can use the weigh-in method described on previous page.

differences of more than 1 kilogram (2.2 lb), then you are likely to be starting the day dehydrated. For example, one rower I advised started the day between 77 and 79 kilograms (170 and 174 lb). He thought the difference was fat loss and was disappointed when I told him that 79 kilograms was his true weight and 77 kilograms was his dehydrated weight.

Is That Clearish?

A simple guide to your fluid levels is the colour of your urine. As a general rule, if it is pale yellow or clear, you're well hydrated. If it is dark orange, you need to drink more fluids now. If you can't remember the last time you had a pee, you desperately need fluids.

The colour of your urine is not always a good indicator of hydration. After high sweat losses, you can still produce clear urine even when still dehydrated. How can this happen? If you have sweated a lot during activity, then you will have lost some sodium too. Only when you have replaced this sodium are you fully rehydrated.

Let's say you have lost 2 litres of sweat during activity. You then drink 2 litres of water over the next half an hour. The water is absorbed into the blood, but the blood needs both water and sodium to replace sweat losses. Just providing water makes the blood dilute. So now we have a situation in which the blood volume is low (dehydration) and the blood is diluted. To reduce dilution, the body produces urine, which will be clear in colour even though you are still dehydrated.

You can increase your sodium levels by doing the following:

- Take a sports drink during and after activity. This will help replace the sodium lost in sweat.
- Eat a meal soon after finishing your activity because the meal will contain sodium. You will still need to drink fluids to replace the fluid lost as sweat.

Taking vitamin supplements is likely to make your pee bright orange all the time because the urine is where a lot of your vitamins end up. If you take a daily vitamin supplement, you need to drink fluids until you pass copious urine (say, once an hour) to be sure you have enough fluids on board. Or weigh yourself before and after exercise as described earlier to gauge your hydration status.

Rehydration and Rapid Stomach Emptying

Any fluid you drink needs to pass from the stomach to the small intestine before it can be absorbed and replace sweat losses. Fluid replacement is not a case of how fast you can drink, but of how fast the fluid gets from your mouth to your blood.

It can take 10 to 20 minutes for fluids to travel from your stomach to your skin for sweating. Sports dietitians recommend drinking fluids early to allow for this delay. People vary greatly in their rates of stomach emptying and intestinal absorption. Factors that may influence stomach emptying include fluid volume, exercise intensity and fluid concentration.

Fluid Volume

Larger volumes empty from the stomach at a quicker rate. Athletes should begin exercise comfortably full with fluids.

Try drinking 300 to 500 millilitres in the 15 minutes before exercise (about 2 glasses). Then drink around 150 to 250 millilitres every 15 minutes during exercise in warm weather. The idea is to keep a reasonable volume of fluid in your stomach because this improves the rate the fluid empties from the stomach into the intestines and then into your blood. Unfortunately, large volumes may also increase gastrointestinal distress and the risk of stitch, so you need to get the balance right.

Exercise Intensity

The rate of stomach emptying decreases in very high intensity exercise, such as sprinting and cycling uphill. It should be noted that not many endurance sports require athletes to maintain a high intensity. At a lower intensity, stomach emptying occurs at near-normal rates.

Fluid Concentration

If the sugar content of a drink is too high, the fluid will empty slowly from the stomach. Sports drinks are especially formulated to empty quickly from the stomach. They have a sugar content of 6 to 8 per cent (i.e., 6 to 8 g per 100 mL). Soft drinks (sodas) have a sugar content of 10 to 14 per cent in most cases, too high for rapid emptying from the stomach. Some energy drinks are 18 per cent sugar. (See chapter 7 for more information on digestion and stomach emptying.)

Sports Drinks

Sports drinks have been around for a while now, following a huge market growth in the 1990s. They were originally based on the theory that because sweat tastes salty, we need a salty drink. That's guesswork, not science. The sports drink has come a long way since then.

There is widespread scientific agreement that sports drinks are of great benefit in replacing both fluid and carbohydrate (sugar) burned during sport. Although frequently cited as being most useful during endurance events, sports drinks can also enhance performance during intermittent, high-intensity exercise such as occurs in most team sports. Sports drinks also provide sodium to replace the sodium lost in sweat.

Before we look at the advantages of a sports drink, I want to give a plug for water. For a lot of active people, water should be the fluid of choice. Water is ideal for gardening, bushwalking, hiking, all light exercise and most exercise taking less than an hour. Water is ideal for children involved in sport, too. Water with meals aids hydration. In fact, water has been nature's hydrator for thousands of years. However, many of us engage in more strenuous and longer exercise, which is when sports drinks come into play.

Advantages of Sports Drinks

This section details the advantages a sports drink can offer the athlete, with a summary of the benefits of water and sports drinks listed in table 5.1 on page 84.

Carbohydrate

The carbohydrate in sports drinks, mainly in the form of the sugars glucose and sucrose, delays fatigue by topping up blood glucose levels to provide glucose for the active muscles. It may also spare muscle and liver glycogen stores, which is very important in exercise exceeding 90 minutes.

Most sports drinks are 6 to 8 per cent carbohydrate (i.e., 6 to 8 g of carbohydrate in every 100 mL). It was once thought that a drink that was

TABLE 5.1 Comparison of the Benefits of Water and Sports Drinks for Fluid Replacement

Benefits of water	Benefits of sports drinks
Very good for rehydration	Excellent for rehydration
Ideal for sports lasting less than 45 minutes	Ideal for sports lasting more than 45 minutes, especially intense activity
Empties quickly from the stomach and is quickly absorbed into the blood	Empties quickly from the stomach and is quickly absorbed into the blood
Cheap and convenient	Low cost, especially if made from a powder
Good for most children's sports	Good for teenage and adult high-intensity or endurance sport
Is neutral, therefore does not damage the enamel of teeth	Taste preferred by most athletes; therefore, often consumed in larger amounts than is water
Good for rinsing out the mouth after a sports drink or when mouth is dry	Is acidic; therefore, should be swallowed without washing around the mouth
	Helps avoid hyponatremia in ultra-endurance events

more than 2.5 per cent carbohydrate slowed the rate at which fluids left the stomach. Additionally, researchers believed that glucose polymers (chains of glucose molecules, sometimes called maltodextrins) were more suited to sports drinks because they emptied from the stomach faster. Now, sports drinks just have the simple sugars, and usually at least two types (e.g., glucose and fructose) because that improves sugar and water absorption in the intestines (Jeukendrup 2010; Shi et al. 1995). Different sugars have different transport systems across the intestines. With two monosaccharide sugars, the body uses two transport systems rather than just the one with, say, glucose. It's like having two doors to one room. The range of sugars normally found in sports drinks is shown in figure 5.5.

More recent research has revealed that a drink with up to 8 per cent carbohydrate empties quickly from the stomach and it doesn't really matter what form the carbohydrate takes, although those with mainly glucose are less

sweet so may be better suited to some people's taste. Once the carbohydrate level is higher than 8 per cent, fluids empty more slowly from the stomach, which means that water is available to the body at a slower rate. During sport, avoid drinks that are over 8 per cent carbohydrate. See table 5.2 on page 88 for a comparison of fluid replacement drinks.

▶ A sports drink should be used to provide the 30 to 60 grams of carbohydrate burned per hour of endurance exercise. The body can burn up to 90 grams an hour if the drink has more than one monosaccharide sugar, allowing quicker absorption. If your sports drinks is 6 per cent carbohydrate, then you will need to drink 500 millilitres (30 g sugar) to 1,500 millilitres (90 g sugar) to get 30 to 90 grams of carbohydrate in an hour.

Concentration

Most sports drinks are labelled 'isotonic', which means that the fluid has a similar concentration as blood. *Isotonic* fluids empty quickly from the stomach into the small intestine where they can be rapidly absorbed into the bloodstream.

Hypertonic fluids are more concentrated than blood and cause water to move from the blood back into the intestine to dilute the fluid. This effectively causes a transient dehydration before the fluid can be absorbed. Generally, drinks with more than 8 per cent carbohydrate (e.g., regular

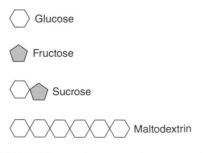

Glucose

Fructose

Sucrose

Maltodextrin

FIGURE 5.5 The main sugars in sports drinks.

soft drinks, fruit juice and energy drinks) are hypertonic.

A *hypotonic* fluid has a lower concentration than blood. Water is a common example, and some sports drinks are slightly hypotonic. Hypotonic and isotonic solutions are absorbed more quickly than are hypertonic solutions.

Salt (Sodium)

Salt (or sodium) is added to sports drinks not just to replace the salt lost in sweat but also to enhance the fluid absorption from the intestines, although carbohydrate concentration may be a more important influence on absorption. Some drinks include magnesium, which doesn't seem to improve fluid absorption. It is true that small amounts of magnesium is lost in sweat, but not to the detriment of health or sports performance.

Added sodium also improves the taste of sports drinks, which generally contain 160 to 800 milligrams (7.0 to 35 mmol/L) of sodium per litre. For comparison, milk has a sodium content of 29 mmol/L, and low-fat natural yogurt has 36 mmol/L.

The more important benefit from the sodium in sports drinks is in helping to maintain plasma volume. In the recovery period after exercise, full rehydration doesn't occur until all sodium losses have been replaced. The sodium in sports drinks helps the body retain ingested fluids rather than just renting them and then losing a lot as pee. After sport, the body needs more fluids than what it lost in sweat because some fluid will be converted to urine even if the body is still dehydrated. Without sodium, much of the ingested fluid passes via the urine.

Fit people generally have a higher blood volume than those who are sedentary. Taking a sodium-containing drink before exercise can further increase blood volume, leading to an improvement in endurance.

If, during ultra-endurance sports, sweat losses are replaced solely by a low-sodium beverage such as water, the athlete may suffer from hyponatremia (low blood sodium). All ultra-endurance athletes should include a sports drink with sodium to avoid this condition.

Added Protein in Sports Drinks

Sports drinks with added protein, usually in the form of whey protein, are currently on the market. Are they a novelty to try to take market share from the well-established carbohydrate sports drink, or is there some substance to their claims of being an improved drink? Protein taken in a drink during exercise may reduce muscle damage, slow muscle protein breakdown and enhance the replacement of glycogen stores after exercise. A protein–carbohydrate drink has the potential to speed up muscle repair when consumed just after exercise. On paper, there appears to be an argument for a sports drink with a mix of protein and carbohydrate.

One study (Saunders, Kane and Todd 2004) showed that endurance cyclists were able to ride for 29 per cent longer when their sports drink contained 1.8 per cent protein (1.8 g per 100 mL). That's an impressive improvement. What must be remembered is that this research was on well-trained cyclists who rode to exhaustion. The effect may not be the same for recreational athletes who train and play for fitness and enjoyment.

Other studies have shown a mixture of results in endurance athletes, some showing no benefit and others showing a small improvement in performance. One study showed no performance advantage of a sports drink with added protein; however, the authors found that it was effective in reducing muscle damage and fatigue after two consecutive two-hour bouts of exercise (Skillen et al. 2008). Compared to commercial sports drinks, the drinks used in the experiment were relatively low in carbohydrate (4.6 per cent), and the added protein was also low (1 per cent). If the protein content had been twice as much (2 per cent), muscle damage may have been lower.

A meta-analysis of the studies to date was done by the University of Connecticut (Stearns et al. 2010). A meta-analysis crunches the numbers from a number of studies to get a clearer indication of the overall effect of a product. The authors of the meta-analysis concluded: 'Based on the results of the meta-analysis, protein may be consumed by endurance athletes during exercise and will most likely not have a detrimental effect on performance. In fact, protein ingestion during exercise may have the potential to improve performance during exercise; however, further evidence is needed before a clear conclusion can be made as to if this effect is because of greater calories or the protein itself' (p. 2201).

Stearns and colleagues (2010) found that the protein–carbohydrate drink offered no benefit in time trials (doing a set amount of work in a set time), but it did extend the time to exhaustion in endurance trials. Testing time to exhaustion is not always practical because few athletes train or perform until they can't go further. A time trial is a better way to observe a potential improvement in a drink. When a small amount of protein is added to the existing amount of carbohydrate in a drink, it appears to improve performance, probably as a result of the extra kilojoules being provided by the protein, allowing the athlete to go for longer. When a carbohydrate drink was compared to a protein–carbohydrate drink that had the same amount of kilojoules per 100 millilitres, there was little difference in performance.

So, that means that adding 2 grams of protein to a 100-millilitre sports drinks (i.e. 2 per cent protein, the amount usually added to a protein–carbohydrate sports drink) does have an ergogenic effect, somewhere around 9 per cent, because there are more kilojoules for the muscle to burn as fuel in endurance events in which athletes go to exhaustion. It may not be due to any special benefit of the protein compared to carbohydrate, and probably won't help you unless you end your events totally exhausted. This suggests that just taking a little extra sports drink or even a gel could have a similar endurance effect. Could the protein in a sports drink diminish muscle damage in elite endurance athletes? We are not certain of that. All the same, there is enough speculation about protein in sports drinks to encourage a lot more studies on how we might manipulate the contents of sports drink to help endurance athletes.

Recovery drinks with a mix of protein and carbohydrate are on the market. Taking one of these drinks after a workout will provide protein, carbohydrate and water, three important nutrients for your recovery. One popular recovery drink provides 3.2 grams of protein per 100 millilitres. Whether the protein component will be useful depends on how soon after finishing you plan to have a meal. If you are having milk, yogurt, meat, fish or eggs within an hour of completion, then your postexercise protein needs will be covered. If you won't, or can't, have a meal for a couple of hours after exercising, then a recovery drink with protein will be useful in helping to repair any minor muscle damage.

Other Considerations for Sports Drink

Although the carbohydrate concentration and sodium levels are very important aspects of sports drinks to athletes, other considerations will influence your choice of sports drink and your enjoyment of it.

Drink Temperature

It's best to keep your drink cool unless you are competing in very cold conditions. A cold drink in warm weather seems to help lower core body temperature and prevent overheating, and thereby may even improve performance (Burdon et al. 2010). If you can't refrigerate your drink during sport, then freeze it prior to the event so it has just thawed by the time you get to drink it. The drink temperature doesn't appear to affect the speed at which the drink empties from the stomach and is absorbed by the intestines. If you exercise in cold temperatures, you may prefer a drink at a warmer temperature.

Taste

Research on athletes shows that they will generally drink more of a flavoured drink than just plain water both during exercise and after exercise. Sometimes 50 per cent more. This holds true for children, adolescents and adults alike. So if you are at risk of dehydration because of the intensity of exercise, the air temperature or the length of the event, you will be better off with a flavoured drink that you enjoy. (Note: The flavour you enjoy when rested may be different to what you enjoy when you are exercising, so choose your favourite flavour when you are hot and sweaty.)

Carbonation

I do not recommend fizzy (carbonated) drinks during sport. Fizzy drinks are absorbed at a much slower rate than non-fizzy drinks, such as water and sports drinks. One research group found that fizzy drinks empty from the stomach three times slower than flat drinks. Fizzy drinks are also difficult to drink quickly and give you the burps (Passe, Horn and Murray 1997). There are still people who swear by drinking flat cola during endurance events; however, the sugar content is really too high. Some people feel a benefit from flat cola near the end of an endurance event because, if their glycogen levels are very low, they will get a boost from the sugar. Likewise, the small amount of caffeine present in flat cola may help improve endurance.

Who Should Take a Sports Drink?

Now that you understand the potential benefits of a sports drink to athletes, let's take a look at which athletes would benefit most under various circumstances.

- **Recreational athletes.** The sugars in sports drinks can be useful in continuous, moderate- to high-intensity aerobic activity that lasts longer than 90 minutes (if glycogen stores are well stocked before exercise). The sports drink may have value in shorter events for athletes who haven't eaten enough carbohydrate before the event.

- **Elite athletes.** Elite athletes may train for two or three hours continuously, or have two or more training sessions in a day. A sports drink can be handy to get them through the demands of training and help replace glycogen stores postexercise.

- **Endurance athletes.** Because of the very high kilojoule needs of endurance athletes, sports drinks can be very helpful in getting them through long training sessions and endurance events. Sports drink help maintain normal blood glucose levels near the end of endurance events or long training sessions. They also improve sprint times at the end of endurance session. This can be particularly important in some events such as long-distance cycling, which can end with a sprint to the finish. Endurance athletes should start drinking early to get the most benefit.

- **High-intensity training athletes.** When the sessions are fast and furious, such as during high-intensity sprint training, glucose and glycogen are burned at a faster rate and may run out after 45 minutes. A sports drink helps athletes in high-intensity sports train longer. They should drink as often as possible throughout training.

- **Tired athletes.** A common cause of tiredness in athletes is not eating enough carbohydrate. All athletes should make sure they are eating enough carbohydrate before and after training. A sports drink will provide additional carbohydrate during sport.

- **Recovering athletes.** Following long and exhausting sessions, a sports drink can help athletes rehydrate and restock glycogen stores quickly. It's great for endurance and elite athletes who must replace lost fluids and carbohydrate quickly, especially if the next event or training session is less than eight hours away.

- **Athletes who don't like water.** Athletes generally prefer a flavoured drink over plain water both during and after exercise.

- **Athletes exercising in the heat.** Glycogen is burned up at a faster rate during exercise in the heat, possibly as a result of an overheated cardiovascular system that is unable to provide enough oxygen and fat to the muscles.

- **Cramping athletes.** Some athletes lose a large volume of sweat during sport. The sodium losses can accumulate over a couple of hours, and the resulting low blood sodium can initiate cramps. Some athletes have very high sweat sodium levels, making them even more prone to cramping. The sodium in a sports drink helps replace lost sweat sodium.

- **Thin athletes.** Athletes who lose too much weight during their sport season may find that the carbohydrate in a sports drink reduces the body's tendency to use its own fat and muscle as fuel.

Which Sports Drink Is for You?

Choose a sports drink that suits your taste and budget and has 6 to 8 grams of carbohydrate in 100 millilitres. Table 5.2 on page 88 shows a comparison of the various drinks on the market. Under warm to hot conditions, it must also be one you can drink 800 millilitres or more of in an hour. If you sweat a lot, I suggest one with more than 15 mmol/L of sodium. For economic reasons, I also suggest you buy the powdered version of sports drinks. Cordial and fruit juice may be diluted 50:50 and used as a sports drink if you wish, but they will be low in sodium and are not ideal for the serious adult athlete.

Other Types of Drinks

Apart from water and sports drinks, other drinks are popular with athletes, although some do not deliver all the benefits they promise. None are harmful in sensible amounts, but they each have some angle you need to consider.

Energy Drinks

A number of so-called energy drinks are on the market. These are not sports drinks and are not recommended before or during most sports.

TABLE 5.2 Comparison of Fluid Replacement Drinks

Drink	Carbohy-drate (g) per serve	Carbohy-drate (g) per 100 mL	Sodium (mg) per serve	Sodium (mmol/L)	Potassium (mg) per serve	Caffeine (mg)
SPORTS DRINKS						
Gatorade, 240 mL	15	6	128	22	56	0
Gatorade Bolt, 240 mL	15	6	128	22	56	0
Gatorade Endur-ance, 240 mL	15.6	6.2	207	36	37.5	0
Gatorade G Series: Prime, 118 mL	25	21	110	40.5	35	0
Gatorade G Series: Perform, 300 mL	18	6	153	22	68	0
Gatorade G series: Recover, 240 mL	7	2.8	125	22	48	0
Powerade Isotonic, 240 mL	19	7.6	70	12	35	0
Staminade, 240 mL	18	7.2	69	12.6	40	0
100 Plus Isotonic, 330 mL	22.4	6.8	158	20.9	46	0
Accelerate pb During, 240 mL	17	6.8	200	34	45	0
Lucozade Sport, 240 mL	16	6.4	125	21.7	n/a	0
Oral rehydration solutions, 240 mL	4	1.6	265	46	200	0
SPORTS WATERS						
Powerade sports water, 240 mL	6.2	2.5	30	5.2	n/a	0
Mizone sports water, 240 mL	9.3	3.7	57.5	10	n/a	0
Waterplus (Sanitarium), 240 mL	0	0	15	2.6	n/a	0
ENERGY DRINKS						
Red Bull, 240 mL	27	11	100	17.4	n/a	80
Lucozade Energy, 300 mL (10 oz)	53.7	17.9	<5	0.2	n/a	0
V Isokinetic, 240 mL	17.5	7	66	11.6	37.5	42
Mother 500 mL	52	10.4	260	22.6	n/a	160

Drink	Carbohydrate (g) per serve	Carbohydrate per 100 mL	Sodium (mg) per serve	Sodium (mmol/L)	Potassium (mg) per serve	Caffeine (mg)
WATERS						
Water, mineral water, soda water	0	0	Variable	Variable	Variable	0
Coconut water, young, 240 mL	16.5	6.6	13	2.2	465	0
Coconut water, mature, 240 mL	11.8	4.7	42	7.4	500	0
SOFT DRINKS AND CORDIALS						
Soft drinks, average, 375 mL	45	12	53	6	4	0
Cola soft drinks, regular, 375 mL	40	11	41	4.8	4	35
Diet soft drinks, 375 mL	0	0	41	4.8	7	0
Diet cola soft drinks, average, 375 mL	0	0	41	4.8	4	45
Flavoured mineral water, 375 mL	35	9.3	56	6.5	19	0
Cordial, 240 mL	25	10	7	1.3	10	0
JUICES						
Fruit juice, average, 240 mL	25	10	20	3	350	0
Fruit juice drinks average, 240 mL	25	10	20	3	80	0
Tomato juice, average, 240 mL	10	4	550	95	500	0

Note: Some drinks in this table have different serve size volumes. Not available = n/a.

They are popular with some athletes who spend many hours in cruise control during endurance events in mild weather. Many contain caffeine (often in the form of guarana) and have a sugar content similar to that of soft drinks (10 to 15 per cent), so they are absorbed more slowly than sports drinks are. Although the sugars slow down fluid absorption, that may not present a problem when sweat rates are low. Most provide 40 to 80 milligrams of caffeine in a 240-millilitre (8 oz) can—the equivalent to a cup of coffee or 2 cups of tea. The caffeine may improve endurance. (See the section on caffeine in chapter 9.)

Please remember that energy drinks are not designed to be sports drinks, no matter the impression you get from advertising. If you drink one after an event, wash it down with other drinks more suited to recovery, such as water or a sports drink.

Oral Rehydration Solutions (ORS)

Oral rehydration solutions (ORS) were originally formulated for infants suffering diarrhea and are widely used by anyone needing to rehydrate after vomiting and diarrhea. Are they suitable for athletes? They differ on three fronts to the sports drink. First, they are quite low in sugars (about 1.6 per cent, a lot lower than the 6 to 8 per cent in sports drinks), so they won't be useful in endurance events. Second, they are much higher in sodium—around twice that found in sports drinks. This could be useful for athletes who lose a lot of sweat and are prone to cramping, although success is not guaranteed. Third is the taste. Sports drinks are designed to taste good during sport. An ORS may not. An ORS is a helpful drink for a dehydrated body, there is no doubt, but it won't be the best drink during endurance events.

Sports Waters

Since the birth of the sports drink and the energy drink has emerged the sports water. As a general rule, sports waters are low in carbohydrate and sodium; hence, they are not a true sports drink. Enjoy them as a refreshment, not as a fluid replacement drink during training or competition.

Vitamin Waters

As discussed in chapter 4, vitamins do not improve sports performance unless you have a clear vitamin deficiency. If you do have a deficiency, you need to improve your food choices, not rely on drinks such as vitamin waters. Vitamin D is the only vitamin that may be low in the diet, and a little sunlight each day will provide your vitamin D needs, except possibly in winter. I really don't see any value in vitamin waters for healthy people.

Coconut Water

At the time of this writing, coconut water had gained public interest as a refreshment, especially with the allure of being a natural drink, not a concocted soft drink. Some have suggested that coconut water would make a good sports drink substitute.

Coconut water is the water from within the cavity of a coconut and is not to be confused with coconut milk from coconut flesh or coconut oil used in food manufacture. People in tropical countries have enjoyed coconut water for centuries. The water of the young coconut is prized the most, partly because it is sweeter than the water of older coconuts, having a much higher fructose content. Coconuts are grown in about 90 tropical countries.

You can see from table 5.2 that coconut water has a similar carbohydrate content as sports drinks. It also has a very small amount of protein and virtually no fat. It empties quickly from the stomach and is absorbed readily by the small intestine. It is low in sodium and a good source of potassium, like fruit juice. The sodium content is higher when the water is taken fresh from the coconut, around 30 to 100 milligrams in 100 millilitres.

Because coconut water is low in sodium, it isn't similar to a sports drink, yet it is very well suited as a regular drink with about half the sugar found in soft drinks. One small study indicated that coconut water was a good postexercise rehydration drink, although it was rated as less enjoyable as a sports drink. If you are doing plenty of training, a sports drink beats coconut water; however, if you are looking for a lower-kilojoule refreshment compared to soft drinks, then chilled coconut water could be the answer. Be aware that commercial coconut water may not be pure coconut water; it may contain added flavouring in the form of juice or sugar and added sodium. Check the nutrition information panel for the details of commercial coconut waters.

I suggest you be really skeptical of any marketing health claims for coconut water. It does have a small amount of minerals and vitamins, but not really enough to get excited from a nutrition standpoint. Enjoy coconut water as a drink and a way to keep well hydrated during activities that result in mild sweat loss; just note that it is not a substitute for a sports drink in endurance events.

Alcohol

Most elite athletes now give alcohol a miss during their sport seasons. Some coaches have a 'no alcohol' policy during the season, whereas others prefer a more lenient 'no alcohol in the 48 hours before competition' policy. Most of the high-level coaches I know also have a 'no alcohol if injured' policy. In 1990 Australian Commonwealth Games swim coach Don Talbot placed an alcohol ban on all swimmers, coaches and officials throughout the Auckland Games. This is accepted policy now for sports tournaments. Despite the myth, alcohol is not sweated out. Only 2 per cent of alcohol appears in the sweat; over 90 per cent of it is metabolised by the liver, which can be damaged by too much alcohol. So can the brain. That's why alcohol needs to be respected.

You have heard that alcohol can be good for your health. Sensible amounts appear to reduce the risk of heart disease and possibly dementia. One or two standard drinks (10 to 20 grams of alcohol) maximum each day can provide some health benefits, but more than that is linked to increased risk of stroke and liver and brain damage. See table 5.3 for the alcohol units

▶ Watch Those Fangs

Any fluid with a pH below 5.5 has the potential to damage the enamel on the outside surface of your teeth. The pH is a measure of acidity of food and drink. Examples of fluids with a low pH are fruit juice, soft drinks (regular and diet) and sports drinks, all of which have the potential to dissolve the enamel of teeth. Sports drinks have been targeted as a cause of tooth enamel erosion, especially in young athletes (Milosevic 1997). This is unfair, because most people drink far more fruit juice and soft drinks than they do sports drinks. If you drink lots of juice, energy drinks, soft drinks, cordials or sports drinks, see your dentist every six months and specifically ask for your tooth enamel to be checked.

Although sports drinks have a low pH, the pH on the surface of the tooth returns above pH 5.5 within five minutes as a result of the buffering action of saliva, thereby halting enamel erosion (Millward et al. 1997). Eating carbohydrate snacks frequently during the day also increases the risk of tooth decay. Any carbohydrate (sugar or starch) that is left in the mouth after swallowing is consumed by resident bacteria in the mouth. The bacteria produce lactic acid, which erodes tooth enamel. To minimise tooth enamel erosion, follow these guidelines when drinking juice, energy drinks, soft drinks or sports drinks:

- Drink cold fluids (cold reduces acidity).
- Don't swish fluids around the mouth; swallow them quickly.
- Drink by the mouthful rather than constantly sipping small volumes.
- Consider using a straw or a squirt bottle so that the liquid doesn't come into contact with teeth.
- In addition, practise good dental hygiene (brushing and flossing), and see your dentist every six months. Although athletes are fit and healthy, their teeth are more vulnerable to decay than the teeth of most adults because of frequent contact with food and drink through the day.

TABLE 5.3 Standard Drinks and Alcohol Units

STANDARD DRINKS (1 = 10 G ALCOHOL)

Drink	One standard drink (approx.)
Low-alcohol beer (2–3% alcohol)	570 mL (1 pint [UK]; 20 oz)
Mid-strength beer (3.5% alcohol)	375 mL (13 oz)
Regular beer (4–5% alcohol)	285 mL (half pint [UK]; 10 oz)
Wine (14% alcohol)	100 mL (3.4 oz)
Fortified wine (e.g., port, sherry; 20% alcohol)	60 mL (2 oz)
Spirits (e.g., whisky, gin, rum; 40% alcohol)	30 mL (1 oz)
Pre-mix spirits (5% alcohol)	250 mL (8.5 oz)

ALCOHOL UNITS (UK) 1 UNIT = 8 G ALCOHOL

Drink	One alcohol unit (approx.)
Low-alcohol beer (2–3% alcohol)	Two-thirds pint
Regular beer (5-6% alcohol)	One-third pint
Wine (14% alcohol)	90 mL (3.0 oz)
Fortified wine (e.g., port, sherry; 20% alcohol)	50 mL (1.7 oz)
Spirits (e.g., whisky, gin, rum; 40% alcohol)	25 mL (0.8 oz)

of standard drinks. In Australia, the National Health and Medical Research Council (2009, 14) stated that the long-term risk associated with alcohol rose when men consumed four or more standard drinks a day and when women consumed two or more standard drinks a day. Lower amounts are recommended to women because they metabolise alcohol more slowly and have a smaller body mass than men do. Naturally, women who are pregnant or planning pregnancy should avoid alcohol altogether.

> During competition I myself once received incalculable help from beer. The race was the 1977 Thanksgiving Day 25 km Turkey Trot in Poughkeepsie, New York. I had been pursuing a runner for 10 or 12 miles and, unable to gain a yard, had despaired of catching him. Without warning he stepped off the road, rummaged in a pile of leaves, withdrew a can of beer he had apparently secreted there earlier, popped open the top, and stood drinking it as I passed. I never saw him again until he came across the finish line a minute or more after I had arrived.
>
> *James Fixx (1978)*

Following are five reasons to respect alcohol:

- **It is dehydrating.** Alcohol has a dehydrating effect on the body. It reduces the ability of antidiuretic hormone (ADH) to regulate urine production. As the name implies, this hormone stops you from producing too much urine. With ADH out of action, you can drink six glasses of wine but pass a greater volume of pee. Smart athletes don't drink alcohol in the 48 hours before an event, nor straight after the event until they are well hydrated. Beer with an alcohol content less than 2 per cent doesn't seem to act as a diuretic. I suggest that you fully rehydrate before you drink any alcohol, but a light beer or two later probably won't be of any harm.

- **It slows injury recovery.** Alcohol increases the diameter of blood vessels to the skin, arms and legs (hence the red eyes and flushed face afterwards). The increased blood supply will make any injury bleed and swell more than normal. Conversely, an ice bag, compression and eleva-

tion of the injured part will reduce swelling and bleeding. Smart athletes don't drink alcohol in the 24 hours after injury.

- **It is fattening.** Although it is not as fattening as fat and fatty foods, alcohol still has the ability to make you gain extra body fat. Excess alcohol is also often associated with a greater consumption of greasy snack foods, chips and take-aways. Smart athletes drink only sensible amounts of alcohol so they stay in control of their eating.

- **It weakens your thinking.** Alcohol can encourage you to do some silly things and stops you from thinking smart. It can also distract you from eating and drinking for optimal recovery after training, when you need to rehydrate and replace your glycogen stores before the next workout. Alcohol also slows the rate of glycogen replacement after sport, giving you a longer recovery time.

- **It is not a good source of carbohydrate.** Beer has a reputation for being a high-carbohydrate drink. This is not true. One can of beer (375 mL) provides around 10 grams of carbohydrate. As a pre-event meal you would need 10 to 20 cans to get enough carbohydrate. Those left standing shouldn't present too much of a problem to the opposition. Beer has around 3 mmol/L of sodium—far less than the recommended 15 to 20 mmol/L in today's sports drinks. Beer is not a suitable sports drink.

Tea, Coffee and Cola

It is often said that caffeine-containing drinks are diuretics and, like alcohol, should be avoided before and after sport. There is little evidence to back this view. All three drinks are good sources of fluids. This is backed by a statement from the U.S. Institute of Medicine (2004), which said the following:

> 'While concerns have been raised that caffeine has a diuretic effect, available evidence indicates that this effect may be transient, and there is no convincing evidence that caffeine leads to cumulative total body water deficits. Therefore, the panel concluded that when it comes to meeting daily hydration needs, caffeinated beverages can contribute as much as noncaffeinated options'.

However, as mentioned earlier in this chapter, these drinks aren't the best choices during sport or immediately after. Cola and other fizzy drinks should not be consumed during sport, but once you have rehydrated, they can be refreshing and contribute to your fluid needs. Tea, coffee and colas shouldn't be discounted simply because of their caffeine content, but they aren't the optimal fluids to use before, during or after exercise because the rate of absorption of fluid into the body will not be as fast as that of sports drinks or water. See the section on caffeine in chapter 9 for more information.

Cramps

OK, put up your hand if you have ever experienced cramps during sport. When I ask this question at talks, about 80 per cent of people put up their hands. You would think with that kind of response there would be a lot of research and knowledge on cramps. There is next to nothing. Let's have a look at what little we do know about it.

> I just have cramping in my leg, that's all.
>
> *Rafael Nadal, commenting at his press conference after he had fluids and stretching administered. Nadal had grimaced and slid down his chair during a press conference after he had won a game during the 2011 U.S. Tennis Open.*

So many of us have experienced that excruciating knot of painful involuntary muscle spasm that can stop us dead in our tracks. About two out of three athletes have experienced the cramp. It commonly occurs in the calf, thigh or foot. It can affect athletes in both cool and warm environments.

In 2002 I was fortunate to accompany Brett Lee, Australian fast bowler, to the Gatorade Sports Science Institute in Chicago, USA. In the laboratory Brett was subjected to sweat sodium measurements. His sweat was quite high in sodium, around 1,300 milligrams per litre, and those losses became a potential problem over a six-hour day of fielding and sweating in which he often lost 6 litres or more of sweat. Brett often suffered cramps in the last hour of play, but once he took a sodium supplement (Gatorlytes), the cramping didn't return.

More recently, studies have shown no difference in blood sodium levels or levels of hydration between crampers and non-crampers (Schwellnus 2009), leading to the view that cramping is due to a tired muscle losing coordination of its contractions. If low levels of salt in the body are the cause of cramp, it does not explain why only certain muscles get cramp or why rest 'cures' cramp in many people. The best explanation to date is that muscle cramp is due to a tiring muscle losing its ability to control its contractions and going into involuntary spasms.

The truth is that we don't fully understand muscle cramp, nor do we know how to avoid it. You may have your own solutions that work for your body. More tips for avoiding cramp can be found in chapter 7.

FINAL SCORE

- It's easy to lose 1 litre or more of sweat during each hour of exercise. Sweating is a very good cooling mechanism. Try to replace sweat losses during sport.
- Grab that drink. Don't wait until you're thirsty. Thirst is not a good indicator of fluid needs during high-intensity sport. Drink before, during and after exercise. Be well hydrated before you start exercising.
  - *Before:* 300 to 500 millilitres (two to three glasses) in the 15 minutes before exercise
  - *During:* 150 to 250 millilitres every 15 minutes
  - *After:* Replace all lost fluids and more (you'll probably need at least 500 millilitres)
- Practise drinking at training. In warm weather, aim to be able to drink 800 millilitres or more each hour. Don't miss an opportunity to drink.
- Thirst is a good guide to your fluid needs normally. The thirst sensation is delayed in exercise, so don't wait until you are thirsty. Thirst during sport means you are very likely already partially dehydrated.
- After sport, rehydrate *before* drinking alcohol. Water is a good choice. Athletes with high energy needs may choose sports drinks, fruit juice, cordials or soft drinks. Drink non-alcoholic fluids until you are properly hydrated before you consider drinking any alcohol.
- Drink fluids until you pass clear urine. If you take vitamin supplements, your urine is likely to be a darker colour anyway. In that case, drink until you pass copious urine frequently.
- Don't overdrink; doing so can result in hyponatraemia. Do not drink more fluid than you lose as sweat during sport. In other words, don't gain weight through excess fluid consumption during exercise.
- For more information on fluids in sport, download the free fluid fact sheets from Sports Dietitians Australia (www.sportsdietitians.com) or from the Australian Institute of Sport (www.ausport.gov.au/ais/nutrition).

PART II

Practical Sports Nutrition for Athletes

Food Choices for the Athlete's Kitchen

> It used to be standard practice that the pre-match meal consisted of eggs, steak and chicken. But I talked them into changing to complex carbohydrates. So now they will sup on porridge, pasta or wild rice.
>
> *Craig Johnston, Liverpool Football Club, England*

Back in the 1980s, Craig Johnston was one of the athletes who adopted the concept that good eating was a key to good performance. A crucial step to making wise food choices is understanding food labels. This chapter will arm you with the skills to decipher food labels (no easy task) and negotiate a supermarket. Even if you are already a skilled grocery shopper, you may get a few extra tips from this chapter.

Food Labels

Food labels are designed to get you to purchase the food. They will promote all the positive aspects, but may not mention some of the negative ones. Contrary to a popular viewpoint, food labels cannot lie to you, and very few do. They can, however, play on your emotions and word things to make you feel better about the product. For example, you might see 'baked, not fried' on the label, suggesting that it is lower in fat. Often this means 'baked in a lot of fat, not fried in a lot of fat'. You see, the word *fried* is not good for sales. That's why, in the early 1990s, Kentucky Fried Chicken became KFC.

Some canned food labels state that they have no added preservatives, so you feel a warm glow when you purchase them. What they don't tell you is that canned foods do not require preservatives because canning is a means of preserving food in itself and has been for over 200 years. Although sugar and salt are preservatives in high enough quantities, they may not come under the definition of a preservative in the food laws. You might see that a high-salt food is labelled as preservative-free. It is the high salt level that is acting as a preservative. All canned food sold in Australia and New Zealand is preservative-free yet may still contain sugar and salt.

What Must Be on Food Labels?

Each label must include an ingredient list (and identify any potential allergen); the name and address of the manufacturer, distributor or importer; and the weight or volume of the food, along with a description of what you can expect to find in the packet. By law, the ingredients are listed on every food label in descending order—that is, the ingredient in the highest proportion is listed first. Some foods such as tea and coffee don't have to have an ingredient list because they contain only tea leaves or coffee beans.

The only ingredient that doesn't have to be listed in descending order is water. The expression 'water added' may be placed at the end of the list. The proportion of any characterising ingredient needs to be given in some countries. For example, an apple pie must give the proportion of apple in the pie, say, '30% apple'. Virtually all labelled foods will have a 'Best before' or 'Use by' date to give you an indication of the shelf life under proper storage conditions. There are quite a few pieces of information provided on a food label, and they are briefly described in table 6.1.

Virtually all food labels in Western countries now include a nutrition information panel (NIP) or a nutrition facts table with details on, for example, protein, fat, sodium and kilojoules. Some foods may not be legally bound to have an NIP; bread bought fresh from a bakery, for example, can be sold without a wrapper. Many franchise bakers provide nutrition information on their range of products at their store or online. Fast foods also do not have NIPs, although the larger franchises post their nutrition information online. Some post information in-store, such as listing the kilojoules on the menu.

By the way, if you want to convert kilojoules to kilocalories (we say calories for short), divide by four. If you want to be more accurate, divide by 4.18 (400 kJ = 96 cal).

Countries have their own labelling peculiarities. Some use a traffic light guide to indicate whether a food is low or high in key nutrients such as saturated fat or salt. Others allow endorsement programs, such as the Tick program by the Heart Foundation in Australia; a Tick endorsement signifies that a food has met the Heart Foundation's criteria for nutrients such as salt, total fat, saturated fat and fibre. When it comes to specific nutrient claims such as low fat or low salt, there are small differences between countries. These are detailed in table 6.2 on page 100.

Nutrition Claims

Any label making a nutrition claim definitely has to provide a nutrition panel. The panel includes information on the protein, fat (including saturated fat), carbohydrate (including the sugar component), kilojoules or calories, fibre, sodium and any nutrient for which there has been a nutrition claim. For example, if the food label states that the food is a good source of calcium, then it must tell you how much calcium per serve is present.

Nutrition claims, such as low fat, are defined in many countries, and food companies must adhere to those definitions. The nutrition claim definitions are stipulated by the Canadian Food Inspection Agency; the U.S. Food and Drug Administration; the Ministry of Agriculture, Fisheries and Food (UK); and the Food Standards Australia New Zealand Code of Practice. Europe is also becoming more uniform in its food labelling. More information can be found at the European Food Information Council website: www.eufic.org/. Following is a summary of the nutrition claims made on labels (more comprehensive information can be accessed from government agencies in your country).

A reduced-fat or less-fat product must be at least 25 per cent lower in fat than the regular item. It doesn't mean it is low fat. A food that that would normally contain 40 grams of fat per 100 grams but is reduced to 30 grams of fat is 25 per cent lower in fat, but this is hardly low fat. If it were truly low in fat, it would be classified as a low-fat food, which is as follows:

TABLE 6.1 What Is on Food Labels

On the food label	Explanation
Ingredients	• Ingredients will be listed in descending order (most to least). For those with food allergies, the label will stipulate the presence of common allergens such as nuts and wheat.
Weight/volume	• Total weight or volume will be declared. Some countries even give the cost per 100 g or 100 mL so you can do a direct comparison of the cost with other similar products.
Manufacturer, importer or distributor	• Contact details of the manufacturer, importer or distributor in the country of sale must be provided, should you wish to make an enquiry or complaint (or even send a compliment).
Nutrient panel	• Virtually all labeled foods have a nutrition information panel (nutrition facts panel) providing the calories or kilojoules, protein, fat (including saturated fat), carbohydrate (including sugars) and sodium. In some countries, the amount of cholesterol and fibre is also provided. • The panel should also give nutrient details for any nutrient claim; for example, if the food has been calcium fortified, the calcium content must be declared. • Information is provided per serve and per 100 g (or 100 mL) in the UK, Australia and New Zealand, whereas just serve sizes are given in the United States and Canada. • Labels now are more likely to include the percentage of your daily needs for certain nutrients in a single serve, based on the needs of an average adult. The % Daily Intake is on the front of the pack in Australia; the % Daily Value is in the Nutrition Facts in the US; the Guideline Daily Amounts are used in the UK and Europe.
Percentage of main characterising ingredient	• In the UK, Australia and New Zealand the label should also state the percentage of the main characterising ingredients, such as the percentage of strawberry in strawberry yogurt.
Percentage of daily values	• In Australia and New Zealand, on many foods there appears the % Daily Intake, giving you the percentage of a nutrient provided per serve based on an average 8,700 kJ adult diet. In the United States, as well as the amount of each nutrient present, the percentage of the day's requirements for each nutrient is given based on a 2,000-calorie (8,400 kJ) or 2,500-calorie (10,500 kJ) diet. In the UK, guideline daily amounts are based on 2,000 calories for women and 2,500 calories for men. In both cases, they should not be confused with the recommended intakes of nutrients. In Canada, each vitamin or mineral listed will be shown as a percentage of the recommended daily needs.
Description of product	• Well, you've got to know what you are buying (although it doesn't always look the same as the picture on the label).
Country of origin	• Information on the country of origin of the entire food, or its ingredients will be detailed.
'Use by' or 'best before' date	• These dates can be on any food with a shelf life less than two years. Most foods will carry 'best before' dates. It doesn't mean that the food is 'off' once the best before date has passed by a day or two (usually it isn't if it has been stored correctly). The 'use by' date will be used mainly on foods that can go "off" quickly e.g. milk, where it is likely that past the use by date the food will not be at its best. Sometimes you may see a 'display until' date; this date is for shop staff to ensure proper stock rotation. You only need to note the 'use by' or 'best before' dates.

TABLE 6.2 Summary of Food Label Terms

On the food label	What does it mean?
Fat free	• Less than 0.15 g of fat per 100 g of food (Australia and New Zealand) • Less than 0.15 g of fat per 100 g of food (UK) • Less than 0.5 g of fat per serve (United States and Canada)
Reduced fat	• The interpretation in most countries is that the amount of fat should be reduced by at least a quarter (25% reduction) compared to the standard food.
Low fat	• Less than 3 g of fat per 100 g in solid foods and less than 1.5 g of fat in liquid food (Australia and New Zealand) • Less than 3 g of fat per serve (for serves under 30 g), or less than 3 g fat per 100 g for pre-packaged meals (Canada) • Less than 3 g of fat per 100 g (UK) • Less than 3 g of fat per serve (United States)
X% fat-free	• Should be used only when a food is classified as low fat. For example, if a food is 97% fat-free, it will have no more than 3 g of fat in 100 g of food. X% fat-free claims are discouraged in the UK.
Low saturated fat	• Less than 1.5 g saturated fat per 100 g of solid food and less than 0.75 g saturated fat per 100 g liquid food. It must also comply with conditions for a low fat claim (Australia and New Zealand) • Less than 2 g of saturated and trans fatty acids combined per serve (Canada) • Less than 1.5 g saturated fat per 100 g and not more than 10% of the kilojoules (calories) of the product (UK) • Less than 1.0 g of saturated fat and less than 15% calories from saturated fat per serve (United States)
Low cholesterol	• Less than 20 mg cholesterol in 100 g (Australia and New Zealand) or in a serve (Canada and United States). In most countries you can make a low-cholesterol claim only on a food that is low in saturated fat. Check the label as there is little advantage in eating low-cholesterol foods that are high in saturated fat and salt. There is no definition of low cholesterol in the UK and low cholesterol claims are no longer recommended.
Cholesterol-free	• Less than 3 mg of cholesterol per 100 g and meet the conditions for low fat or saturated fat to be less than 20% of the total fat (Australia and New Zealand) • Less than 5 mg of cholesterol per 100 g (UK), although it is recommended that cholesterol-free claims no longer be made • Less than 2 mg of cholesterol and 2 g or less of saturated fat per serve (Canada and United States)
Fibre	• At least 1.5 g of fibre for a 'source of fibre' claim, or at least 3 g of fibre for a 'good source of fibre' claim, per serve (Australia and New Zealand) • At least 2 g of fibre for a 'source of fibre' claim, or at least 4 g of fibre for a 'high source of fibre' claim, per serve (Canada) • At least 3 g of fibre for a 'source of fibre' claim, or at least 6 g fibre for a 'high fibre' claim, per 100 g (UK) • At least 2.5 g of fibre for a 'good source of fibre' claim, or at least 5 g fibre for 'high source of fibre' claim, per serve (United States)
Low salt/sodium	• Less than 120 mg of sodium per 100 g of food; less than 40 mg per 100 g of food for a 'very low sodium' claim (Australia and New Zealand) • Less than 140 mg of sodium per serve; less than 5 mg sodium per serve for a 'sodium-free' claim (Canada) • Less than 40 mg of sodium per 100 g; less than 5 mg of sodium per 100 g for a 'sodium-free' claim (UK) • Less than 140 mg of sodium per serve; less than 35 mg of sodium per serve for a 'very low sodium' claim (United States)

On the food label	What does it mean?
Salt reduced	• The interpretation in most countries is that the amount of sodium has been reduced by at least a quarter (25% reduction) compared to a common reference food
Light, lite	• This label should tell you what it is 'light' in, such as light in salt, light in flavour, light in colour. It may not be light in fat, calories or kilojoules, although food manufacturers are encouraged to use the term 'light' only when a food is low fat, low calorie or low joule.
Low joule Calorie-free	• Virtually free of kilojoules or calories • Fewer than 80 kJ per 100 mL of liquid foods and fewer than 170 kJ per 100 g of solid or semisolid foods (Australia and New Zealand) • Fewer than 40 cal per 100 g and fewer than 40 cal per serve (UK) • Fewer than 5 cal per serve (Canada and United States)
No added sugar	• No added sugars such as sucrose, glucose, dextrose, maltose, fructose, honey, molasses
Sugar-free	• Less than 0.2 g of sugar per 100 g of solid food and less than 0.1 g of sugar per 100 g of liquid food (Australia and New Zealand) • Less than 0.2 g of sugar per 100 g (UK) • Less than 0.5 g of sugar per serve (Canada and United States)
Natural	• There is no definition for this term. Most manufacturers use the term to mean they have not used additives in the product.

• 3.0 grams of fat per 100 grams, or less, in a solid food, and 1.5 grams of fat per 100 grams, or less, in a liquid food in Australia and New Zealand

• 3.0 grams of fat, or less, per 100 grams in the United Kingdom

• 3.0 grams of fat, or less, per serve in the United States and Canada

So, it follows that a reduced-fat food may not be a low-fat food.

You can see in table 6.2 that although fat-free foods can have some fat, the amounts that are allowed are next to nothing in fat terms. The same holds true for the term *low saturated fat*, the definition of which varies in different countries from 1 to 2 grams of saturated fat per serve or per 100 grams. Although each country has its own definition, the expression *low saturated fat* does indeed mean low in saturated fat.

The expression *X% fat-free* should be used only on foods that meet the requirements for a low-fat or fat-free designation, and it must carry a statement of the total fat content (expressed as a percentage of the food) in close proximity to the claim. So, a food can be labelled *97% fat-free*, meaning it is 3 per cent fat and therefore a low-fat food. This style of claim is no longer recommended for use in the UK.

A claim for low cholesterol can be made only if the cholesterol content is not more than 20 milligrams of cholesterol per 100 grams, or in a serve, depending on the country. The term *low cholesterol* can be a bit distracting because the cholesterol content of a food is not a major health issue; the type of fat has the biggest effect on health and heart disease risk. For this reason the Food Standards Agency in the UK recommends that low cholesterol claims no longer be made on food labels.

The important thing to know is that the cholesterol content of a food is not related to its fat content. So, *cholesterol-free* means low in cholesterol and does not mean low in fat. A cholesterol-free food can still be high in fat (e.g., cholesterol-free oils are 100 per cent fat), so check the label. In most countries, any reference to cholesterol should be made only on a food that is either low fat or low in saturated fat. See table 6.2 for more specific details.

The fibre content of a food can be a useful selling point. If the food is claimed to be high fibre, it will have around 3 to 5 grams of fibre per serve. Table 6.2 gives more details for each country. Because adults should consume around 25 to 30 grams of fibre a day to avoid constipation and keep the gut healthy, any food providing 4.0 grams of fibre in a normal serve size will help you meet your fibre needs. You will see some foods labelled as whole grain, which refers to a grain that has the endosperm, germ and bran layers still intact as you would have in a wheat grain or oats. Brown rice, rolled oats, rye, corn and wheat are all whole grains. Don't confuse whole grains with fibre. Although whole grains do provide fibre, there can be fibre in foods that don't have whole grains. Some processed food manufacturers add fibre to a product to meet the criteria for high fibre. For example, some breads have added corn or maize that has resistant starch, and some yogurts have chia seeds added. These can all contribute to your fibre intake.

There is a legal definition for a 'low-salt' food in all countries (table 6.2). Salt is sodium chloride, and it is the sodium component that is of most interest to us from a health perspective. Excessive sodium intake can raise blood pressure and leach calcium from bones. To determine whether a food is low in salt, you need to check the label for the sodium level. Do not rely on taste as a guide. Plenty of foods are high in salt, yet do not taste salty. Some breakfast cereals have as much salt as salted potato crisps. Many food companies are now actively working to reduce the sodium levels of their products to give us more low-salt and reduced-salt choices.

A reduced-salt food must be at least 25 per cent lower in sodium than the same quantity of the reference food. Salt is a learned taste and can often detract from the natural flavours of food (or mask the lack of flavour in food!). We generally consume far more salt than we need, so I suggest you choose lower-salt foods.

The expression 'light' or 'lite' is not defined in any country, although the product should specify what it is referring to (e.g., light in flavour or texture). It does not necessarily mean the food is light in kilojoules or calories. For example, light olive oil is only light in taste and still 100 per cent fat, and light potato crisps are reduced in salt, although often still high in saturated fat.

A low-kilojoule or calorie-free food is truly that—low in kilojoules or calories. Many low-kilojoule foods contain a sugar substitute such as aspartame (Nutrasweet). Eating low-kilojoule foods may make little difference to your weight or your appetite, so don't assume they will automatically result in weight loss. There is not a shred of evidence that any sugar substitute (artificial sweetener) causes cancer in the amounts consumed by humans. The rumour that Nutrasweet causes multiple sclerosis is one of many e-mail nutrition hoaxes.

'No added sugar' means that the food manufacturer did not add sucrose, honey, glucose, molasses, malt, and so forth. Big deal. Sugar is not as evil as the pop nutritionists try to make it out to be. It doesn't give you pimples, heart disease or diabetes. If not cleared from the mouth, sugar can contribute to tooth decay, but then so can any starchy food (e.g., bread or those potato crisps I just mentioned). Be mindful that 'no added sugar' foods may not be low in kilojoules, although they may have fewer kilojoules than the regular product with sugar. For example, a flavoured yogurt without sugar (artificially sweetened) will have fewer kilojoules than regular flavoured yogurt. Sugar is often replaced in confectionery (candy) and chewing gum by other sweetening agents to reduce the risk of tooth decay. Other than that, enjoy sugar if you wish and concentrate on bigger nutrition issues, such as the type of fat, salt content, fibre levels and whether the food is a good source of other essential nutrients.

Natural is a great marketing word, but it has no legal definition under food law. Most companies use it to mean 'no additives' or 'minimally processed'. I suggest you read the ingredient list and see if the food meets your definition of natural. (Note that beef fat and salt are 'natural', but I don't think you want to see them at the top of the ingredient list.)

Shopping Tips

Some simple tips can make you a more efficient and wiser grocery shopper. Naturally, you may already have shopping down to an art form, but those who still have some difficulty may find these tips useful.

Be Fat Aware

Be aware of the fat content of foods. As a general guide, a food needs to be less than 10 per cent fat before it can be considered relatively low in fat. In other words, it must have less than 10 grams of fat per 100 grams of food. (In reality, a food must be less than 3 per cent fat to be called low fat, but nutritionally, foods consisting of less than 10 per cent fat are considered low in fat.) Many foods are fat-free, such as fruit, vegetables, pasta and rice. Bread and breakfast cereals generally have little fat. Muesli is 10 to 15 per cent fat because it has nuts and seeds. Even the oats provide a little fat. But don't use the 10 per cent guide as law because some nutritious foods are more than 10 per cent fat, such as avocados, nuts, peanut butter and good-quality chocolate (and there should always be room in your diet for a little good-quality chocolate).

What Type of Fat?

Saturated, monounsaturated and polyunsaturated are all types of fat. The unsaturated versions are generally the healthier choices because they don't raise blood cholesterol. Remember, though, that all fat is high in energy (kilojoules/calories), so you need to use fat wisely. Be aware that any reference to the cholesterol content (e.g., cholesterol-free) may not be linked to the amount of fat in that product. For example, unsaturated margarines are cholesterol-free, yet also 70 to 80 per cent fat.

Salt of the Earth

Most people would benefit from eating less salt than they currently do. About 75 per cent of our salt intake comes from foods in which the manufacturer has added salt, so not adding salt to your dinner doesn't mean you are on a low-salt diet. I recommend that you choose the salt-reduced or low-salt versions of food so that you taste the taste rather than the salt. A high salt intake is linked to high blood pressure and excess calcium loss from the bones.

Go Fruity

Buy and eat plenty of fresh fruit, which is a great source of carbohydrate, fibre, water, essential nutrients and antioxidants. Canned fruits are also nutritious and are great for dessert or in smoothies, and dried or canned fruits are perfect on breakfast cereal.

Frozen Assets

Frozen foods are exceptionally convenient, especially for single people or couples. Frozen vegetables are very nutritious because they are normally frozen within 24 hours of being harvested; only minor nutrition loss occurs during the blanching before freezing. (Blanching is the process of dipping into boiling water for a short time.) Don't for a moment think that frozen vegetables are less nutritious than fresh. In fact, they may be more nutritious if you have left your fresh vegetables too long before you get around to eating them. Also, check frozen meals for their nutrition profile. Many promote their benefits,

such as being low in fat, but you need to check that they are also a reasonable source of fibre (6 grams or more of fibre for a medium meal would be expected) and are not too high in sodium (I suggest less than 300 milligrams for a medium meal). Some meals are quite small because they are designed for weight watchers so you could need two or three to get a decent feed.

Rice and Beyond

Asian meals are usually a good value for health. Stock up on rice and veggies for a stir fry high in carbohydrate for periods of heavy training. Add some lean meat, chicken or seafood for protein, iron and zinc.

Consider experimenting with other grains, such as spelt flour, millet or quinoa. Spelt is an early form of our current wheat, and its flour can be used in place of wheat flour. Spelt bread and pasta may be found in some specialty shops. Millet is a type of grass seed with a long history of human consumption, too. The most common form is pearl millet, and it can be used to make a porridge. Although not a true grain, quinoa is gaining popularity. Quinoa flakes also can be cooked into a porridge, added to homemade muesli or be a substitute for rice. Unlike spelt, millet and quinoa are gluten free. There is more to the world of grains than just rice, oats and wheat.

Pasta Blasta

Pasta can be the base of so many simple and inexpensive meals. The carbohydrate is great for replacing glycogen stores. There are lots of pasta sauces on the market—just add your own extra vegetables for fibre and antioxidants.

Simple Fare

Buy a precooked chicken, take it home, remove the skin and serve with microwaved vegetables. Or get a low-fat frozen meal from the supermarket; add extra potatoes, vegetables or rice if it doesn't look filling enough. Or buy a prepackaged rice or pasta dish. Check the label to make sure you aren't getting too much fat or salt. Simplicity is the friend of the tired and hungry athlete.

Lunch Cereals

Who said that breakfast cereals should be eaten only at breakfast? Cereal and milk are great any time of the day, and are popular with young athletes after school.

Oooh Yeah!

If your baseline diet is good, there will always be room for some of your very favourite foods such as ice cream, chocolate, confectionery and pizza. Two things to keep in mind regarding these foods are balance and moderation. Yes, it is a cliché, I know, but it is the essence of eating for performance and a long life.

FINAL SCORE

- Familiarity with your local supermarket will make shopping easy and quick.
- A simple knowledge of food labels allows you to compare products and make more nutritious choices.
- If you forget everything else, always remember to choose the week's groceries with the view to keeping the saturated fat and salt to a minimum.
- The least processed foods are generally the most nutritious. Canned and frozen fruits and vegetables retain most of their nutrients.
- When you are fit and active, and eat well, you have room for the occasional treat without worrying about your waistline.

Digestion and Timing of Meals

Nearly 200 years ago, way back in 1822, French Canadian Alexis St. Martin accidentally received a gunshot wound to the stomach. Fortunately, U.S. Army surgeon William Beaumont was able to save his life, although on healing there remained a hole in St. Martin's abdomen through which Beaumont could place his fingers and see inside his stomach! For the next few years Beaumont did a series of 238 'physiological experiments' in which food was introduced through the opening and observed for the rate of disappearance and production of hydrochloric acid by the stomach. Beaumont discovered that all foods and all combinations of food were digested. He wrote his findings in 'Experiments and Observations on the Gastric Juice and the Physiology of Digestion', published in 1833.

St. Martin said that he went through a lot of pain to teach the world about digestion. I'm sure that you too have gone through some pain learning about your digestive system. Have you ever suffered nervous diarrhea right before a big competition, or been slowed down by the pain of heartburn during exercise? They can be just as debilitating as the cramp or stitch discussed in chapter 5. In this chapter we take a look at the digestive system, where food and drink are broken down into small molecules that are then absorbed into the blood. We travel through the digestive tract and see what happens to our meals as they go from mouth to south. Along the way, I tackle some myths of digestion and show how our knowledge of the digestive system is relevant to active people. By the end of the chapter, you will have a good idea of what happens to your food once you eat it and how you can control some of the most common gastrointestinal upsets.

Stage 1: The Mouth

Chewing is a very important part of your enjoyment of food. Although most of your taste buds are on your tongue, saliva is necessary for experiencing the flavours from food. Try dabbing your tongue dry with a paper towel and sprinkling some sugar on your tongue—you can feel something there but you can't taste the sugar until you mix it with saliva.

Saliva also lubricates food to facilitate swallowing, and it starts digesting starch carbohy-

Sports that involve blows to the body have a higher risk of heartburn unless the stomach is empty from the start.

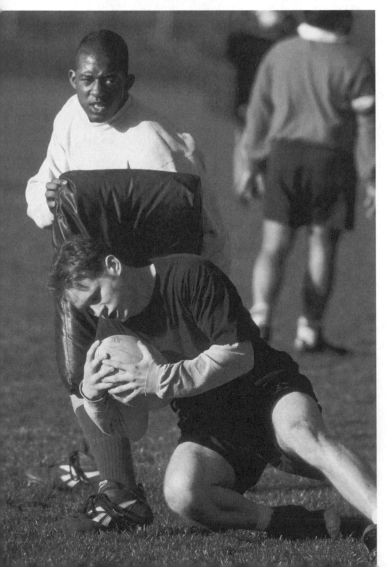

drate through the action of the enzyme amylase. Remember from chapter 3 that amylose is a type of starch.

Finally, saliva plays an important role in protecting your teeth from decay. When a food is eaten and some carbohydrate remains in the mouth, oral bacteria feed on the carbohydrate and produce lactic acid. This acid can break down tooth enamel and begin the process of decay. Saliva then comes to the rescue. The minerals in saliva (calcium, fluoride and phosphorus) help remineralise teeth after each snack or meal as long as at least two hours pass between meals or snacks. Naturally, brushing your teeth regularly also helps. Athletes who are constantly dehydrated may not produce enough saliva to keep their teeth healthy. This is a good reason to keep well hydrated during and between sporting events.

Stage 2: The Stomach

Once chewed and mixed with saliva, the food goes down the throat and lands inside the stomach after passing the gastroesophageal sphincter. The stomach plays the role of a food warehouse with a capacity of around 1,000 to 1,200 millilitres in adults. Only a small amount of digestion happens here, and no nutrients are absorbed from the stomach. The two main functions of the stomach are as follows:

- To add hydrochloric acid to the food to kill some of the nasty bacteria you may have eaten along with your food.
- To liquefy everything you have eaten, because the small intestine (it follows the stomach) can digest food only in a liquefied form.

The stomach does secrete a little protease enzyme to help kick-start protein digestion, but this is only a minor function. The majority of digestion doesn't occur in the stomach, but in the small intestine.

Now, you might think the food inside your stomach is inside your body. This is not so. The lining of your digestive tract is just an extension of your skin; the cells of the skin 'specialise' to become lips, tongue, throat, stomach and intestinal lining before exiting via the anus to return to being normal skin again. In a fashion, you are like a giant doughnut; the hole in the middle is your digestive system. Whatever is inside your stomach and intestines is still really outside your body. Food is not technically inside the body until it has been digested and absorbed into the blood, which happens mainly in the small intestine, the next stage of the digestive system. The importance of this concept will become evident soon.

A low-fat meal empties from the stomach faster than a high-fat meal does—in fact, usually within two hours. That's why a fatty meal can make you feel sluggish—it can take three or four hours to exit the stomach. Sports dietitians suggest that athletes eat a moderate-carbohydrate, low-fat meal two to three hours before exercise or training, to allow time for it to empty from the stomach. This is especially important in running-based sports in which comfort depends on an empty tummy.

Drinking water with meals also helps your stomach to empty faster. It is a misconception that drinking water with meals slows down the rate of digestion. Food that has been diluted by water empties more quickly into the small intestine than food that has not. In addition, the digestive enzymes produced by the pancreas work far more efficiently on diluted food.

During sport, fluids in the form of water or sports drinks empty the most quickly from the stomach, as explained in chapter 5. Because fluids cannot be absorbed from the stomach, they must move from the stomach to the small intestine as quickly as possible. It is here that virtually all liquids are absorbed to replace sweat losses.

Stage 3: The Small Intestine

When the stomach contents have been liquefied, the liquid from the stomach then trickles into the first part of the small intestine at around 1 or 2 teaspoons per minute. Most of the digestion and absorption of food and water happens in the 6.5 metres (21 ft) of the small intestine, especially in the first part called the duodenum (see figure 7.1). The process of digesting a meal in the small intestine generally takes about two hours. (This is in addition to the two to three hours it can take to empty from the stomach.)

As shown in figure 7.2 on page 108, during digestion, protein is broken down to short chains of amino acids, fat is broken down to fatty acids, and carbohydrate (sugar and starch) is broken down to its sugars, primarily glucose and fructose.

Now that the food is broken down into smaller molecules, it can be absorbed into the blood, where it is officially inside your body. This concept is important to remember when

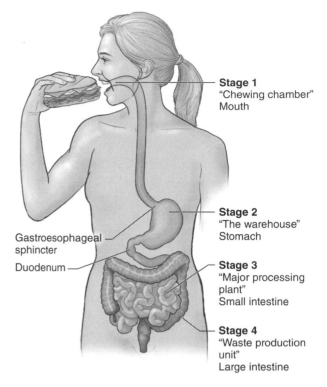

FIGURE 7.1 The digestive system comprises four main stages, with each stage playing an important role in digesting and absorbing nutrients.

you are taking fluids. Concentrated fluids such as soft drinks take some time to empty from the stomach and be absorbed from the intestine, whereas sports drinks and water will be absorbed much more quickly.

Because of the natural delay between the time fluid enters the stomach to the time it is absorbed from the intestine, I tell athletes to start drinking fluids before they begin training or competing. With 250 millilitres (8.5 oz) of fluid taking about 15 to 20 minutes to empty from the stomach, this delay before absorption needs to be considered. Drinking early means that fluids are being absorbed around the same time fluid is being lost as sweat. Waiting until, say, 30 minutes into sport until you drink means that your body may not start replacing sweat until the 45- to 50-minute mark, and in that extra 15 to 20 minutes you may have lost another 300 millilitres (10 oz) of sweat.

If food is too concentrated for the small intestine to deal with immediately, it requests water to dilute the contents. There are two ways this happens. Either you drink more water with your meals, or the intestines take some water from your blood temporarily to perform the dilution. The first way is smart. The second way creates mild dehydration, which is not a problem if you are just watching TV. It could be mildly

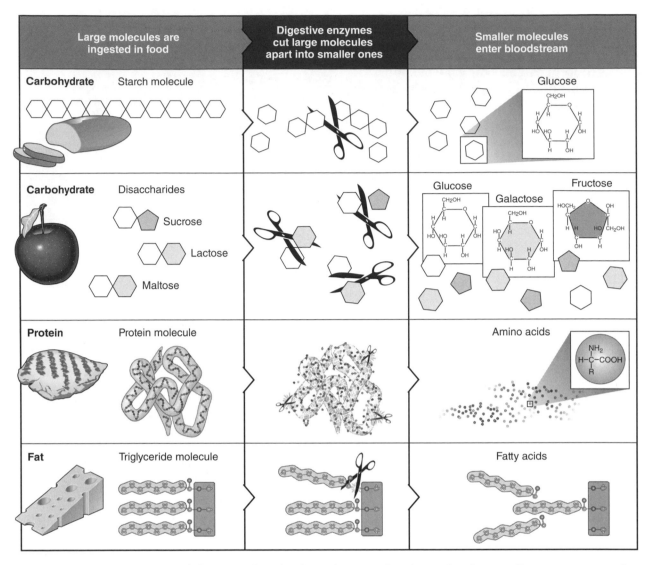

FIGURE 7.2 The process of digestion breaks down large molecules in food to smaller components that can be absorbed into the blood to nourish the body.

problematic, however, if you are going to train in the following two or three hours.

If your exercise is of a lower intensity, say, walking or recovery training, then digestion and absorption will continue during exercise. It will stop only during intense exercise, which may only be occasional in your sport (e.g., short sprints in netball or football). If your sport involves sprint work or high-intensity work such as circuit training or hill climbing, then you will definitely need an empty stomach, or the contents may revisit your mouth and burn your throat. Virtually everyone has experienced heartburn (a misnomer because it is your throat that is burning), and it is extremely common in running-based sports. Undigested food that has mixed with hydrochloric acid in the stomach is forced up through the gastroesophageal sphincter and into the throat. The stomach is designed to accommodate acid; the throat isn't.

Generally, your aim is to get food from the stomach to the small intestine as soon as possible so that nutrients and fluids can be absorbed to fuel active muscles and replace fluids lost during sweating. That is, only when food and fluid have moved from within the tube inside your body to within your blood can we say it is truly inside your body.

Stage 4: The Large Intestine

The remaining bits and pieces of your meal (mainly fibre and a little starch and protein that is resistant to digestion) move past the appendix and enter the large intestine, so called because it has a wider diameter than the small intestine. Here, water absorption is completed and healthy bacteria that naturally reside in the large intestine have a feast on the fibre and leftovers to produce protective compounds against bowel cancer.

▶ Can You Eat Protein and Carbohydrate Together?

You may have heard that you should not eat high-protein and high-carbohydrate foods in the same meal because together they won't digest and will ferment in the stomach. There is no scientific evidence of this. It is perfectly OK to eat protein and carbohydrate together. Another myth is that it is not possible to digest meat and vegetables when they are in the same meal. This notion, too, is quite false. Your digestive system has the capacity to digest and absorb nutrients no matter the combination of foods or when you eat them. William Beaumont's experiments on poor Alexis taught us that almost two centuries ago. Also, since 1935 we have known that the pancreatic enzymes that digest protein and carbohydrate are secreted simultaneously regardless of the type of food eaten. Why do people say that protein and carbohydrate eaten together won't digest and will ferment in the stomach? I'm not sure, but they are way, way, way out of date, and there isn't a dietitian or physiologist in the world who will back that claim.

Of course, if you couldn't digest protein and carbohydrate together, then most of the world's population would be in trouble. The most popular food on the planet is rice, a delicious combination of protein and carbohydrate. Likewise, bread, pasta, legumes, milk, yogurt and many vegetables have both protein and carbohydrate. Breast milk is the perfect blend of protein and carbohydrate, along with some fat. Women don't have one breast labelled protein and the other, carbohydrate! And don't believe the old story about meat taking six weeks to digest. Meat generally requires about four hours to travel from the stomach and be fully digested in the small intestine.

The waste spends about 18 to 30 hours in the large intestine if you have chosen a healthy diet with adequate fibre (much longer if you haven't eaten enough fruit, vegetables and whole-grain cereal foods). If the diet contains plenty of fibre, the bacteria proliferate to make the waste soft and bulky and easy to pass. The normal range for bowel motions is once every three days to twice a day. Once a day is common for most people, although it may not be normal for everyone.

The Quickest Way From the Stomach to the Small Intestine

It is not comfortable to have food in your stomach during competition or training. So how do you get valuable nutrients quickly from your stomach into your small intestine to be digested and absorbed and into your blood? Consider the factors shown in figure 7.3 on page 110 and expanded on here.

- **Avoid concentrated foods.** Foods with a high kilojoule concentration such as high-fat foods or high-sugar drinks empty slowly from the stomach. Avoid soft drinks and energy drinks just before, or during, sport because they are very concentrated and empty slowly from the stomach. The fluids that empty the most quickly from the stomach are water and sports drinks. A meal of fish and chips could take four to five hours to empty from the stomach, whereas a meal of steamed rice, stir-fried vegetables and lean meat may take only two hours to empty. It's best to eat high-carbohydrate meals with little fat because they empty from the stomach in about two hours. Low-fat snacks such as a banana or low-fat yogurt empty in about an hour or so. Drinking some water with meals dilutes the kilojoules and facilitates quicker emptying from the stomach and quicker digestion in the small intestine.

- **Consider liquid foods.** Liquids empty from the stomach more quickly than solids do. Sometimes athletes prefer not to have solid foods before sport because it makes them feel uncomfortable, so a liquid meal such as a smoothie, Sustagen Sport, AktaVite, low-fat flavoured milk or a low-fat soy beverage is ideal.

- **Keep topping up.** The more fluid you have in your stomach, the faster it will empty into the small intestine for absorption. When drinking fluids during exercise, don't let fluid empty completely

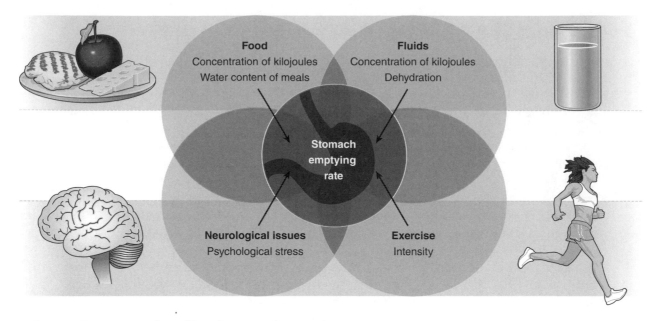

FIGURE 7.3 Factors that affect the rate of stomach emptying.

from the stomach before you have another drink, if possible. Keep topping up with fluids every 10 to 15 minutes.

- **Don't dry out.** Dehydration during exercise slows stomach emptying. This can be a problem for the athlete trying to replace lost fluids as quickly as possible. This is the reason athletes are told to start drinking very early in exercise, well before they are thirsty or have a dry mouth.

- **Relax.** When you are hurried and anxious, food empties more slowly from the stomach. Sometimes a bit of anxiety can't be helped, especially before important events, job interviews and exams. If you are the nervous type, allow a little more time between the pre-event meal and the event—say, three to four hours. (Unfortunately, anxiety can have the opposite effect on the large intestine, giving you the squirts. If you get turbulent insides during sport, see the following section.) Physical pain can also slow down stomach emptying.

- **Consider your exercise intensity.** The stomach empties normally during low-intensity exercise (e.g., walking, jogging), but as the intensity increases, the emptying rate slows down. This rarely presents a problem because high-intensity exercise is not maintained for long periods. Games that involve intermittent high-intensity exercise (e.g., soccer, basketball) can cause a slight slowing in stomach emptying.

Note: There is some evidence that women have a slower stomach-emptying rate than men do and therefore may be more prone to heartburn. There is also a great deal of variation among people in their stomach-emptying rate; what works for you may not work for others.

Gastrointestinal Upsets: Solid, Liquid or Gas?

It's happened to just about all of us. There we are, deep into a training session, and our insides start playing a strange symphony. It's usually athletes involved in running-based or endurance sports who suffer the problems of tummy upsets, wind and diarrhea. Such conditions are also more common during high-intensity exercise and as the training schedule becomes longer and harder. During high-intensity exercise, blood is shunted from the gut to the muscles and to the skin to help with cooling the body. Some believe that the gastric trouble athletes experience is due to that drop in blood flow to the gut. Let's examine some common problems and potential solutions. Table 7.1 (page 115) shows a summary of gastrointestinal problems and their solutions.

Urgency

The need to have a bowel movement in the middle of training or competition can be quite distressing. It's also quite common. Some people even have to arrange their training so they are close to a toilet.

The urge is more likely to occur when exercising just before the normal time of toileting. It occurs most in running-based sports, possibly because the constant pounding of feet on the ground quickly pushes waste through the descending colon of the large intestine.

Possible Solutions

- If possible, train yourself to have a bowel movement before exercising. Conversely, schedule your training after the time you would normally have a bowel movement.
- Warm liquids can have a gentle laxative effect. A hot cup of coffee or tea before an event can stimulate the movement of waste through the large bowel.

Stomach Cramps, Intestinal Cramps, Abdominal Bloating and Diarrhea

About half of all triathletes and long-distance runners suffer some kind of intestinal trouble during events and training. Swimmers, rowers and cyclists are less likely to experience such trouble, probably because they are in weight-supported sports and don't jangle their insides around as much as those in running-based sports do.

There isn't a simple answer that will solve everyone's problems. If none of the following suggested remedies solve your problem, or if you see blood in your stools or vomit, see your sports physician immediately.

Possible Solutions

- Avoid highly concentrated drinks and supplements. Some high-kilojoule drinks (e.g., soft drinks, energy drinks) and supplements (e.g., amino acid powders) are very concentrated and will drag water from your blood into the bowel, resulting in cramps, bloating and possibly loose stools.
- Eat two hours before sport, which will increase your likelihood of having an empty stomach when you start. People who vomit or get stomach cramps during exercise usually have eaten too close to training or the event.
- Drink plenty of fluids. Gut problems are more common in people who are dehydrated. Blood flow to the intestines is reduced in exercise by 70 to 80 per

cent. This is normal. But when an athlete is dehydrated, this blood flow is further reduced, possibly causing a disturbance in the normal function. Drinking water or sports drinks during sport is unlikely to be a cause of stomach cramps, unless large volumes are drunk at once.

- Beware of fructose. Fructose is a sugar appearing in most carbohydrate foods, notably fruit and fruit juices. The intestines have a limit as to how much fructose they can absorb. If too much fructose is eaten in one hit, some ends up in the large intestine where resident bacteria use it to produce substances that cause diarrhea. Large amounts of fructose can be taken by drinking lots of apple juice, grape juice and the juices in many canned fruits, so limit yourself to 2-3 glasses a day; less or none if you suspect these high fructose fluids are causing a problem. Eating up to 4 or 6 pieces of fruit a day is unlikely to cause fructose problems.

Nervous Diarrhea

Almost everyone has experienced the need to have a bowel movement just before an event. The long queues at the toilet before the start gun at triathlons and fun runs are testimony to the fact that many people experience this reaction. The cause is probably anxiety and stress causing quicker movement of food through the gut.

Possible Solutions

- There is no simple solution. If you can find a way to relax, you may just solve this problem.
- Take a spare toilet roll to events, just in case the public toilets are unreliable.
- Remember that diarrhea can have a number of causes such as food poisoning or celiac disease.
- If diarrhea persists beyond the pre-event time, see your physician.

Nausea and Vomiting

Nausea and vomiting during sport occur more frequently in athletes who eat close to the event (less than one hour), have too much fat in their pre-event meal or have taken highly concentrated fluids such as soft drinks or energy drinks just before sport. In all cases some contents of the food or drink remain in the stomach.

Possible Solutions

- Eat at least two hours before sport so that you start with an empty stomach. Make sure the meal is low in fat and high in carbohydrate.
- Try liquid meals. They tend to empty more quickly from the stomach and minimise problems with nausea or vomiting.
- Avoid highly concentrated foods such as fatty foods and regular soft drinks.

Muscle Cramp

What triggers a cramp? Nobody knows for sure. Surprisingly, this topic is poorly covered in most sports medicine books and is not well researched. Cramps tend to occur more frequently with age. It has long been suspected that the most common causes in athletes are dehydration, heavy salt losses or, more recently, muscle fatigue leading to a loss of muscle control.

Heavy sweat losses can cause significant salt (sodium) losses from the body, and this may trigger a cramp if the sodium isn't replaced. To combat the threat of cramp, athletes add some extra salt to their meals and take a sports drink throughout training and competition. A study of a tennis player who regularly got cramps revealed that he lost more sodium through sweat than he ate in his diet (Bergeron 1996). By taking a sports drink and increasing the sodium in his diet, he was able to reduce the cramps to rare occurrences. A study of footballers showed that those losing the most sweat were the most cramp-prone (Stofan et al. 2005).

Possible Solutions

- Drink plenty of fluids to avoid dehydration. A dehydrated body may be more prone to cramping.
- If you lose a lot of sweat during exercise, especially over an hour or more, drink a sports drink to replace the lost sodium. People who sweat heavily are more prone to get cramp.
- Be fit. Cramps are less common in athletes who are well trained.
- Eat well. Cut the fat that clogs arteries. Cramps occur in muscles that have a reduced blood supply as a result of narrowed arteries.
- Stretch before and after exercise. If you suffer night cramps, stretch before going to bed.

- Wear proper clothing. Loose, comfortable clothes are best. Tight-fitting clothes can reduce blood flow to muscles, making them more susceptible to cramps.
- Acclimatise to the environment in which you will perform.

If you do get a cramp, stretching the cramped muscle is the best way to reduce the pain. If it happens in the calf, grab the toes and ball of your foot and pull them toward the kneecap. This helps the muscle to relax. Applying ice can also stop the spasm and reduce the pain.

▶ Let me give you a tip from an experienced athlete called Susan. First a word: *philtrum*. The philtrum is the vertical groove below the nose and above the upper lip. Susan told me that if you strongly squeeze the philtrum during a calf cramp, the cramp will disappear in 30 seconds. Sounds like an old wives' tale to me, just a wonderful way to distract you from cramp pain. Tell me if it works for you.

The Stitch

As with the cramp, very little research has been done on the stitch, yet so many of us have suffered sharp pain in the abdominal region at some stage during exercise. The stitch is now referred to as exercise-related transient abdominal pain (ETAP). The stitch occurs most commonly in the midabdominal region and, strangely, more often on the right side than on the left. Younger people are more prone to the stitch, and fitness provides some protection against it. However, the stitch still occurs in many fit people. Different sports have different rates of the stitch. One study showed that each year about 70 per cent of runners and swimmers experienced the stitch, whereas the stitch occurred in only one third of cyclists and about half of basketballers and aerobics participants.

It is unclear as to what exactly is 'the stitch'. One theory is that blood flow to the diaphragm drops and the lack of blood causes pain. Another theory is that the pain emanates from stress on the ligaments from the diaphragm to organs in the abdomen as a result of the jolting motion of sport, but that can't explain why swimmers get the stitch. The third theory, and the one that best fits the symptoms, suggests that stitch pain is due to the two membranes of the parietal peritoneum rubbing together and causing a friction pain (see figure 7.4). The outer layer attaches to the abdominal wall, and the inner layer covers the organs inside the abdomen (stomach, liver, spleen). Between the two layers is lubricating fluid, so that the two layers can move across each other during any movement of the torso. The parietal peritoneum can get irritated from the following:

- Dehydration, reducing the fluid level between the two membranes, promoting friction
- Distension of the stomach pushing the two membranes together
- Increased movement in the abdominal region during some sports

It is believed that the two membranes of the parietal peritoneum rubbing together generate the pain experienced as the stitch. Based on our current knowledge, the best advice for avoiding the stitch is as follows:

- Don't eat in the two hours before sport. This will allow ample time for the stomach contents to empty into the small

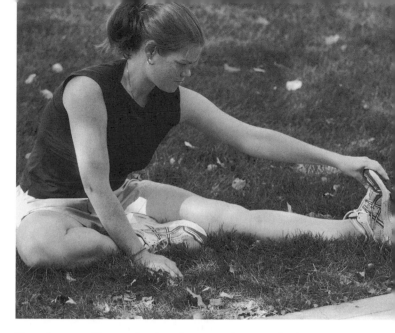

To relax a calf muscle that is cramping, grab the toes and ball of your foot and pull them towards yourself.

intestine. Eating a big meal close to the event increases the chance of stitch.
- Don't become dehydrated.
- Don't drink soft drinks or energy drinks just before sport because this often provokes the stitch.
- Drink small amounts of fluid frequently during exercise. This will help avoid stomach distension and large volumes of fluid bouncing around inside the stomach.
- Drink only water or sports drinks as these empty more quickly from the stomach than other fluids do.

Possible Solutions
- Bend forward and push on the affected area.
- Breathe out with pursed lips.
- Wear a wide cloth belt (like a cummerbund) that can be attached firmly around the waist.
- Slow down or stop. This is about the only sure-fire way to stop the stitch.

Have you ever had a shoulder stitch? If you have, you know exactly what I mean. If you haven't, then, like me, you may be thinking: How can you have a shoulder stitch? Well, it seems that parts of the parietal peritoneum are linked to the phrenic nerve. When the parietal peritoneum experiences pain, it sometimes 'refers' the pain up to the shoulder. Weird, isn't it? In a study of a community fun run, around 7 per cent of runners experienced shoulder stitch (Morton, Richards and Callister 2005).

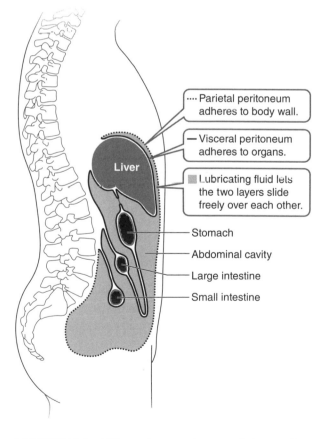

Parietal peritoneum adheres to body wall.

Visceral peritoneum adheres to organs.

Lubricating fluid lets the two layers slide freely over each other.

Liver

Stomach

Abdominal cavity

Large intestine

Small intestine

FIGURE 7.4 When the two layers of the peritoneum around the abdominal cavity rub together you feel the sensation of the 'the stitch'.

Heartburn

A sphincter at the bottom of your throat called the gastroesophageal sphincter closes after swallowing to keep your food inside your stomach. During exercise, this sphincter can weaken and allow the movement of food into your throat. Heartburn during sport is caused by a combination of food being in the stomach and a weaker sphincter at the time of exercise. The acidic contents of the stomach come up past the gastroesophageal sphincter and into the throat, giving a burning sensation. Note: Heartburn has nothing to do with your heart.

Possible Solution

- Ensure that your stomach is empty before you start exercise or sport. You can usually avoid heartburn by eating a high-carbohydrate, low-fat meal at least two hours before the event.
- Eat a liquid meal (e.g., Sanitarium Up&Go; Sustagen Sport) before sport because it will empty quicker than a solid meal.

Endurance Diarrhea

Stomach cramps, diarrhea and sometimes fecal incontinence can occur near the end of a marathon or triathlon. During intense exercise, blood supply to the intestines is reduced. If exercise continues for a long time, and especially if dehydration occurs, the intestines can lose control over their contents.

Possible Solutions

- Drink sufficient fluid to avoid dehydration. Diarrhea is much more likely to happen during endurance sport if you are dehydrated. Keep those fluids up!
- If you suspect there is blood in your stools, or if diarrhea is a persistent problem, please see your doctor.

Burping

Burping is not usually a hazard on its own, just more of a nuisance. It commonly occurs when drinking fizzy drinks or eating food so quickly that lots of air is swallowed with the food. The gases accumulate in the stomach, to be released later as a burp.

Possible Solutions

- Choose non-fizzy drinks such as water and sports drinks.
- Eat and drink slowly in a relaxed setting to avoid swallowing air with food and drink.
- Avoid speaking and chewing at the same time to reduce air swallowing.

Flatulence

A bit of wind is quite normal but can become an ill wind that blows no good if abdominal cramps are also present. It is caused by gas being pushed through the last part of the colon. Sometimes athletes suffer flatulence and abdominal pain due to undiagnosed lactose intolerance or celiac disease.

Possible Solutions

- Avoid wind generators such as cabbage, Brussels sprouts and legumes (e.g., baked or kidney beans) in the two meals before the event.
- See your doctor if flatulence is associated with gut pain, diarrhea or unanticipated weight loss.

Constipation

Constipation is uncommon in athletes because moderate exercise is usually very good for getting waste to move efficiently through the digestive system. Constipation may occur during travel across time zones or between countries, or if you are forced to change from your regular diet.

Possible Solutions

- Choosing higher-fibre versions of carbohydrate foods (whole-grain breads, fresh fruits, baked beans, vegetables) will definitely help relieve constipation.
- If constipation is caused by travel, you can expect your bowel habits to return to normal after about 48 hours.

TABLE 7.1 Summary of Gastrointestinal Problems in Athletes

Problem	Possible solution
• Urgency	• Have a bowel movement before exercise.
• Stomach cramps, bloating, diarrhea	• Eat at least two hours before exercise. • Avoid dehydration. • Avoid concentrated drinks such as soft drinks and fruit juice.
• Nervous diarrhea	• Try relaxation methods.
• Nausea and vomiting	• Start exercise with an empty stomach. • Avoid concentrated drinks such as soft drinks and fruit juice.
• Heartburn	• Start exercise with an empty stomach.
• Endurance diarrhea	• Avoid dehydration during the event.
• Burping	• Eat slowly and avoid fizzy drinks.
• Flatulence	• Avoid 'windy' foods.
• Constipation	• Eat higher fibre foods.
• Cramps	• Drink plenty of fluids. • Stretch before and after exercise.
• Stitch	• Don't eat two hours before sport. • Drink small amounts of fluid frequently during exercise.

FINAL SCORE

- The main function of the digestive system is to break down the large molecules in your food into small molecules that can be absorbed into the body.
- Protein is broken down into amino acids.
- Carbohydrate (both sugars and starch) is broken down into sugars, mainly glucose and fructose.
- Fat is broken down into fatty acids.
- Athletes should allow a couple of hours for the stomach to empty before they engage in sport and should be familiar with the factors that influence stomach emptying.
- If food remains in the stomach while exercising, athletes have a much higher risk of heartburn, nausea and possibly vomiting.
- Common causes of stomach cramps are dehydration or drinking very concentrated fluids. Choose water or a sports drink, and drink to replace fluid loss during sport.
- A common cause of 'the stitch' is dehydration or stomach distension, so drink small amounts of fluid frequently during sport.

What to Eat and Drink Before, During and After Exercise

> I came out with high energy, which I have been lacking in the last couple of games. I think it was the baked beans on toast for pregame.
>
> *Basketballer Lauren Jackson during the women's world basketball championships (2002)*

Dietary advice to athletes has changed over the years. In the beginning it was purely speculation and experimentation, before science gave us a better understanding. We now know that what you eat, and when you eat it, will make a big difference to how you perform. It can be a bit tricky for some people to work out what and when to eat on the big day. This chapter will help you to be your best at event time.

Nutrition Before the Event

Before exercise, a meal or snack should provide sufficient fluid to maintain hydration, be relatively low in fat and fiber to facilitate gastric emptying and minimize gastro-intestinal distress, be relatively high in carbohydrate to maximize maintenance of blood glucose, be moderate in protein, be composed of familiar foods, and be well tolerated by the athlete.

Position of the American Dietetic Association, Dietitians of Canada and the American College of Sports Medicine: Nutrition and Athletic Performance (2009, 510)

Some people eat far too close to an event or training session and find themselves feeling quite unwell soon after the start of exercise. Others can leave too long between a meal and the start of their sport. I met a footballer who wouldn't eat after his 8:00 a.m. game-day breakfast because he thought he might vomit during the game. His problem was that he was hungry and tired by game time. 'Any ideas?' he asked. Well, because the game didn't start until 3:00 p.m., I introduced him to the concept of lunch. He thought that the stomach took over a day to empty.

Some of the concepts mentioned in chapter 7 on digestion are relevant when discussing the best food and fluids to consume around sport. The following sections address key issues regarding eating before exercise.

High Carbohydrate and Low Fat

The preexercise meal needs to be high in carbohydrate to top up your glycogen stores for endurance. The glycemic index (GI) of the foods will probably have little bearing on your performance unless that performance is longer than 120 minutes, but you might want to experiment with the low GI foods mentioned in chapter 3. For a guide to how much carbohydrate you need just before, during and just after exercise, take a look at table 8.1. For example, a light meal of 75 to 150 grams of carbohydrate will suit most people (about 1 to 2 g per kg of body weight) as a preexercise meal. The same amount of carbohydrate will be needed after exercise to start the process of replenishing muscle glycogen stores. After a moderate amount of exercise (e.g., a 60- to 90-minute workout), you will need 5 to 7 grams of carbohydrate per kilogram of body weight in the following 24 hours, which is 350 to 490 grams for a 70-kilogram (154 lb) person (probably less for females or if the exercise is low intensity).

The preexercise meal should also be low in fat so that it empties as quickly as possible from the stomach and into the small intestine where it will be digested and absorbed into the blood. Food remaining in the stomach when you begin your activity is likely to make you feel uncomfortable, especially in running-based sports because the food can joggle up and down inside the stomach. Remember, only absorbed food can fuel the body. See chapter 3 for examples of high-carbohydrate, low-fat eating.

Moderate Protein

Some people will tell you that you should eat plenty of protein before a workout or a hard training session. Unfortunately, there is no evidence that this is helpful. Of course, there is a very good chance that your preexercise meal will contain a reasonable amount of protein anyway because it is likely to include milk, cheese, cereal, bread, pasta, rice, meat or fish.

TABLE 8.1 Approximate Carbohydrate Needs for Sport

Timing	Carbohydrate intake
Before exercise	• 1–2 g per kg body weight about 2–3 hrs before exercise
During exercise	• 30–60 g per hr of endurance exercise (e.g., 500–1,000 mL [17–34 oz]) sports drink per hr • Up to 90 g per hr in high-intensity exercise
After exercise	• 1.0 g per kg body weight soon after exercise finishes • 5–7 g per kg body weight during 24 hrs after moderate exercise • 7–12 g per kg body weight during the 24 hrs after heavy exercise

Note: Women may require the lower end of the carbohydrate range given.

You may prefer a food bar as part of your pre-event meal, and most of these contain some protein. As long as you are eating enough protein over the day, your body and muscles will be happy. See chapter 2 for more information on protein.

Timing of Meals and Snacks

Two to three hours is usually enough time for the stomach to empty before the event. Most low-fat, light meals empty from the stomach within two hours. Almost all meals are out of the stomach within three to four hours. How close you eat to an event is up to you, but consider the following:

- You generally need to allow more time for digestion in running-based sports, such as football, netball and hockey, because any food remaining in the stomach will bounce around and make you feel uncomfortable. The food may also rise through the sphincter at the top of the stomach and burn the lining of the throat (heartburn).

- You can eat closer to the event in sports in which your body weight is supported, such as swimming, rowing and cycling. Put another way, weight-supported sports may be performed with a small amount of food in the stomach and not upset the athlete.

- Any sport that involves physical contact to the stomach such as boxing, rugby or wrestling requires an empty stomach to avoid embarrassing moments.

- Allow more than three hours between meals and sport if you get nervous. Anxiety slows the rate at which the stomach empties. This is usually an important consideration before important sport events.

- Liquid meals, such as fruit smoothies and low-fat flavoured milk, tend to empty more quickly from the stomach than solid foods do. This is a very efficient way to get food into your body if you don't want solid foods or you get nervous before events.

- Sometimes it isn't convenient to eat a couple of hours before exercise, such as when you have an early morning training session. In that case, ensure that your meal and snacks before you go to bed are high in carbohydrate. Consider diluted fruit juice or a sports drink on waking before a long early morning training session. These will top up your glycogen stores before you start.

Sugar Before Sport

Many claim that eating sugar, or a sugar-containing food, before sport can ruin your performance. The premise is that the sugar causes high blood glucose levels, which causes high levels of insulin to be released into the blood, resulting in low blood glucose levels and poor performance. This assumption is based on one study published in 1979. Although this study showed a reduction in performance after eating carbohydrate in the hour before sport, most subsequent

The pregame meal needs to provide carbohydrate to boost glycogen stores, fluid to ensure you are well hydrated and a modest amount of protein.

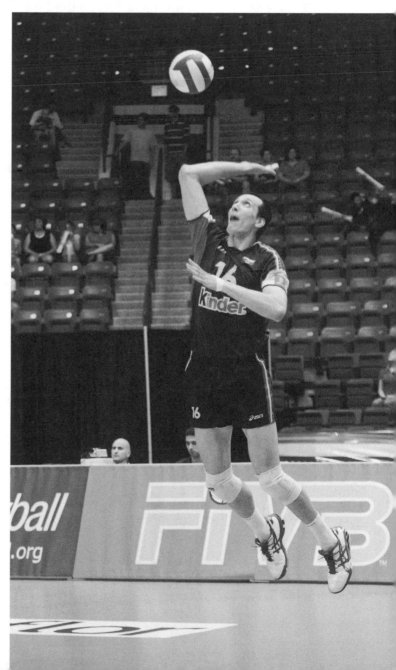

studies have shown either a neutral effect or a performance boost of 7 to 20 per cent. It's interesting that these haven't received as much publicity as the study over three decades ago. (You will recall that a sharp rise in blood glucose levels probably doesn't occur, because sugar, or sucrose, has a moderate glycemic index.) A glass of soft drink (240 mL [8 oz]), for example, has a moderate glycemic load of 14, so it probably won't cause a high blood glucose level.

So, don't take the old truism as natural law. Experiment with foods and fluids and find out what feels best for you. If you believe sugar is a 'downer', then avoid it; if you think it's your 'upper', then please enjoy a small sugar boost. It's your body.

Carbohydrate Gels

Conveniently packaged, and popular with runners and triathletes, is the carbohydrate gel (e.g., Carboshotz, Roctane, High5 EnergyGel). Most sachets are around 30 to 45 grams (1-1.6 oz) providing 20 to 30 grams of glucose in the form of maltodextrin (medium chains of glucose molecules). Many athletes slip these inside their shorts or bike tops and retrieve them when required. Because they are a concentrated source of carbohydrate (50 to 70 per cent carbohydrate in most cases), I strongly suggest that you experiment with them during training. Although they can be consumed on their own, it makes physiological sense to dilute them by washing them down with water (around 400 to 500 mL [13.5 to 17 oz] for every 30 grams of carbohydrate). The dilution will encourage the glucose gel to leave the stomach and enter the intestine more quickly than if it were eaten alone. As a guide, have one sachet in the 10 minutes before the start of an event, and then one or two sachets per hour of sport depending on intensity. Carbohydrate gels are of most benefit to endurance athletes. For the nutrient profile of some gels, see table 8.2.

Lack of Appetite Before Sport

Even if you aren't hungry before exercise, it is still smart to eat some form of carbohydrate food, especially if you are endurance training or playing sport in the morning after a sleep. If you don't fancy a solid meal, think liquid. A smoothie (see recipes in chapter 12), fruit juice,

TABLE 8.2 Carbohydrate Gels

Gel brand	Protein (g)	Fat (g)	Carbohydrate (g)	Sodium (mg)	Caffeine (mg)
Shotz Energy Gel 45 g (1.5 oz)	0	0	30	36	0
Shotz Energy Gel with caffeine 45 g (1.5 oz)	0	0	30	36	80
GU Roctane 32 g (1.1 oz)	1	0	25	125	0
GU Energy Gel with caffeine 32 g (1.1 oz)	0	0	25	55	20
Endura Sports Energy Gel 35 g (1.23 oz)	0	0	26	9	8.5
High5 EnergyGel Plus 38 g (1.34 oz)	0	0	23	40	35
High5 EnergyGel 38 g (1.34 oz)	0	0	20	20	0
High5 IsoGel 60 mL (2.0 oz)	0	0	22	30	0
Pb energy gel 35 g (1.2 oz)	0	0	27	31	0

AktaVite, Sustagen Sport and other commercial low-fat liquid meals are good choices. Low-fat liquid foods generally empty from the stomach within two hours.

Special Foods

As yet, there is no specific food that can be taken just before sport that is guaranteed to improve your performance. But many athletes truly believe that a certain food makes a big difference, and if that is your belief, then eat it. It may give you a psychological advantage. It's also called the placebo effect. A footballer once told me that he always eats bananas before a game because the first time he had a pregame banana he was judged best on ground. Just as the cricketer puts the left pad on first for good luck, you should choose whatever food or drink you think is lucky for you.

Relaxation

A lot of people get nervous before big events. Relaxing can be a difficult task for many athletes concerned about an impending event. Some feel nauseated; others suffer loose bowels or frequent urination. If you get tummy trouble, read chapter 7 for advice. Anxiety can slow the rate of stomach emptying, so you may benefit from taking a liquid meal.

Fluids

Avoiding dehydration is crucial to your performance. You should be well hydrated before you start an event. I suggest you drink an extra 300 to 500 millilitres (10 to 17 oz) in the 10 minutes before you start, even if you don't feel thirsty. Why this can be a distinct advantage is covered in chapter 5 on fluids. Water is an excellent sports drink. Use a commercial sports drink if you don't fancy water, if the session is of high intensity, or if the event is likely to last more than an hour.

Nutrition During the Event

During exercise, primary goals for nutrient consumption are to replace fluid losses and provide carbohydrates (approximately 30-60 g per hour) for maintenance of blood glucose levels. These nutrition guidelines are especially important for endurance events lasting longer than an hour when an athlete has not consumed adequate food or fluid before exercise, or if an athlete is exercising in an extreme environment (e.g., heat, cold or high altitude).

Position of the American Dietetic Association, Dietitians of Canada and the American College of Sports Medicine: Nutrition and Athletic Performance (2009, 510)

There is no doubt that you need fluids during exercise. Try to drink around 150 to 250 millilitres (5 to 8.5 oz) every 15 minutes during exercise, the bigger amount in warm weather. Don't wait until you are thirsty. If you feel thirsty, you are already too dehydrated to perform at your best. If your event lasts over an hour, it is wise to take some carbohydrate in with your fluid (e.g., a sports drink or sports gel) because it improves performance, especially near the end of an event.

Scientists aren't certain how carbohydrate consumed during an event improves endurance, but it's probably due to the following:

- Sparing muscle glycogen. Carbohydrate ingested during low-intensity exercise can be remade into glycogen for later use.
- Sparing liver glycogen. The extra glucose taken orally means that the liver doesn't have to produce as much glucose to maintain blood glucose levels.
- Keeping blood glucose (sugar) levels normal during moderate- to high-intensity exercise and providing extra fuel for empty muscles.

Near the end of an endurance event, blood glucose levels gradually drop and can get low, making you feel faint or tired. Consuming carbohydrate during sport keeps blood glucose levels up, providing glucose for muscle energy and thereby delaying fatigue. Of course, you will feel tired eventually during sport depending on your training and muscle glycogen stores before the event. Guidelines for eating and drinking vary depending on the type of event.

Team Sports and Shorter Events

Most team sports and individual events are completed within 90 minutes (e.g., netball, squash, football, soccer, field hockey or a 10

▶ Pasta, Pizza and Pancake Power

It was reported that U.S. swimmer Michael Phelps consumed over 42,000 kilojoules (10,000 cal) every day to sustain his five-hours-a-day training schedule in the lead-up to winning eight gold medals in the 2008 Beijing Olympics. His daily menu was as follows:

Breakfast: Three fried-egg sandwiches loaded with cheese, lettuce, tomatoes, fried onions and mayonnaise. One five-egg omelet. One bowl of grits. Three slices of French toast topped with powdered sugar. Three chocolate-chip pancakes. Two cups of coffee.

Lunch: 500 grams of enriched pasta with carbonara sauce. Two large ham and cheese sandwiches with mayo on white bread. Energy drinks packing 1,000 calories.

Dinner: 500 grams of pasta. One huge pizza. More energy drinks.

When his diet was reported, it created quite a stir because, on the face of it, it was high in saturated fat and low in vegetables. In truth, we don't have enough information. He has tomato and lettuce in sandwiches. Veggies could feature elsewhere, too. If I were his dietitian, I would recommend that his omelettes include tomatoes, mushrooms, onions and other vegetables and that the pasta sauce and pizza include vegetables and lean meat, seafood or chicken. I would also definitely be pushing some fruit for energy and health. Michael very likely needs all those kilojoules, too. If he started losing weight, he would start losing speed, too. Of course, it made headlines because he eats three or four times more than the average adult. Well, the fitter you are and the more you train, the less likely you are to be average. Try some of the suggested meals and snacks listed in table 8.3 to provide you with high-carbohydrate- and protein-rich foods that are much lower in fat than those in Michael Phelps' training diet.

TABLE 8.3 High-Carbohydrate Meals and Snacks

Meal or snack	Protein (g)	Fat (g)	Carbohydrate (g)
1 medium baked potato 1/2 cup baked beans 1/2 cup mushrooms	9	1	30
200 mL (7 oz) low-fat yogurt 1 tbsp dried fruit	10	1	35
Fruit smoothie (made of 200 mL non-fat milk and banana)	10	0	35
1 cup breakfast cereal 150 mL (5 oz) low-fat milk 1/2 cup canned fruit	11	1	55
2 slices raisin bread 2 tbsp ricotta cheese 1 tbsp jam	7	5	45
45 g (1.6 oz) lean ham and salad 1 bread roll 1 fresh fruit	15	3	45
1 cup spaghetti or baked beans 2 slices toast	12	3	60
2 cups breakfast cereal 200 mL (7 oz) low-fat milk 1/2 cup canned fruit	17	2	90
2 slices toast 1 tbsp honey 240 mL (8 oz) fruit juice	6	2	65
1 1/2 cups steamed rice 1 1/2 cups stir-fried vegetables 100 g (3.5 oz) lean meat	35	6	90

km [6 mile] jog). There is little advantage in eating solid foods during these sports because there is not enough time to digest and absorb the food. Besides, solid food will probably feel uncomfortable in your stomach. Having said that, many tennis players eat a banana or a food bar between sets and still feel comfortable. The trick is to experiment during training and see what works best for you.

Fluids are very important in all exercise and should be taken during these sports. To replace glycogen stores and blood glucose, many athletes eat jelly beans or other soft confectionery at the half-time break of many sports. They need to be washed down with water to assist absorption. It can be helpful to take a sports drink to provide some carbohydrate and delay fatigue in a short event, but proper nutrition before the event is the best move to avoid fatigue.

B ananas are a really good fruit aren't they? I mean they, if you're on the bike for instance they give you a great surge of energy, the bananas. Mmm. They're really, really fantastic the bananas.

Tony Abbott, triathlete and Australian Liberal Party Leader, on PM (ABC radio program), 20 July 2010

Endurance Events

Events over 90 minutes long are generally considered endurance events. You can go along easily for 90 minutes if you were well fuelled before you started. Unfortunately, because we don't have a never-ending supply of glycogen fuel, in endurance events you should try taking more carbohydrate fuel on board while on the move, like a jet fighter taking a mid-air refuel.

The carbohydrate found in a sports drink or a sports gel will help delay fatigue. If you decide to eat solid food, choose one you know will not upset your digestive system. For example, jelly beans, jelly snakes, muesli bars (low-fat, of course) and bananas are popular solid foods with long-distance athletes.

▶ Experimentation on athletes shows that around 30 to 60 grams of carbohydrate per hour should be consumed in an endurance event to delay fatigue (the lower amount for smaller athletes, or lower-intensity exercise). This is the equivalent

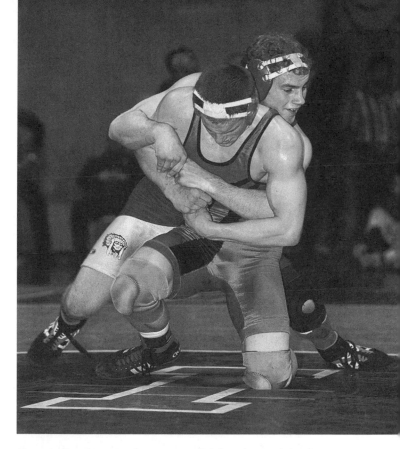

Generally you need to eat solid food two hours before sport so you play with an empty stomach and minimise the risk of gut discomfort, especially in body contact sports.

to 500 to 1,000 millilitres (17 to 34 oz) of sports drink or 10 to 20 jelly beans. There is evidence that consuming up to 90 grams of carbohydrate in an hour is helpful in continuous, high-intensity sports such as cycling (Burke and Deakin 2010, 335)

Ultra-Endurance Events

Ultra-endurance athletes who take part in events that last over four hours train and compete at a lower intensity than athletes who compete in short-distance events and team sports. Because an exercise intensity that requires less than 70 per cent maximum heart rate may not interfere with digestion, ultra-endurance athletes can consume high-carbohydrate foods with small amounts of protein and fat such as muesli bars, breakfast bars, jam sandwiches and hot soups (if the event is held in cold conditions). They may find foods with a higher glycemic index preferable because of their more rapid digestion.

Liquid meals are popular with ultra-marathoners. If this is your sport, try commercial food drinks such as Sustagen Sport during training to see whether they agree with your constitution.

Ultra-endurance athletes should enlist the help of an experienced sports dietitian because of their very high energy and nutrition requirements.

Many need over 21,000 kilojoules (5,000 cal) a day just to maintain their body weight and get the energy they need. Ultra-marathoners who completed a 100-kilometre (62-mile) run consumed an average of 4,200 kilojoules (1,000 calories) with a range of 1,970 to 8,000 kilojoules (470 to 1,905 cal) during the run. Their favourite solid foods were potatoes and bananas, and their favourite drinks were sports drink, water and soft drinks (Fallon et al. 1998).

When glycogen stores get low, the body begins to use protein as a muscle fuel. Even if glycogen stores are reasonable, a small amount of protein is used as a fuel source near the end of endurance events. This implies that endurance athletes need more protein. This is true, but see chapter 2 for more details.

Nutrition During Recovery

You may be exhausted and too tired to eat or even think of food after exercise. Or you may have a hunger you could photograph. In both cases your body is crying: Give me carbohydrate and give me fluid! The answer for some athletes is to drive into the nearest take-away or chug down a few beers. Whoops! Fried chicken and fries, or alcohol, are not what your body needs to recover from the exertion of sport. You have exercised for performance, fun and fitness, not to endure 48 hours of feeling tired and lethargic. What you eat and drink can greatly enhance your recovery.

After exercise, dietary goals are to provide adequate fluids, electrolytes, energy and carbohydrates to replace muscle glycogen and ensure rapid recovery. A carbohydrate intake of 1–1.5 g/kg (0.5–0.7 g/lb) body weight during the first 30 minutes and again every 2 hours for 4–6 hours will be adequate to replace glycogen stores. Protein consumed after exercise will provide amino acids for building and repair of muscle tissue.

Position of the American Dietetic Association, Dietitians of Canada and the American College of Sports Medicine: Nutrition and Athletic Performance (2009, 510).

General Principles

After exercise, drink at least the amount of fluid that you have lost as sweat. See chapter 5 for instructions on figuring out the correct amount. You also need to replace your energy stores. Muscle glycogen can generally be replaced at 5 per cent per hour, so it takes about 20 hours to replace all the glycogen used after a long training session or an endurance event. Generally, carbohydrate is converted to glycogen faster than normal in the two hours straight after exercise because muscles are ready to take up glucose. An enzyme called glycogen synthase is activated with the specific job of making more glycogen, and muscle cells have an increased ability to absorb glucose from the blood. But, you must remember to eat; without carbohydrate, glycogen replacement is very slow.

Take advantage of this increased speed of glycogen replacement. Eat food and fluids high in carbohydrate. Try to eat 50 to 100 grams of carbohydrate in the two hours after exhausting exercise. You may prefer to take in carbohydrate in liquid form such as fruit juice, soft drinks, sports drinks, commercial meal replacement drinks or your own liquid concoction such as

▶ Tour de France

Over three weeks, competitors in the Tour de France cover around 4,000 kilometres (2,485 miles), climbing altitudes of up to 2,700 metres (8,858 ft). It is considered one of the most strenuous sporting events in the world. In fact, during this race one of the highest daily energy expenditures by a human was recorded—a massive 32,700 kilojoules (7,786 cal).

Researchers from the University of Limburg, The Netherlands, found that the cyclists ate an average of 24,280 kilojoules (5,781 cal) and 850 grams of carbohydrate a day. On some days they ate up to 32,400 kilojoules (7,714 cal); that's more than most people eat in three days. Fluid consumption was frequently over 10 litres (2.6 gallons) a day (Saris 1990; Lucia, Earnest and Arribas 2003). Be glad you don't have to pay for their groceries!

▶ World Record a Huge Drag

Tour de France riders have been recorded at over 31.4 megajoules (7,500 cal), and cross-country skiers at 29.3 megajoules (7,000 cal) daily. That was impressive until Mike Stroud from the Institute of Human Nutrition, Southampton, England, and a mate pulled sledges, initially weighing 222 kilograms (489 lb), almost the entire width of Antarctica and through the South Pole (Stroud et al. 1997).

Using the isotope-labelled water technique, their individual daily energy expenditure was measured at a whopping 44.6 megajoules (10,650 cal) and 48.7 megajoules (11,630 cal) during the toughest part of their journey when they had to drag their heavy sledges uphill. During the first 50 days of the trek, the two men burned a daily average of 38.3 megajoules (9,150 calories) and 28.6 megajoules (6,830 calories) each. This dropped down to 26 megajoules (6,200 cal) a day in the latter part of their journey when the sledges were lighter and some of the terrain was downhill.

It's no surprise that the men lost more than 25 per cent of their body weight, despite eating an average of 21.3 megajoules (5,100 cal) a day, 57 per cent of that as fat (330 g fat) and 35 per cent as carbohydrate (around 450 g). Probably the only weight control program that could honestly boast 'All you can eat . . . and still lose weight'. It also demonstrates a rare endurance feat that needed a high fat intake.

The walk had to be abandoned on the 95th day because both men were clearly suffering from severe malnutrition and struggling in high winds and temperatures of –45 °C to –10 °C (–49 °F to 14 °F). The expedition was the first to successfully complete a crossing of Antarctica without the use of aircraft to ferry food and equipment. It was the longest unsupported walk ever made at the time, a distance of 2,300 kilometres (1,429 miles).

a smoothie. The bonus here is that the fluids you are taking with your carbohydrate are also replacing fluids lost through perspiration. To recover quickly, you need to drink non-alcoholic fluids until you pass clear urine.

You may choose high glycemic index (GI) foods, but if you have at least 24 hours before the next training session, it probably won't matter what form of carbohydrate you choose, just as long as you eat enough of it. Eat enough carbohydrate and you will refill your muscle glycogen fuel tank within 24 hours. (The GI of food is covered in more detail in chapter 3.)

Although some have suggested that eating some protein with the carbohydrate after exercise quickens the remaking of muscle glycogen, this process seems far more dependent on carbohydrate than on protein. One study showed that consuming a liquid supplement providing about 50 grams of protein and 160 grams of carbohydrate (half straight after finishing exercise and half two hours after exercise) resulted in one and a half times more glycogen being stored (Zawadski, Yaspelkis and Ivy 1992). Other studies indicated that when athletes eat enough carbohydrate after sport, glycogen is replaced quickly. If athletes eat only a small amount of carbohydrate with protein, the protein seems

to enhance glycogen stores more than expected (Burke, Collier and Beasley 1995).

Be aware that there is a good chance that you will eat both protein and carbohydrate together in the next meal after sport. High-carbohydrate foods such as bread, rice, potatoes, pasta, breakfast cereals and food bars contain protein, and you might combine them with high-protein foods such as milk, yogurt, meat, eggs or fish. Recreational athletes training one hour a day can rely on good nutrition to replace protein and carbohydrate needs. Elite athletes who train twice or more a day, for a total of four plus hours per day, could benefit from a posttraining supplement that offers both carbohydrate and protein in addition to what they get from meals.

Multiple Events

If you are competing more than twice in one day or competing two or more days in succession, how well you eat will make a huge difference to your recovery and performance in subsequent events. The common question is this: What do I eat between events? Following is a simple guide to food and drink choices. Choose one or more items to match your appetite, your sport and the time you have before the next event. For example, if you have 90 minutes before the next event, you

▶ Tired? Not Hungry?

Not surprising, especially if you have had a hard training session or completed a tough event. Exercise tends to increase satiety hormones, making you less likely to want to eat. This helps control your weight if you do a moderate amount of exercise each day. If you do a lot of training, then a reduced appetite could result in gradual weight loss over a season, which can impair performance. How quickly you recover from exercise will depend on your choice of food and drink. Skimping on carbohydrate is the most common nutritional cause of tiredness in athletes. See the fatigue guide (table 4.3 on page 60) in chapter 4 for causes and remedies of tiredness.

might choose a sports drink, a handful of jelly beans and a banana. If you have two and a half hours before you are active again, a sandwich or a tub of yogurt, with a piece of fruit, a cup of coffee and a bottle of water could be ideal.

Less Than One Hour Between Events

Try a combination of one or more of the following:

- Water (provides fluid only)
- Sports drink (fluid and carbohydrate)
- Soft confectionery such as jelly beans (carbohydrate)
- One small banana (carbohydrate)

One to Two Hours Between Events

Try a combination of one or more of the following:

- Water (provides fluid only)
- Sports drink (fluid and carbohydrate)
- Fruit juice, fruit juice drinks (fluid and carbohydrate)
- Soft drink (fluid and carbohydrate)
- Smoothie (fluid, carbohydrate and protein)
- Piece of fruit such as a banana or apple (carbohydrate)
- Soft confectionery such as jelly beans (carbohydrate)
- Liquid meals (fluid, carbohydrate and protein)

Whatever you choose, don't overfill yourself, or you may feel sluggish for the next event. Fluids exit more quickly from the stomach than solid foods do. If your events are short (e.g., swimming 50 to 400 metres), then you might find you need only water or a sports drink between events.

Two to Three Hours Between Events

In this situation you have more time to relax and digest your chosen meal. If you are really hungry, consider a banana sandwich; pasta, rice or potato salad; a muesli bar; a breakfast bar; a fruit bar; and other low-fat, high-carbohydrate snacks such as canned or fresh fruit. Use the Nutrient Ready Reckoner in the appendix on page 215.

Again, don't overeat, and make sure you have fully replaced your fluid losses from the previous event. (This is a good reason to weight yourself before and after events; the weight lost is mainly in the form of sweat.) Your fluid replacement can include tea and coffee, as well as other non-alcoholic drinks. The meal should be small and provide mainly carbohydrate, protein and fluid, and be low in fat for quick digestion. This is not the time to eat large meals or fatty take-aways. As always, you know your body best, so try some ideas of your own.

More Than Three Hours Between Events

The eating advice for meals between events that are more than three hours apart is similar to that offered in the section on pre-event eating earlier in this chapter:

- Replace all your fluid losses.
- Eat to replace the muscle and liver glycogen used during the previous event.
- Include protein-containing foods to help repair any muscle damage.

FINAL SCORE

- Meals in the 48 hours before sport should be high in carbohydrate and low in fat so the meal is digested quickly and maximises muscle glycogen stores.
- Aim for 1 to 2 grams of carbohydrate per kilogram of body weight in your presport meal.
- Sugar-containing food or drinks can be eaten or drunk in the hour before sport. In most cases they will improve performance.
- Fluid is all that is required during most sporting events and training sessions. A sports drink has many advantages in sessions longer than 45 minutes.
- During long events and training sessions, aim to consume 30 to 60 grams of carbohydrate per hour of exercise. Sports drinks are a simple way of achieving this.
- It is important to refuel your body after exercise. High-carbohydrate food and drinks are good choices. Aim for 50 to 100 grams of carbohydrate (around 1 gram of carbohydrate per kilogram of body weight) soon after finishing sport.
- The body relies on adequate carbohydrate intake after sport to quickly replenish glycogen stores. There is some evidence that protein eaten with carbohydrate foods and fluids after sport enhances glycogen restoration. It also helps repair any minor muscle damage.
- If you are constantly tired, check your carbohydrate intake and make sure you are well hydrated.

Nutritional Supplements

> Iron tablets, wheat germ oils and vitamins are known to be consumed by some young sportsmen and women keen to improve their performances. With the majority of them, there is not the slightest scientific evidence to suggest that they do have beneficial effects. At best, they can be regarded as forms of placebo, with more psychological than physiological benefits.
>
> *Warren and Dettre 1974, 94*
>
> Those athletes who are under particular strain have to drink the fresh blood of soft shelled turtles, which I myself have beheaded.
>
> *Ma Junren, Chinese athletics coach, 1993*

The first person to seek a nutritional ergogenic aid could have been Dromeus of Stymphalus, who, in 450 BC, thought that eating muscle could increase his own muscular strength. Aztec warriors ate the hearts of brave foes in the belief that it would add to their own bravery. A crazy idea, maybe, but some of the supplements on the market are based on similar logic. As you can see from the opening quotes to this chapter, athletes have been seeking a benefit from supplements for many decades.

Most athletes have experienced illness, fatigue or a performance slump that is difficult to pull out from. If they can't pin down the cause, many consider a nutritional supplement as a possible solution. Athletes who train hard are always on the search for a supplement to give them the edge over the opposition. Why wouldn't they? If performance improves after taking the supplement, it is easy to assume that the supplement did all the work.

A scientist would now step in and remind us that improvement is not proof that the supplement worked. It may be just a convenient coincidence. Proof only comes when the same result can be repeated time and time again. It's well known that just giving an athlete a pill can improve performance; this is known as the placebo effect. A review of 11 studies on the placebo effect in athletes showed that the placebo improved performance, usually by 1 to 5 per cent, sometimes more (Beedie and Foad 2009). A 5 per cent improvement is huge. Imagine if you could improve your time by three minutes in every hour of a marathon or a triathlon.

In one study (Piantadosi 2006) runners were told of the performance boosting effects of super-oxygenated water and then were given either water or water labelled super-oxygenated. When they believed they were taking the special water, their performance improved 8 per cent over a 5 kilometre (3.1-mile) run. The belief in the suggested benefits suddenly had a high-octane result.

The question remains with many supplements: If there is a change in performance, what caused the change—the supplement or the psychology? In this chapter, we explore answers to this question. I also identify supplements that have potential benefits, supplements that don't have enough evidence for or against them and some supplements that are not recommended.

> The logical conclusion from any study in which an athlete performs to a higher level as a result of receiving a sham treatment is that there is untapped psychological potential in that athlete.
>
> *C.J. Beedie and A.J. Foad,*
> *(2009, 327)*

In the Mind or in the Pill?

Manufacturers of most nutritional supplements tell you how their product *will* improve your performance. As soon as you believe in the supplement, the placebo effect may come into operation as a psychological ergogenic aid, and your performance may improve. Science attempts to separate the true physiological ef-

fect of a supplement from the perceived effect. This is best done with a double-blind trial in which athletes are given either the supplement or an inactive placebo that looks and tastes like the supplement. Neither the researcher nor the athletes know what is being taken (hence 'double-blind') until the very end of the trial when an independent person provides the code. If those taking the supplement improve and those taking the placebo do not, or if those on the supplement improved a lot more than those on the placebo, then the researchers are onto something big. If both groups improve, then the improvement is likely to have come from the mind or be just an effect of regular training. If there is no effect with either, then we can assume the supplement is not providing a benefit.

Unfortunately, determining the benefits of nutritional supplements is never as cut and dried as performing a double-blind trial. Scientists can spend years researching the worth of a supplement and still not get an answer. The difficulty comes in trying to measure the benefits. Current equipment may not be sophisticated enough to record a slight improvement in performance, or the improvement may be in only certain athletes under certain circumstances. Males may differ in response to females; the untrained could differ in response to the trained. Considering that even a placebo can deliver a 1 per cent improvement in performance, the difference between gold and fifth, it's no surprise that athletes will grab at anything that gives a hint of a performance edge.

Assessing Nutritional Supplements

When assessing the potential value of a nutritional supplement, consider the following:

- **Has there been any independent research on the supplement?** You will be surprised to find that many supplements have not been researched in healthy athletes, or that the research has been done only in-house and not been independently assessed.

- **If research has been conducted, has it been published in an independent, peer-reviewed, scientific journal?** The marketing of some supplements relies on magazine or online articles written about the product. Articles are not research. Before research is published in scientific journals, experts in the field review it to make sure it is up to a high standard and that any conclusions are valid. Research is more reliable than publicity.

- **Is the research relevant to athletes?** Many supplement manufacturers cite research articles that are unrelated to the claims for the product. One food bar claimed to assist body fat loss, yet none of the references cited to support its claim were about weight loss. If you can't assess the research yourself, ask a sports dietitian or go to a reputable website (see the resources section on page 241) for their opinion on the research.

- **Is the supplement patented?** If a product has been patented, then the patent holders usually do most of the research because they will directly benefit from future sales. Truly independent research is rarely published in such circumstances.

- **Is the majority of research from one researcher or laboratory?** The value of a supplement can be determined only if many researchers from different laboratories work independently to assess it under varying conditions. This has been done, for example, in the case of creatine and sports drinks.

- **Has the research been performed on athletes under normal training or competition conditions?** Just because a product has benefits for people with certain conditions such as heart disease or a nutrition deficiency, it doesn't follow that the same benefits hold for fit and healthy athletes.

- **Although there may be research suggesting a benefit of a supplement, is there any research showing no effect or possible dangerous side effects of using the supplement?** If one research paper shows a positive effect, but 10 others show no effect, then it is disingenuous to mention the positive result and not to say that the balance of evidence is for no effect.

- **Is the product suited to your sport and your level of training?** Taking supplemental creatine can benefit sprint and power athletes, but it is unlikely to benefit marathon runners. If research shows a positive effect for elite athletes, will you get the same benefit when training purely for health and fitness?

- **Have other independent scientists, sports dietitians, sports institutes or sports medicine groups offered supporting comments about the supplement?** Check out what organisations such as the International Society of Sports Nutrition, the National Sports Medicine Institute of the UK, the Australian Institute of Sport or Sports Dietitians Australia have to say about a supplement to get a more balanced opinion. Their websites, listed in the resources section at the back of the book, have information on most nutritional supplements promoted to athletes.

Only when you start asking questions will you be able to determine the value of a supplement. Be aware that many supplement providers will not like you asking questions (because they won't have credible answers) and will rely on a testimonial from an athlete or a bodybuilder as proof. If all you get from a supplement company is essentially promotional brochures and personal stories from athletes, then you know that science has not been able to support the implied benefits of the product. At least your decision to use, or not use, the product will be an informed one.

Frequently, the argument for a supplement is based on flawed logic. A good example of this logic is royal jelly. It was assumed that what is good for queen bees is also good for humans. We were told that the queen bee is fed on royal jelly, a mixture of pollen and secretions from the glands of worker bees. This is why she grows to be twice as large as the regular bees and lives for four or five years, compared to 45 days for the worker bees. That is fine for the bee, but who's to say that it's any good for humans?

Based on this logic, we should be eating antelope, because the fastest land animal is the cheetah (96 km/h, or 60 mph), which feeds on antelope. The fastest marine animal is the killer whale (55 km/h, or 34 mph). More plankton for swimmers! Going back to the insect world, it would make far more sense to eat like a flea, which can jump up to 130 times its own height, or dine like a tropical cockroach, which can travel 40 times its body length in one second. Royal jelly is definitely not recommended for asthma or allergy sufferers because it has triggered fatal asthma attacks. Thankfully, royal jelly has lost favour as a supplement.

Testimonials From Famous Athletes

A common, and very powerful, marketing technique is to get an endorsement from a famous athlete. Most elite athletes get their talent and prowess from intense training, coupled with healthy eating, positive mental attitude and favourable genes. Because they often train for many hours a day, elite athletes often don't have time to earn money to pay for all their training and travel expenses. They are then willing to try supplements and endorse them to earn some cash. It certainly doesn't mean that they have checked or understood the science, if any, behind the product.

Be also wary of network marketed products. Supplement companies recruit private citizens to promote their supplement to, and through, a network of family members, friends, work colleagues, sports clubs and individual athletes. The supplement companies often market their product on the basis that it is being used by a famous athlete or sporting team, rarely on the basis of being proved to be useful. The Australian Institute of Sport website says: 'Network marketed supplements are not recommended or endorsed by the AIS'. Now that is a strong message to consumers.

Flawed Ingredients Lists

You can never be sure that supplements contain the ingredients stated, in the amounts stated. More alarmingly, some have ingredients that are not declared on the label. This is of great concern to elite athletes who have to undergo drug testing. The World Anti-Doping Agency (WADA) says that around 20 per cent of nutritional supplements have undeclared ingredients that could lead to a positive doping result (WADA 2004). The WADA website states: 'The use of dietary supplements by athletes is a concern because in many countries the manufacturing and labelling of supplements may not follow strict rules, which may lead to a supplement containing an undeclared substance that is prohibited under anti-doping regulations. A significant number of positive tests have been attributed to the misuse of supplements and taking a poorly labeled dietary supplement is not an adequate defense in a doping hearing'.

WADA warns that taking a poorly labelled nutritional supplement is not a defence if an elite athlete is asked to attend a doping hearing. In 2008, Canadian bobsledder Serge Despres was banned for two years after testing positively for the steroid nandrolone. It was an undeclared ingredient in a supplement. Your local sporting authority will provide information on the safest source of a supplement should you decide to take one. In the past, WADA warned that supplement manufacturers make claims about their products that are not backed by valid scientific research, and they rarely advise the consumer about potential adverse effects. The supplement industry is a money-making venture, and athletes should get proper help to distinguish marketing strategies from reality.

Current Findings

We will see many sports nutritional supplements more vigorously researched, and, no doubt, there will be breakthroughs such as supplemental creatine. Most nutritional supplement research has been done on fit young men. The future could see nutritional supplements offering genuine performance benefits to certain subgroups of people, such as young women or people over 55.

We will now look at some examples of the common supplements on the market, and you can judge whether they are worth your money. Not all supplements are covered. You can find more information online from the Australian Institute of Sport, Sports Dietitians Australia,

▶ Warning: Children, Women and Supplements

Women who are planning a pregnancy, are pregnant or are breastfeeding should not take any nutritional supplement without their doctor's advice. I do not recommend any nutritional supplement (including creatine) to people under 18 years old because most have not been tested on their long-term effects on growth and development. This is also the view of national institutes of sport. Again, seek the advice of your doctor or sports physician, or contact the sports medicine association in your country.

the British Dietetic Association, Dietitians Association of Australia and the U.S. Food and Drug Administration.

The supplements discussed here have been divided into three categories:

- **Those with potential benefits.** These offer benefits to some athletes under certain conditions. (A supplement will rarely benefit every athlete.)

- **Those for which it's too early to tell.** These supplements look promising on the basis of early research, but it is too early to be certain of the benefits, if any, to athletes.

- **Those that are not recommended.** The research for these supplements is either non-existent or indicates that the supplement has little benefit in sports performance.

Supplements With Potential Benefits

A few supplements can help some athletes, yet not one of them will definitely help you personally all the time. For example, the sports drink is excellent because every athlete sweats and uses glucose as a fuel, but the sports drink is only generally useful if you are doing more than 60 minutes of exercise. The other supplements discussed here (in alphabetical order) may help you to get a little extra out of your body. You will need to experiment on yourself with an open mind. Naturally, if you exercise purely for health, fitness and pleasure, then good, wholesome eating and water are likely to provide you with all your body needs.

Antioxidants

Without oxygen, you would die. Yet the very oxygen that is keeping you alive is also contributing to your death because oxygen is toxic in the long term. Inhaling oxygen naturally produces harmful free radicals as a consequence of normal metabolism. Free radicals are unstable molecules or fragments of molecules that can cause gradual damage to body cells. The free radicals are made much less harmful by being neutralised by antioxidants produced by the body and those eaten in the diet.

Exercise can create a 10- to 20-fold increase in oxygen consumption and therefore a subsequent increase in free radical production. It has evoked

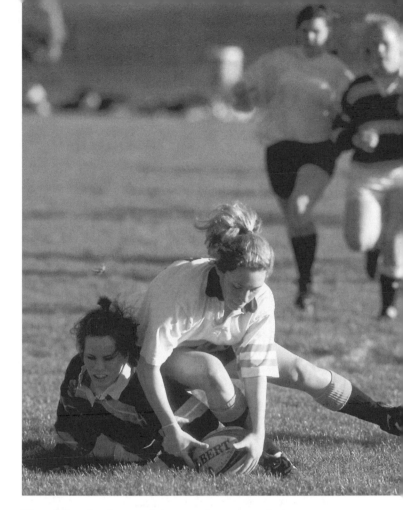

First check the opinions of national sports institutes, the World Anti-Doping Agency or an accredited sports dietitian before taking a supplement.

the idea of the 'oxygen paradox'—that is, exercise (proven to be good for you) increases the level of free radicals (proven to be bad for you).

Does the bad outweigh the good? The answer is no. Research strongly suggests that regular exercisers have a much higher level of natural antioxidant enzymes in their body to help protect against the free radicals produced in exercise. In addition, regular exercisers eat more food such as fruits and vegetables, which are abundant natural sources of antioxidants, including the vitamins C and E. This has led to the theory that the weekend warrior most requires antioxidant supplements because his or her antioxidant enzyme levels are lower than someone who exercises regularly throughout the week. It should also be noted that regular exercise reduces the risk of bowel cancer, diabetes, heart disease and becoming overweight, so there are benefits to exercise beyond producing more antioxidant enzymes.

A small number of studies have shown a decrease in free radical damage in physically active people who take vitamin E and vitamin C supplements, but most data shows no protective effect on muscle damage from taking these vitamins as a supplement. The message may well be different depending on whether the athlete is strength training, speed training or endurance training. Indeed, long-term supplementation with vitamin E at high doses may increase the risk of early death. At the moment, some scientists favour the use of vitamin E as a supplement, especially when increasing training or moving to different climates, whereas others see no value in promoting vitamin E supplements to athletes. One review article (McGinley, Shafat and Donnelly 2009) suggests that, because there is little advantage in taking antioxidant supplements, and because vitamin E supplements can cause harm, 'The casual use of large doses of antioxidants by athletes and others should be curtailed' (1012). Despite the varying views on antioxidant supplements, everyone is unanimous in the belief that athletes need to eat plenty of fruits and vegetables to get extra antioxidants.

No one seems to be certain about the amount of an antioxidant supplement needed, or how much exercise warrants a supplement. As suggested, the regular exerciser is least likely to need a supplement when training, but anyone involved in hard training or competition for 10 hours or more a week may benefit from a low-dose supplement. A daily supplement of 10 to 15 milligrams of alpha-tocopherol equivalents (vitamin E) covers the daily intake recommended by most countries and may be a useful adjunct to a normal diet that, for many people, provides only 8 to 10 milligrams daily. Vitamin E appears safe at doses of 200 milligrams or less daily. Vitamin C is abundant in fruits, fruit juice and vegetables, but a supplement of 100 to 200 milligrams daily is unlikely to cause a problem (unless you have haemochromatosis—see chapter 4 on iron). There does not seem to be a benefit to—and in fact, there appears to be possible harm from—taking higher-than-recommended amounts of vitamins E and C.

Following are some good food sources of antioxidants:

- **Vitamin E**—Vegetables, fruits, nuts, vegetable oils, wheat germ, oily fish (such as salmon, mackerel, tuna and herring)
- **Vitamin C**—Fruits, vegetables (such as orange, Kiwi fruit, bananas, strawberries, grapefruit, capsicum [peppers], broccoli, cabbage and peas)
- **Carotenoids**—Yellow-orange fruits and vegetables, dark green vegetables, tomatoes, fruit and vegetable juices

If you prefer to get your antioxidants through good eating, then, as a guide, you need to eat at least two fruit serves a day (about 300 g) and at least 2 to 3 metric cups of vegetables a day (about 400 g). This is not a lot of food and should be a simple task for any healthy, active adult. Unfortunately, only 1 in 10 adults is eating that much today. Although healthy eating, a supplement, or both, may reduce oxidative stress, there is no evidence that this will also improve sports performance.

Bicarbonate

During high-intensity anaerobic exercise such as sprinting, lactic acid is produced more quickly than it can be metabolised and can reach a level that causes fatigue. If this lactic acid can be neutralised (buffered) quickly, then high-intensity exercise can continue for an extended time. Athletes have taken a neutralising alkaline salt such as sodium bicarbonate (baking soda) or sodium citrate before sprint events as an ergogenic aid.

Sodium bicarbonate may be useful in elite athletic events of one to seven minutes' duration, but it doesn't appear to be of any value in events shorter than 30 seconds. Some studies have shown a benefit to athletes in endurance events of 60 minutes (McNaughton, Siegler and Midgeley 2008). This is a rare example of a legal, effective and medically safe nutritional ergogenic aid. A typical dose is 300 to 500 milligrams of bicarbonate per kilogram of body weight, mixed with water, taken about one to two hours before the event. Some have tried a chronic loading program of 500 milligrams per kilogram of body weight per day of bicarbonate for five days broken up into four doses over the day.

Although many studies show the value of sodium bicarbonate supplementation, the effective dose can have a number of unpleasant side effects, such as nausea, vomiting, flatulence, diarrhea and muscle cramps. The higher the dose, the more likely is gastrointestinal discomfort. For this reason, it is wise to experiment under the supervision of a sports scientist. Drinking plenty of water with the bicarbonate may alleviate the side effects. If the dose is reduced to, say, 200 milligrams per kilogram of body weight, the side effects diminish, but the ergogenic effect is lost, too.

Sodium bicarbonate is not banned by the International Olympic Committee, although some say it could be considered in violation of

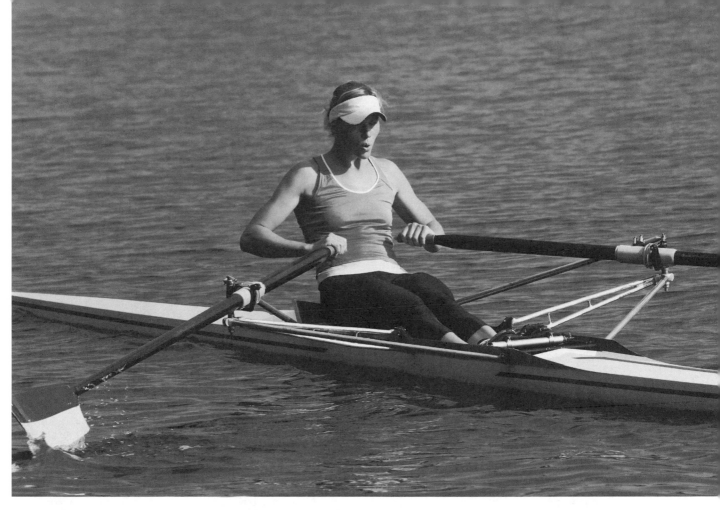

Caffeine found in tea, coffee, guarana, cocoa and the kola nut may improve alertness and increase endurance in athletes.

the IOC anti-doping rule, which states that athletes shall not use any physiological substance taken in an attempt to artificially enhance sports performance.

Caffeine

Most of our caffeine comes in drinks made from the coffee bean, tea leaf, kola nut and cacao bean, all of which contain caffeine naturally (see table 9.1 on page 136). Plants contain caffeine and the related compounds theophylline and theobromine in their leaves as natural insecticides. Caffeine also appears in guarana, energy drinks and some medications. The chemical name for caffeine is 1,3,7-trimethylxanthine.

Guarana (*Paullinia cupana*) is a Brazilian plant naturally high in caffeine and claimed to reduce stress and depression and increase sports performance. It is a popular soft drink in Brazil, where the guarana paste is mixed with fizzy (carbonated) water and sugar. Any value to athletes is probably more related to its caffeine content. The amount of caffeine present in guarana-containing products is not always stated; therefore, it can be difficult to judge the dose you are taking.

There is so much confusion about caffeine, which is a common ingredient in the Western diet. The brain is the part of the body most sensitive to caffeine. As a stimulant to the central nervous system, caffeine can keep the brain alert. Excessive consumption of caffeine can cause increased urination, nervousness, upset stomach, tremors and irritability. Withdrawal, in those accustomed to high caffeine intakes (500 or more mg per day), is associated with headaches, lethargy, irritability and muscle pains, which are usually relieved by a caffeinated drink. Insomnia may occur at 1,000 milligrams a day (about 14 cups of coffee or 8 litres of cola drink).

Is Caffeine a Diuretic?

Technically, caffeine is a diuretic, but that doesn't mean that a cup of coffee will make you urinate excessively or cause dehydration, which is the impression you get from some quarters. In a review of the literature on caffeine and diuresis, Armstrong concluded that: 'The literature indicates that caffeine consumption stimulates a mild diuresis similar to water, but there is no evidence of a fluid-electrolyte imbalance that is detrimental to exercise performance or health' (Armstrong 2002, 201).

Reviewing the evidence on the effect of caffeine on pee production, Dr. Ron Maughan and Jane Griffin, of Loughborough University in

TABLE 9.1 Approximate Caffeine Content of Various Foods and Drinks

Drink	Approximate caffeine content
Instant coffee (1 tsp/cup)	60–80 mg/240 mL
Percolated coffee	60–120 mg/240 mL
Drip method coffee	110–150 mg/240 mL
Ground/instant coffee (1 tsp/cup)	25–30 mg/240 mL
Decaffeinated coffee	2–5 mg/240 mL
Coffee substitutes	Caffeine–free
Iced coffee	50–100 mg/300 mL
Short black or espresso (café)	25–210 mg/serve
Tea (1-minute brew)	10–30 mg/240 mL
Tea (5-minute brew)	20–50 mg/240 mL
Tea bag	40–70 mg/240 mL
Green tea	50–80 mg/240 mL
Herbal tea	Caffeine–free
Cocoa powder	4 mg in 1 tsp
Drinking chocolate	2 mg in 2 tsp
Milo, Nesquik	1 mg in 2 tsp
AktaVite	2 mg in 2 tsp
Ovaltine	Negligible
Horlicks	Negligible
Hot chocolate	5–10 mg in 240 mL
Milk, coffee flavoured	45 mg in 300 mL
Regular cola soft drinks	30–50 mg/375 mL
Jolt Cola	50 mg/375 mL
Diet cola	40–60 mg/375 mL
Caffeine-free cola	Negligible
Non-cola soft drinks	Negligible
Energy drinks	50–80 mg/240 mL
Caffeinated sports gels	8–80 mg/sachet
Milk chocolate	20 mg/100 g
Cooking chocolate	27 mg/100 g
Dark chocolate	60 mg/100 g
No Doz tablets	100 mg/tablet

Note: The large variation in the caffeine content of teas and coffees is due to the variety of beans or leaves, the processing method and infusion times.

the UK, estimated that 1 milligram of caffeine produces 1.1 millilitre of urine (Maughan and Griffin 2003). So, if you have a 200-millilitre cup of tea containing 50 milligrams of caffeine, you will be obligated to produce 55 millilitres of urine, with the remaining 145 millilitres being part of your fluid intake. 'Single caffeine doses at the levels found in commonly consumed beverages have little or no diuretic action' (416), said the authors. People who regularly consume caffeinated drinks are least likely to respond to any mild diuretic effect of caffeine. Only single large doses of 250 to 300 milligrams seem to cause any significant diuretic action.

Researchers at the University of Connecticut in the United States tracked 10 athletes for three days while they trained for four hours per day (Fiala, Casa and Roti 2004). The athletes drank water during the training sessions and only cola for the rest of that day, unaware that in one trial the cola had caffeine and in another trial the cola was caffeine-free. Although they drank the equivalent of seven cans of cola each day, there was no difference in their hydration levels on the days they drank cola with caffeine and the days they drank caffeine-free cola.

In a review paper on caffeine and sport, Burke (2008) stated that: 'Many studies that have examined caffeine supplementation and fluid balance have found that doses of caffeine that are within the range proven to be ergogenic do not alter sweat rates, urine losses, or indices of hydration status during exercise' (1329). So, enjoy sensible amounts of tea, coffee or other caffeine-containing drink—they won't dehydrate you.

Please note that the caffeine figures given in table 9.1 are only approximate. Drinks such as tea and coffee vary greatly in their caffeine content. For example, the caffeine content of a cup of espresso varied from 25 to 210 milligrams among different cafés in one area (Desbrow et al. 2007). In a second study, it varied from 130 to 280 milligrams per cup of coffee purchased from the same store (McCusker, Goldberger and Cone 2003). The caffeine content of a cup of tea depends on how long the pot brewed or the teabag was dangled.

Caffeine and Sport

The consensus is that caffeine has an ergogenic effect in many events, ranging from short-duration, high-intensity events (1 to 5 minutes), to team sports (60 to 90 minutes), to endurance events (90 to 180 minutes), to ultra-endurance events (4+ hours). There may not be much benefit for strength workouts or very brief events such as the 100-metre sprint.

How caffeine benefits performance is not clear. We know that it increases adrenaline levels and that this extra adrenaline is thought to be useful by improving alertness and reaction times. It was thought that caffeine might also enhance the use of fat as a fuel and thereby spare glycogen stores, although this has not been seen with all athletes. This action would mean that the body would be able to exercise for longer. Not all researchers agree with this theory, because exercise alone makes the body more efficient at using fat. Many athletes find that caffeine reduces the perception of exertion, fatigue and pain, and this alone might be its greatest effect in getting them to perform better.

Previously, researchers found that giving endurance athletes doses of 5 to 6 milligrams of caffeine per kilogram of body weight (350 to 420 mg in a 70 kg person) improves performance. The view now is that doses as low as 2 or 3 milligrams per kilogram of body weight (about three cups of coffee in a 70 kg person) provides maximum performance benefits. There doesn't appear to be any extra benefits from exceeding 3 milligrams per kilogram of body weight.

Caffeine has different effects on different people. Its effect depends on how much caffeine the person regularly takes during the day, the person's level of training, the amount of caffeine taken before exercise and genetics. In someone who has very little caffeine normally, two cups of coffee or an energy drink might give such a zing to the brain that it dramatically reduces performance. Someone else may find that exercise is easier and endurance is improved after drinking a caffeinated drink.

Because there is a huge variation in the response to caffeine, you will have to determine whether there is a personal benefit to you. For example, if caffeine disrupts your sleep, the negative effect of sleep deprivation will probably outweigh any ergogenic effect. My advice is to give caffeine a try if you wish and gauge your personal performance both with and without it. Try a daily dose of 2 to 3 milligrams per kilogram of body weight—a level now used by endurance athletes and those in team sports. Whatever you do, experiment during training sessions, not during sporting events. The consensus is that caffeine has an ergogenic effect in endurance sports without any negative effect on hydration.

The International Olympic Committee (IOC) used to state that the maximum permitted level of caffeine in the urine was 12 milligrams per litre. Above that amount was considered doping and resulted in disqualification of the athlete. In January 2004 caffeine was removed from the list of tested compounds by the World Anti-Doping Agency because caffeine was so widespread in the general diet of many athletes.

Carbohydrate Supplements

Supplemental carbohydrate can come in many forms: meal supplements (as powder or liquid), food bars, gels and even confectionery. They can be a very useful adjunct to healthy eating especially when regular food is not available or not suitable. It is much easier to eat some jelly beans on a long bike ride than a sandwich. Mixing up some Sustagen Sport or AktaVite in water or skim milk can be a great snack or meal substitute when time is short or you are on the road. Food bars are a favourite of athletes needing something to dampen the appetite before they can get hold of a meal. Although sugar confectionery doesn't provide many nutrients, it is still a very convenient glucose top-up during a break in a game or event and during endurance events. Jelly snakes are very popular with cyclists. Taking extra carbohydrate, other than in regular food, will be of most use to athletes involved in high levels of training, endurance sports and high-intensity sports. For more information, see chapters 3 (carbohydrate) and 8 (carbohydrate gels).

Creatine

Creatine suddenly became popular after it was claimed that British sprint athletes Linford Christie and Sally Gunnell used it to win gold in the 1992 Olympic Games.

About 95 per cent of creatine is found in skeletal muscle as free creatine and creatine phosphate. You may recall from chapter 1 that adenosine triphosphate (ATP) provides the energy for muscle contraction. During intense exercise such as sprinting and weightlifting, ATP lasts only one to two seconds. The role of creatine phosphate is to generate new ATP as quickly as it is broken down. There is enough creatine phosphate in muscle to allow ATP regeneration for the first five to six seconds of sprint exercise before glucose can be used to produce ATP. In other words, creatine phosphate helps create

enough ATP for most of a 100-metre running sprint. Thereafter, glucose is broken down to produce ATP for fuel during exercise.

Creatine has a second function of acting as a buffer to reduce lactic acid build-up in the muscle, which further delays fatigue. Exercise increases the creatine content of exercising muscles, so creatine levels are generally higher in fit people.

Creatine occurs naturally in the diet and in the body. It is manufactured by the kidneys, liver and pancreas from the amino acids arginine, glycine and methionine. Creatine is found in foods with muscle or nerves (e.g., fish, meat, shellfish and eggs), but we eat only 1 to 3 grams of creatine a day through these foods, much less than the experimental amounts used in creatine studies. Unfortunately, cooking tends to destroy creatine. Don't be too concerned if you're vegetarian—although you get less in food, your body still makes creatine.

Fatigue that occurs during very high intensity exercise is associated with the depletion of muscle creatine phosphate. If creatine levels were higher, possibly as a result of supplementation, then creatine phosphate could be remade quickly and plenty would be available for the repeated sprints that occur in sports such as football, rugby, tennis, netball, basketball and soccer, or the repeated muscle contractions in weight training.

Research over the last 20 years shows that creatine supplementation improves high-intensity work output probably because the extra creatine accelerates creatine phosphate resynthesis during recovery from intense muscle contraction. In other words, supplemental creatine helps nature restock creatine phosphate stores.

Creatine should not be viewed as another gimmick supplement; its ingestion is a means of providing immediate, significant performance improvements to athletes involved in explosive sports. In the long run, creatine may also allow athletes to train without fatigue at an intensity higher than that to which they are accustomed. For these reasons alone, creatine supplementation could be viewed as a significant development in sports nutrition.

Greenhaff, 1995, S109

Recreational athletes would probably see little benefit from taking a costly supplement such as creatine. For the serious amateur and professional athlete whose sport involves sprint work and intense muscle contraction, creatine could offer an advantage.

Despite some calls for banning creatine supplementation, it is not banned by the International Olympic Committee or any other sporting body. There appear to be no harmful side effects when taken in the dose needed for an ergogenic effect. In the past, creatine has been linked to cramping, but there is little evidence for this (Dalbo et al. 2010). Despite these assurances, creatine supplementation is not recommended for people under 18 years because no one is sure of its effects on growth and development.

Creatine Loading

If you haven't taken creatine before, the quickest way to get the maximum levels in your muscles is to creatine-load. Take 0.3 gram creatine per kilogram body weight a day (about 24 g for a 80 kg person) for at least three days, followed by a maintenance dose 3 to 5 grams per day to keep creatine stores high (Buford et al. 2007). It is wise to break up the large initial dose—for example, taking 5 grams of creatine four to six times a day. Take the creatine with a meal or snack, because carbohydrate (about 70 g) enhances the absorption of creatine as a result of the stimulatory effect of insulin. This dose seems to increase muscle creatine by about 25 per cent, but it will vary greatly from person to person. You can take a smaller dose (3 to 5 g a day), but it will take longer (about a month) to load the muscles with creatine. When loaded, the muscle creatine content remains elevated for four to six weeks. Figure 9.1 illustrates creatine regimens and their corresponding total creatine levels.

Not all athletes benefit from creatine. Possibly as many as one third do not receive a benefit. Some athletes have naturally high levels in their muscles; others have lower levels. Those with lower levels benefit the most from supplementation. Lower levels are most likely in vegetarians because they don't eat food with the greatest amount of creatine (meat and fish). As always, you will need to see for yourself whether creatine supplementation helps you; don't assume that it will. (You can only know your creatine levels by having a muscle biopsy, which is impractical for most recreational athletes.)

There is no evidence that creatine increases muscle strength or improves performance in endurance events or low-intensity exercise, although it can increase sprint power during, or at the end of, an endurance event, such as a cycling race. There is no evidence that creatine provides a useful ergogenic effect for an endurance athlete.

Creatine seems to work best when there is a short recovery period between sprints, say, between 30 seconds and three minutes, improving performance by 5 to 15 per cent. Creatine is of little value in single sprints such as 100-metre swimming (but it is useful in training when multiple sprint sessions are required).

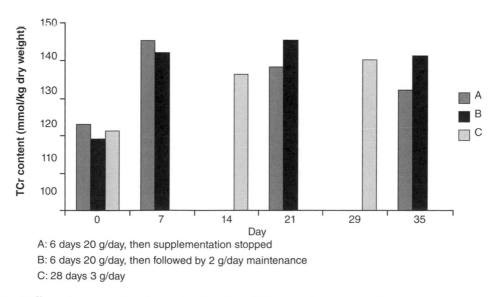

A: 6 days 20 g/day, then supplementation stopped
B: 6 days 20 g/day, then followed by 2 g/day maintenance
C: 28 days 3 g/day

FIGURE 9.1 Different protocols of creatine loading. TCr equals total creatine.

Reprinted, by permission, from A. Jeukendrup, 2010, *Sports nutrition: An introduction to energy production and performance*, 2nd ed. (Champaign, IL: Human Kinetics), 278. Adapted from E. Hultman, et al., 1996, "Muscle creatine loading in men, " *Journal of Applied Physiology* 81(1): 232-237.

Weight Gain

Creatine supplements may cause an initial weight gain of around 1 kilogram (2 lb) in the first 7 to 10 days of usage. This is most likely due to water retention, not an increase in muscle size, as some athletes believe. The extra water weight may be a disadvantage for sprint athletes (e.g., those in 100 m or 200 m track events) if they compete soon after starting creatine supplementation, because they will have to transport that weight in their sprints. Over the next couple of months, weight gain may increase to 5 kilograms (11 lb) or more, which is most likely muscle gain due to the extra weight training the athlete can perform when creatine loaded.

Sports Drinks

Sports drinks are designed to replace lost fluids and provide carbohydrate as an energy source during exercise. They are valuable in endurance events and high-intensity exercise. See chapter 5 on fluids for a comprehensive review of sports drinks.

The use of supplements does not compensate for poor food choices and an inadequate diet, but supplements that provide essential nutrients may be a short-term option when food intake or food choices are restricted due to travel or other factors.

International Olympic Committee Consensus Statement on Sports Nutrition (2010)

Vitamins

Vitamins and antioxidants are discussed in chapter 1 and earlier in this chapter. Because so many athletes take a multivitamin supplement, I will briefly mention their potential value here. Athletes who are travelling a lot and cannot guarantee the quality of their food supply could benefit from a daily multivitamin to ensure they meet their vitamin needs. Athletes who are on very restricted diets for weight loss, or maintaining a low body weight, should also consider a multivitamin supplement. Those experiencing a very heavy training schedule may also benefit. Otherwise, if you eat well, all your vitamin needs will be met. If you do take a multivitamin, choose one that provides 50 to 100 per cent of your daily needs (often listed as RDIs on the label). You do not need vitamin supplements that provide greater than 100 per cent of your daily needs. Always remember that a multivitamin is never, ever a substitute for poor eating habits.

Supplements Without Enough Evidence to Recommend

Some supplements look exciting if you check just some of the research. However, when you look at the balance of all the research, the case for supplementation is less compelling, usually for two reasons:

1. There are very few studies on the supplement.
2. Although some studies may show a positive result, most show no benefit.

These reasons don't mean that we dismiss the supplement, however. Future research may unearth some definite benefits for some athletes in certain situations.

Beta-Alanine

First, let me tell you about carnosine, a compound that acts much like bicarbonate in that it buffers the lactic acid produced during exercise, thereby helping you to exercise at high intensity for longer. (When lactic acid builds up in muscle during exercise, you have little option but to slow down.) Beta-alanine is an amino acid that, when joined to histidine, becomes carnosine, which is found mainly in skeletal muscle. If too little beta-alanine is available, then not enough carnosine can be made by the muscle and the ability to train at high intensity drops; this relationship is supported by the fact that beta-alanine occurs in much higher concentrations in fast-twitch muscle fibres (designed for anaerobic activity with short bursts of strength or speed) than in slow-twitch muscle fibres (designed for aerobic endurance exercise). In fact, sprinters have more muscle carnosine than marathoners do (Derave et al. 2010).

Both carnosine and beta-alanine are found in the diet, mainly in white meat such as chicken breast and fish. Beta-alanine supplements of 5 to 6 grams a day seem to increase muscle carnosine by 60 to 80 per cent over one to two months; in other words, don't expect an instantaneous response. It is recommended that you split the beta-alanine into about four doses of controlled-release capsules (1,600 mg per capsule) over the day and take it with carbohydrate to enhance absorption and to reduce the risk of experiencing the sensation of pins and needles, the most common side effect experienced about 15 minutes after taking beta-alanine. People respond differently to taking additional beta-alanine; some increase their muscle carnosine by 60 to 80 per cent, whereas others respond with an increase of only 10 to 20 per cent. Once beta-alanine supplementation stops, muscle carnosine levels drop at an average of 2 to 4 per cent each week.

Like bicarbonate discussed earlier, beta-alanine is likely to be most useful in high-intensity, short-duration events of one to seven minutes long, such as sprint training or weight training programs. It doesn't appear to be useful in endurance training. Unlike bicarbonate, beta-alanine causes no gastrointestinal discomfort. Because carnosine works inside the muscle and bicarbonate works outside the muscle within the body, carnosine may complement any benefit found with bicarbonate. Because vegetarians generally have lower levels of carnosine in their muscles, they may also benefit from beta-alanine supplementation.

Three reviews of the research (Artioli et al. 2010; Derave et al. 2010; and Sale, et al 2010) were very positive about the potential of beta-alanine in high-intensity exercise, especially early in a training program. Derave and colleagues (2010, 259) made this observation: 'Still, it must be noted that the effects of beta-alanine supplementation on the performance are small and probably only relevant to athletes who have already optimized the other training modalities and who are seeking a minor improvement in performance'.

It is still early to make a song and dance about beta-alanine. Expect a lot more research to be published to refine the advice given on how and when to best use it as a supplement, so keep an eye on the view of recognised authorities such as the Australian Institute of Sport.

Colostrum

Colostrum is milk produced by mammals just after birth. This early milk is rich in bioactive compounds such as immunoglobulins, lymphocytes and growth factors that help the infant get a good start in life. For this very reason health au-thorities encourage mothers to breastfeed their babies. Because calves benefit from cow's milk, someone came up with the idea that colostrum from cows might benefit athletes, helping them stay healthy and possibly reduce fatigue and the risk of infections, and improve performance and recovery times from exercise. Immunoglobulins, or immune proteins, in colostrum are present in amounts that are 100 times greater than that found in regular cow's milk. One of these, immunoglobulin G (IgG) mediates the effects of growth hormone and muscle protein synthesis.

As with many new nutritional supplements, colostrum got attention from athletes hoping for a natural product that would help them. One of the first studies was conducted in Australia and showed that 60 grams of colostrum a day for eight weeks improved the ability to perform a second bout of maximal exercise after an initial maximal exercise effort (Buckley et al, 2002). A more recent study hints that regular consumption of colostrum at 20 grams per day did reduce the depressive effect on athlete's immune function that often follows hard training (Davidson & Diment 2010).

Australian scientists looked at all the research on colostrum supplements and the effect on exercise performance because it has become so popular with athletes (Shing, Hunter and Stevenson 2009). All the goodies in colostrum meant that it could be bolstering the immune system, especially when training and competition became really tough work. Indeed, they found that colostrum was most effective during high-intensity training and the recovery period after by helping the immune system, increasing musculature and improving the muscle ability to buffer any acid build-up. Despite that, they didn't get too excited about it.

There was no obvious benefit for endurance athletes, although colostrum supplements seemed to assist performance during consecutive days of high-intensity training and in the recovery period afterwards. There is still great speculation as to why there may be a benefit.

Although colostrum is not specifically banned for use by elite athletes, please be aware that colostrum will potentially provide the athlete with natural compounds that are banned by the World Anti-Doping Agency such as insulin-like growth factor 1 (IGF-1) which is prohibited at all times in sport. If you are an elite athlete who gets randomly checked, please get advice before taking colostrum.

Sadly, the big hopes pinned on colostrum have not been realised, probably because the components of it vary in amounts across different supplements, resulting in contradictory research findings. The ideal dose is uncertain, although some positive results were seen with doses between 10 and 60 grams per day. There is no broad agreement as to the benefit, and any benefit may be small and only in certain athletes under certain circumstances. More research will help us to refine our advice, but right now I suggest saving your money until we find out a lot more, especially given that colostrum supplements can cost between $50 and $80 (£30 and £50) a week.

Glucosamine and Chondroitin

Whether you are young or old, the worst feeling is arthritis or joint pain that reduces your ability to perform, and enjoy, physical activity. Both glucosamine and chondroitin are normal constituents of joint cartilage. Glucosamine sulphate and chondroitin sulphate are common supplements that have long been used to ameliorate joint pain, especially knee and hip pain. Many athletes believe that they minimise joint cartilage damage during sport, or help repair any damage in the recovery period after sport.

Researchers do not agree about the benefits of glucosamine and chondroitin for the general public or athletes. One meta-analysis of six studies involving 1,500 people found a delay in the progress of osteoarthritis of the knee after daily use of the supplement for two to three years (Lee et al. 2010). (A meta-analysis is the combination of several studies to get a more precise answer on the effectiveness of a treatment.) This analysis was not a study of the pain associated with osteoarthritis, nor did it assess athletes. All the same, it is encouraging news, although the authors state: 'The results of our meta-analysis should be treated with caution' (362). One reason is that six studies are not enough research on which to draw a firm conclusion. Another reason is that the studies used pharmaceutical, prescription-only products with glucosamine sulphate (1,500 mg) and chondroitin sulphate (800 mg). Not all over-the-counter supplements may meet such stringent standards or levels.

To confuse matters, another meta-analysis on glucosamine and chondroitin and their effect on osteoarthritis of the hip and knee came up with a different conclusion (Wandell et al. 2010). They looked at 10 trials in 3,800 people and found that glucosamine and chondroitin did not reduce joint pain or improve joint cartilage. Other reviews of the evidence have been equivocal. The consensus is that glucosamine and chondroitin, whether taken together or separately, have no discernable effect on joint health. If a benefit is noticed, then it is only minor or thought to be a placebo effect. On the other hand, there is broad agreement that neither is harmful in any way, so if you believe that glucosamine and chondroitin help you, go ahead and use them.

Very few studies of glucosamine and chondroitin have been done on athletes without osteoarthritis. A study of young adult soccer players showed that taking glucosamine supplements offered an advantage, but only while the supplement was being taken; any advantage soon disappeared after stopping the supplement (Yoshimura et al. 2009). The players who took either 1,500 or 3,000 milligrams of glucosamine every day for three months had less collagen degradation in their joints. Whether this means that the soccer players will have less joint pain and better joint health in the future remains to be seen.

Be assured that scientists are looking for a natural supplement that will reduce any pain or arthritis associated with exercise because many athletes want to remain active into their 60s and 80s. Fitness doesn't stop at 35 years. One such supplement could be collagen hydrolysate. A study has shown a distinct advantage to nearly 100 athletes taking 10 grams of collagen hydrolysate daily for 24 weeks (Clark et al. 2008). They experienced less joint pain. As you know, one study doesn't provide proof, but it could be one of the new products on the market that extends your knee, hip and athletic life span.

Glutamine

Glutamine is one of the most abundant amino acids in the body and is made by the muscles, liver, kidneys, heart and lungs. Glutamine supplementation has been proposed for increasing muscle mass and reducing the risk of the flu and other bugs that often afflict the athlete who trains hard or overtrains. Because glutamine is involved in muscle synthesis and intense exercise may reduce glutamine levels, it seems plausible that glutamine supplementation would help increase muscle mass. One study revealed that glutamine had a protein-sparing effect at a high dose of 0.9 milligram per kilogram of body weight, although it didn't influence muscle performance during strength training (Candow et al. 2001).

Glutamine is an important fuel source for lymphocytes and macrophages, special cells that are part of the immune system. Athletes involved in endurance sports or intense training with little recovery time seem to be more prone to infections than athletes who are not, probably because intense exercise puts the body's immune system under stress, causing glutamine levels in the blood to fall. Currently, no research shows a consistent benefit from glutamine in reducing the risk of colds or enhancing the immune system. This may, in part, be because fit people generally get fewer colds and flu anyway.

Two reviews of the research on glutamine and sports performance agree that glutamine doesn't have an ergogenic effect, doesn't increase muscle mass, doesn't assist recovery from exercise and doesn't boost immune function (Gleeson 2008; Phillips 2007). Dr. Michael Gleeson from Loughborough University in the UK says: 'The available evidence at present is not strong enough to warrant a recommendation for an athlete to use a glutamine supplement' (2048S).

HMB

Beta-hydroxy-beta-methylbutyrate, or hydroxy methylbutyrate, or just plain HMB, is a popular bodybuilding nutritional supplement introduced to the U.S. market in 1996. It is a metabolite of the branched-chain amino acid leucine and alpha ketoisocaproate, which has also been touted as a bodybuilding aid. The main claims for HMB are that it increases muscle mass, reduces muscle protein breakdown, reduces body fat stores and aids recovery from workouts. The body produces 0.2 to 0.4 gram of HMB each day in the muscle and liver depending on the amount of leucine in the diet, whereas the dose most commonly used in research has been 3.0 grams per day. The amount of HMB used in research studies, up to 6 grams, is often more than is found in HMB supplements.

Although a possible action of HMB is not clear, one hypothesis is that HMB inhibits the breakdown of muscle during strenuous exercise, because there are fewer metabolic by-products of exercise-induced muscle damage in the blood and urine following HMB supplementation. In a review by Steven Nissen at Iowa State University in the United States, the balance of research showed that HMB supplementation of around 3 grams a day enhanced muscle gain and strength when taken in conjunction with a strength training program, doubling the effect of strength training in many cases. This benefit was seen in both men and women, with additional benefits if HMB was taken in combination with creatine (Nissen 2004, 163). More recently, a review of all the evidence showed that for fit, trained athletes there is virtually no benefit to taking HMB (Rowlands and Thompson 2009). There was very little effect on strength and body fat. There was a mild increase in strength for untrained strength athletes in the first one to two months, but a negligible effect in trained strength athletes.

Like most sports nutritional supplements, HMB was released onto the market well before its effectiveness could be assessed. Overall, recent evidence suggests that HMB has little to offer to fit people who include resistance exercise in their training program. It appears to be safe to use at 3 grams a day, taken in 1-gram doses three times a day. Be warned that there are no studies on the long-term effects of HMB supplementation, and it is expensive.

Nitrate

Nitric oxide has number of roles in the body, such as relaxing arteries to improve blood flow and control blood pressure. One source of nitric oxide (NO) is from the nitrates we eat; a major source is vegetables such as green leafy vegetables and beetroot. Eating plenty of vegetables, and therefore nitrates, seems to raise NO levels in the blood, relaxing arteries and reducing blood pressure (Webb et al. 2008).

Could increasing nitric oxide improve blood flow and deliver more oxygen to the muscles and thereby improve performance? This is where beetroot juice comes into the picture. Beetroot juice doesn't provide NO, but it does provide the nitrate that becomes NO. Studies on athletes who have taken beetroot juice have been encouraging.

One small study of eight male cyclists showed that beetroot juice helped them to get more oxygen to their lungs (Bailey et al. 2009). The athletes consumed 500 millilitres of beetroot juice each day for three days. As expected, blood pressure dropped slightly, but the remarkable outcome was that the athletes could go for a lot longer, 16 per cent longer, before they became exhausted.

Because cycling to exhaustion is not a good indication of improved sports performance, the same research group conducted 4-kilometre and 16-kilometre (2.5-mile and 10-mile) time trials with nine male cyclists and again found an advantage with nitrate from drinking beetroot juice (Lansley et al. 2011). All nine cyclists reduced their time trials by 2.7 per cent compared to when they didn't take beetroot juice. It seems that nitrate supplementation makes the body more oxygen efficient, allowing a greater power output. Even people with narrowed arteries have an improved exercise tolerance after taking 500 millilitres of beetroot juice.

If you choose to try beetroot juice, be prepared for red urine and red stools. Oh, and no one raves about the flavour. No doubt, someone will come up with a concentrated version of beetroot juice that is easier to consume and more palatable.

Probiotics (and Prebiotics)

Probiotics is a general term for bacteria that you consume in a food or as a supplement and that survives the passage all the way through the stomach and the small intestine to maintain a healthy bacterial balance in the large intestine. You have most likely seen advertisements for yogurt with Lactobacillus acidophilus or Bifidobacteria, as well as small bottles of supplemental live bacteria; these are examples of probiotics. Having a healthy bacterial balance in the large intestine is linked to normal bowel habits, healthy immunity, improved bioavailability of nutrients and possibly less risk of bowel cancer. With more healthy bacteria in the large intestine, fewer nasty bacteria are able to get a foothold and cause internal turmoil. For example, the good bacteria such as Lactobacillus produce organic acids that retard the growth of nasty bacteria such as Salmonella.

As an athlete's training load increases, so does the risk of illness, such as respiratory tract infections; therefore, anything that can help the immune system (e.g., colostrum, discussed earlier) may keep an athlete healthy through heavy training and competition. The results of the few studies on the effects of probiotics have been either positive or neutral. One study found that a probiotic significantly reduced the severity and duration of respiratory tract illnesses in 20 male elite distance runners (Cox et al. 2010). Another study of male and female athletes found that those taking a probiotic also had a much lower incidence of respiratory tract infections (Gleeson et al. 2011). The authors speculated that this positive outcome might be due to higher levels of immunoglobulin A in those on the probiotic.

Other studies have not seen a significant difference in respiratory symptoms between probiotic takers and non-takers, and a review of all the evidence resulted in authors not being that enthusiastic about athletes taking probiotics, although they did concede that they had potential for athletes undergoing heavy training (West et al. 2009). Less abdominal pain, flatulence, bloating and diarrhea was noted in study of 88 cyclists taking capsules of Lactobacillus fermentum during a high training load (West et al. 2011). Please note that these researchers studied elite or highly trained athletes who are likely to be under greater immune stress; healthy recreational athletes may not receive the same benefits.

Certainly, no harm will come from taking probiotic bacteria as part of your daily diet or as a supplement. In addition, probiotics may be helpful in circumstances other than sport. If you have food poisoning or any condition with diarrhea, then you may have washed out a lot of healthy bacteria. If you have been taking antibiotics, they may kill both the nasty bacteria causing your illness as well as some of the healthy bacteria in your bowel. In both cases taking some probiotics as a supplement or via a food such as yogurt with Lactobacillus bacteria will help re-establish the good bacteria in the bowel and make it difficult for pathogenic bacteria to take hold. Some athletes today take probiotics in the hope that it will prevent travellers' diarrhea.

You may also hear the term *prebiotic*. Prebiotics are nutrients and compounds in food, usually non-digestible bacteria, that are consumed by the healthy bacteria in your large intestine. Inulin and fructo-oligosaccharides are examples of prebiotics that may be naturally present in food (e.g., asparagus, oats, onions and bananas), or added to foods marketed as prebiotic sources. In many ways most wholesome food has some prebiotic action. Fruit, vegetables and whole grains all provide fibre that is later consumed by friendly bacteria in the large intestine. In turn the bacteria help keep us healthy on the inside. At the time of this writing there were no studies on prebiotics and sports performance.

Supplements Not Recommended

Ergogenic aids that do not perform as claimed. The majority of ergogenic aids currently on the market are in this category. These include amino acids, bee pollen, branched chain amino acids, carnitine, chromium picolinate, cordyceps, coenzyme Q10, conjugated linoleic acid, cytochrome C, dihydroxyacetone, gamma-oryzanol, ginseng, inosine, medium chain triglycerides, pyruvate, oxygenated water, and vanadium. This list is by no means exhaustive, and it is likely that other substances would be best placed in this category.

Position of the American Dietetic Association, Dietitians of Canada and the American College of Sports Medicine: Nutrition and Athletic Performance (2009, 522)

When a supplement has received very little research or the research indicates no benefit to the athlete beyond good nutrition, recommending it to athletes is really unethical. Sadly, many of the nutritional supplements on the market fall into this category. This section looks at a small number of these. Remember that many new supplements arrive on the market each year. I suggest that you follow the guidelines given early in the chapter to assess their value to you, or check expert websites, such as the following:

U.S. Food and Drug Administration. Consumer education and general information on dietary supplements. http://fnic.nal.usda.gov/nal_display/index.php?info_center=4&tax_level=2&tax_subject=274&topic_id=1320

World Anti-Doping Agency. WADA promotes, coordinates and monitors the fight against doping in sport in all its forms.

www.wada-ama.org/en/Anti-Doping-Community/Athletes-/QA-on-Dietary-Supplement/

Australian Institute of Sport. Review of supplements. www.ausport.gov.au/ais/nutrition/supplements

International Society of Sports Nutrition. *Sports Nutrition Insider* (journal). www.sports-nutritionsociety.org/sports-supplement-journal.html

Sports Dietitians Australia. The professional body of accredited sports dietitians.

www.sportsdietitians.com

Sports Dietitians UK

www.sportsdietitians.org.uk

Bee Pollen

Bee pollen, like royal jelly mentioned earlier, has been claimed to improve athletic and sexual performance, prevent infection and cancer, prolong life and improve digestion. These assertions never held any weight from the very beginning. Last century, Dr. Melvin Williams said that 'six well-controlled studies reported that bee pollen supplementation had no effect on metabolic, physiological and psychological responses to exercise, VO_2max, or endurance capacity in several exercise tasks' (1998, 135).

Promotion of bee pollen never made any logical sense. An advertisement for bee pollen once stated: 'Bee pollen contains more amino acids than any other natural substance and all the amino acids necessary for human beings. No other natural substance can make this claim'. Except, of course, milk, yogurt, cheese, meat, poultry, seafood and eggs.

Bee pollen offers a glamorous and exotic approach to performance enhancement. However, there is doubt over the real composition of some supplements. This might explain why the controlled trials have failed to find any improvement after taking bee pollen. The balance of studies suggests there is no effect.

Dr. Louise Burke, Head, Department of Sports Nutrition, Australian Institute of Sport (1995, 131)

Because the digestibility of bee pollen is quite low, it is not a particularly useful food supplement. Athletes who are prone to allergies or who have a known reaction to pollen are advised to avoid bee pollen. Like many supplements, those promoted to athletes come and go quite quickly. Bee pollen has been out of favour since the 1990s.

Carnitine

Carnitine came to prominence when Italy won the 1982 FIFA World Cup because their players were supposedly on carnitine. Was it the carnitine that led to success? It seems more likely that Italy won because they were the best team in the tournament.

Carnitine is made in the liver from the amino acids lysine and methionine and stored in the heart and muscles. Carnitine is also in red meat and some dairy foods, with the average non-vegetarian diet providing 100 to 300 milligrams of carnitine each day.

Carnitine is commonly marketed as useful for body fat loss and appears in most products that claim to be fat mobilisers or fat metabolisers. Carnitine is necessary as part of the transport enzyme that carries fat into the mitochondria, the powerhouses of body cells. The theory is that carnitine can mobilise more fat into the mitochondria so it can be used as fuel and improve endurance and spare any protein breakdown as glycogen stores diminish. Taking the theory further, it was thought that increased burning of fat as a fuel could increase the rate of body fat loss. Unfortunately, the theory is not supported by research. Just because you can fill the mitochondria with more fat doesn't mean that the mitochondria will burn more fat. Muscle appears to have enough natural carnitine to work at maximal rates anyway, and carnitine supplements don't increase muscle carnitine levels; the extra is merely excreted.

In their review of the scientific literature, Moffat and Chelland (in Wolinsky and Driskell 2004) concluded that 'the majority of studies reveal that carnitine supplementation does not seem to provide an ergogenic benefit to human performance' (74). Since then, a study at the University of Stirling in Scotland on 20 male endurance athletes found no difference in the protein, fat and carbohydrate burned during the exercise when taking 2 grams of carnitine daily compared to a placebo (Broad, Maughan and Galloway 2008). It means that no extra fat was being burned or that protein stores were being protected by carnitine over the two-week study. Another study on 43 men and women over eight weeks also found no changes in either aerobic or anaerobic performance when comparing those on carnitine to those taking a placebo (Smith et al. 2008). As always, it might be that carnitine

has benefits under different circumstances, such as over a longer duration of supplementation or during recovery from heavy exercise, as other research has suggested.

There is no evidence that the body's supply of carnitine becomes depleted in heavy exercise. Carnitine supplementation does not improve sports performance or help weight loss. Evidence does suggest that supplemental carnitine can improve the work capacity of people with stable angina, but that is hardly useful to fit athletes.

With such disappointing results on sports performance throughout this century, it is no surprise that major sporting authorities do not recommend carnitine. It is likely that very little research will continue to be done on carnitine and exercise and, unless a surprising result is found in the future, interest in carnitine as a supplement for athletes will wane.

Chromium and Chromium Picolinate

Chromium, a metal, is a part of the glucose tolerance factor that helps insulin to work effectively to store glucose in muscles. This spawned the theory that chromium supplements might boost the glucose tolerance factor and improve the rate of glycogen storage after exercise. Because chromium also assists in protein metabolism, it got the attention of those wishing to increase muscle mass and strength. Sold mainly as chromium picolinate, it is also promoted as reducing body fat.

Chromium doesn't boost glycogen storage above normal rates. Giving 600 micrograms of chromium picolinate a day to healthy, but overweight, males did not improve their glycogen synthesis rates even when they were given adequate carbohydrate (Volek et al. 2006). Adding 1.8 grams of conjugated linoleic acid to 400 micrograms of chromium picolinate in a supplement did not change body composition or assist weight loss either (Diaz et al. 2008). Women taking the supplement for 12 weeks did not differ from those on the placebo in respect to total body weight or body fat. The reason for adding conjugated linoleic acid is that there had been some claims that it decreased body fat and increased muscle mass. That wasn't the case in this study.

It is generally agreed that chromium picolinate plays no significant role in weight loss. There is a patent for chromium picolinate. Being patented, however, doesn't mean that it is useful or meets its claims, just that it is different to other items. Even back in 1997 the patent holders in the United States were ordered by the Federal Trade Commission to stop making weight loss claims because they could not be substantiated.

High-quality research studies found no indication of an ergogenic effect in athletes from chromium supplementation. A study of 36 American footballers revealed that chromium picolinate supplements of 200 micrograms a day had no effect on muscle mass or strength or body fat levels (Clancy et al. 1994). This has been supported by all subsequent published research.

> The preponderance of evidence shows that chromium supplements will not increase lean body mass or decrease fat mass. Despite the widespread hype to the contrary.
>
> *Dr. Priscilla Clarkson, University of Massachusetts, USA (1997, 347)*

An adequate intake for chromium has been reliably estimated to be 35 micrograms for men and 25 micrograms for women. Good sources of chromium include meats, cheese, nuts, whole grains and brewer's yeast. Chromium intakes of up to 400 micrograms daily don't appear to be toxic.

As with many essential minerals, chromium supplementation is useful for those with diagnosed chromium deficiency. It appears that more chromium is lost in the urine during exercise than during rest days, but trained athletes may be able to conserve chromium better than non-athletes. Although there is continuing research on chromium as an ergogenic aid, the information gathered to date is not encouraging, and no major sporting authority has given supplements of chromium or chromium picolinate any backing at all.

Fat Mobilisers, Fat Metabolisers and Fat Transporters

Products claimed to be mobilisers, fat metabolisers and fat transporters do not help body fat loss at all. The only way to mobilise fat is to exercise and eat fewer kilojoules than you burn. Even if a supplement could magically mobilise fat, the fat would still need to be burned up with exercise. A tablet cannot get rid of body fat for you. Although such supplements can legally be on the market, you have to wonder how they can ethically be marketed as helping anyone lose weight without a skerrick of evidence to justify their use. Most contain carnitine, inositol, choline and other ingredients with no proven ability

to assist fat loss. Notice that advertisements for these products provide testimonials from people saying they lost weight while using them, along with a kilojoule-controlled diet and exercise. What do you think caused the weight loss? Give them a miss; it's as simple as that.

Ginseng

The root of the plant *Panax ginseng* has been used in China as a tonic for centuries. Its active ingredients are steroid glycosides called ginsenosides. Obtaining authentic ginseng is difficult and expensive; hence, the amount of ginsenosides greatly varies in commercial preparations; some have been found to have none at all.

Large doses of ginsenosides given to animals seem to increase endurance and promote muscle synthesis. This evidence has been hard to reproduce in human performance studies, possibly because commercial preparations of ginseng vary so much in quality and purity, and most research has been of poor quality. Although ginseng appears to be relatively safe, there have been reported adverse effects from its use, such as headaches, disturbed sleep and gastrointestinal upsets.

It was thought that ginseng increases growth hormone, testosterone and insulin-like growth factor and therefore has an anabolic effect on muscle size. There is no evidence that ginseng increases levels of these hormones. It has also been difficult to show any benefit of ginseng on either aerobic or anaerobic exercise, or on the recovery from either type of exercise. Although some research has suggested that ginseng may reduce stress and anxiety in animals, there is no evidence of a similar effect in healthy adults. Ginseng appeared to help with thinking in a laboratory setting, but this doesn't appear to assist athletes to perform better.

In a comprehensive review, Bahrke, Morgan and Stegner (2009) concluded that 'supplementation with ginseng does not improve physical performance and recovery of individuals undergoing exhaustive exercise' (316). This, the authors believe, is because a lot of research has flawed methods and it is difficult to get supplement samples with a guaranteed level of ginseng. There may also be interactions between the ginseng supplements and the diet or medications taken by athletes in the studies.

According to the U.S. Olympic Committee on Substance Abuse Research and Education, no scientific evidence supports the claim that ginseng enhances performance; hence, it is not banned by the International Olympic Committee.

Siberian ginseng is not ginseng at all; it is an entirely different plant called *Eleutherococcus senticosus*. There is no evidence that it is useful to athletic performance.

ZMA

ZMA is short for zinc magnesium aspartate, a concoction devised in the 1990s based on the view that zinc and magnesium in particular may be low in athletes, possibly because of increased losses in the sweat or a poor intake of these minerals. It would make sense that such a supplement would assist performance and, possibly, immune function. It is marketed mainly to athletes who do resistance exercise, especially bodybuilders. Very few studies have been done on ZMA, which makes it difficult to make a detailed assessment of its value to athletes.

The first study on ZMA showed encouraging results in footballers, but it drew criticism because one of the authors owned the laboratory that made ZMA (Brilla and Conte 2000). Later, a well-designed eight-week study of 42 resistance trained young men who were given either ZMA or a placebo, but didn't know which one they were receiving, showed no advantage in taking ZMA (Wilborn et al. 2004). Although blood levels of zinc increased in those given ZMA, there was no difference in body composition, muscle strength or endurance, or even in natural anabolic hormone levels. Both studies were on fit, well-trained men. We don't know whether ZMA may have helped the novice weight trainer. No sports authority would ever recommend a supplement based on two conflicting studies; that is why ZMA is not recommended.

Please remember that under the World Anti-Doping Code, all athletes are responsible for any substance found in their bodies, whether illegal or not, even if they believe it was a contaminant in a perfectly legal supplement. If you are randomly checked, be familiar with not only the World Anti-Doping Code, but also the supplement and drug regulations of your specific sport and your country. For example, the Australian Sports Anti-Doping Authority, the UK National Anti-Doping Policy and Drug Free Sport New Zealand all keep athletes up-to-date on permitted supplements and drug use. Just put those names into a search engine to find the websites for more information.

FINAL SCORE

- People vary greatly in their response to training, environmental conditions, psychological barriers and nutritional supplements, so it will always be difficult to assess the value of proposed ergogenic aids.

- Some products have proven ergogenic properties in some athletes under certain conditions. They are creatine, sports drinks, carbohydrate supplements, caffeine and bicarbonate.

- Based on current knowledge, the best regimen for achieving optimal performance is to avoid excess body fat, drink plenty of fluids to avoid dehydration, eat enough carbohydrate to fuel your training program, eat adequate protein for muscle growth and repair, and eat for good health. Most nutritional supplements do not enhance sports performance in well-nourished athletes.

- Be wary of the 'health assessment' or 'fitness program' that is designed to find faults in your health that can only be rectified by one or more supplements. Supplements are often better at making profits for their manufacturers than they are at enhancing sports performance.

- It is difficult to check the quantity and quality of the ingredients of many supplements that may contain 'natural' ingredients. In many cases, no analytical methods exist for verifying the contents.

- Caveat emptor (let the buyer beware). The current climate is that manufacturers can make claims for products, leaving it up to scientists to spend years of research to determine whether they work, whether they are safe and what the best dose is if they do appear to work.

Nutrition for Vegetarian Athletes

10

> Vegetarian athletes may be at risk for low intakes of energy, protein, fat, and key micronutrients such as iron, calcium, vitamin D, riboflavin, zinc, and vitamin B12. Consultation with a sports dietitian is recommended to avoid these nutrition problems.
>
> *Position of the American Dietetic Association, Dietitians of Canada and the American College of Sports Medicine: Nutrition and Athletic Performance (2009, 510)*

Athletes choose a vegetarian lifestyle for a range of reasons—taste, philosophy, religion, environment, cost and culture. Whatever your reason for being vegetarian, please don't choose to be vegetarian because someone has said that you will be instantly healthier. There is such a thing as an unhealthy vegetarian diet. French fries or chips, onion rings, cakes, biscuits and pastries can all fit into the definition of vegetarian, yet you wouldn't want to be eating too many of those types of food for long-term health. These foods are also high in fat and kilojoules, so vegetarian eating doesn't mean instant weight loss either.

Vegetarians are often proclaimed as being healthier than meat eaters. It is not the avoidance of meat that usually makes them healthier, though; it is their other lifestyle choices. Vegetarians are less likely to smoke or abuse alcohol and are more likely to be active and take an interest in their food and health. Vegetarians generally eat more fibre and less salt and saturated fat, which is part of the reason they have lower blood pressure and lower rates of heart disease than meat eaters do. At least one person in my family has been vegetarian for the last 25 years, so I have enjoyed vegetarian meals for a long time, including the famous beans on toast as a child.

In this discussion we must first determine what *vegetarian* means, because there are many types. If you avoid only red meat and processed meats such as ham and salami, you are not what we consider to be a vegetarian because you still enjoy poultry and fish. The main types of vegetarian follow.

Flexitarian Flexitarians are not classical vegetarians; many people now choose to eat this way. They eat a vegetarian diet for one to five days of the week, usually for environmental and philosophical reasons. The vegetarian days include eggs, milk, cheese and yogurt. The non-vegetarian days might include lean meat, chicken or fish. This has become a very popular style of eating, especially as people embrace the dishes of other cultures or follow trends such as meat-free Mondays. Flexitarian can easily get all their nutrients from the wide range of foods in their repertoire.

Lacto-Ovo-Vegetarian Lacto-ovo-vegetarianism is the most common type. In addition to fruits, vegetables, legumes and grains, lacto-ovo-vegetarians eat dairy products (lacto) and eggs (ovo). This diet is very popular with athletes and young people because it suits their beliefs about the need to safeguard the environment and is inexpensive. Virtually all restaurants and take-away outlets cater for this style of eating, making it easy to dine out. Likely the only nutrient of concern is iron because iron is less abundant and less easy to absorb from plant foods and eggs (dairy foods contain no iron).

Lacto-Vegetarian As the name implies, the lacto-vegetarian diet includes milk, yogurt and cheese, but not eggs. Although eggs are exceptionally nutritious, you should be able to get the nutrients found in eggs from other sources. For example, protein can come from milk, dairy, cheese, legumes, nuts and breakfast cereals.

Ovo-Vegetarian Ovo-vegetarianism is a vegetarian diet with eggs, but no dairy products. In the place of dairy, soy products are often consumed. People on this diet may lack calcium, riboflavin and possibly protein, unless a calcium-fortified soy beverage is substituted for milk. Dairy foods are easily the best source of calcium for humans. If you don't consume dairy products, you will need to take extra care to ensure that you get enough calcium in your diet. See table 10.1 for good sources of calcium for non-dairy consumers.

Vegan A vegan is a person who eats only plant foods (e.g., legumes, mushrooms, fruits, vegetables, nuts, grains, seeds) and does not eat any animal products at all. Vegan athletes are at risk for being low in vitamins B_{12}; the minerals iron, zinc and calcium; protein; and essential fatty acids. I would not recommend a vegan diet to children or teenagers because it could hinder growth and development. Pregnant and lactating athletes should get advice from a dietitian to ensure that both mother and baby are getting enough of the essential nutrients. Breast milk could be low in nutrients such as vitamin B_{12}, which will compromise the baby's development.

Other Styles There are other types of vegetarians, such as fruitarians and people on macrobiotic diets. There is no clear definition of a fruitarian. The diet consists mainly of fruits, nuts and seeds without animal products, vegetables or grains. For some, it includes honey and olive oil (a fruit oil). There is often little agreement as to what constitutes a fruit. Although capsicums (peppers) and cucumbers are fruits, some fruitarians don't eat them. A macrobiotic diet is extremely restrictive and limited to grains and vegetables. Both types of diet have many potential nutrient deficiencies because of their very restrictive nature. Neither is recommended for good health or sporting achievement, and they certainly aren't suited to children or teenagers.

This chapter considers the most common type of vegetarian—that is, the one who avoids animal flesh yet eats dairy foods (or at least calcium-fortified soy drinks) and eggs. I won't cover vegan, fruitarian or macrobiotic diets because athletes on these diets need special advice from a physician and a sports dietitian.

Nutrients and the Vegetarian Diet

The small amount of research on vegetarian athletes indicates that they perform equally as well as meat eaters and will have no trouble in meeting their sports nutrition goals of high carbohydrate, moderate protein and moderate fat. As the quote at the beginning of the chapter suggests, the vegetarian athlete has a slightly higher risk of being low in some nutrients, although in my experience, vegetarian athletes have a greater knowledge of, and greater interest in, nutrition and health, so they eat pretty well anyway. Their diet is usually higher in antioxidants and fibre from a higher consumption of fruit, vegetables

TABLE 10.1 Sources of Non-Dairy Calcium for Vegetarians

Food	Calcium (mg)
Calcium-fortified soy drink, 250 mL	300
Tofu, firm (calcium coagulant) 100 g	300
Tofu, soft (calcium coagulant) 100 g	80
Tempeh (fermented soy) 100 g	75
Bread, 1 slice	20
Bread, calcium fortified, 1 slice	60
English muffin, 1 whole	60
Breakfast cereal, calcium fortified, 40 g	200
Collard, 1/2 cup cooked	70
Tahini, 1 tbsp	65
Baked beans, 1 cup	80
Soybeans, 1/2 cup	65
Pak choi (bok choy), 1/2 cup cooked	80
Almonds, 30 g	70
Kidney beans, chick peas, 1/2 cup	50
Brazil nuts 30 g	45
Peanuts, 30 g	15
Peanut butter, 1 tbsp	10
Sunflower seeds, 20 g	20
Sesame seeds, 3 tbsp, 30 g	20
Egg, 1 whole, 50 g	20
Broccoli, 1 cup cooked	30
Dark chocolate, 50 g	25
Cocoa powder, 1 tbsp	25
Aktavite, Milo 20 g (note Milo has milk powder)	160
Molasses, blackstrap, 1 tbsp	40
Golden syrup, 1 tbsp	60
Bonox beef extract, 1 tbsp	20
Vegemite, 1 tbsp	13
Apricots, dried 20 g	13
Figs, dried 20 g	40
Basil, parsley fresh, 20 g	45
Tomato, sun dried, 20 g	20
Pasta, 1 cup	10
Rice, 1 cup	5

Sources: McCance & Widdowson's *The Composition of Foods*, 6th Summary Edition, Food Standards Agency; NUTTAB 2010 Food Standards Australia New Zealand; food labels.

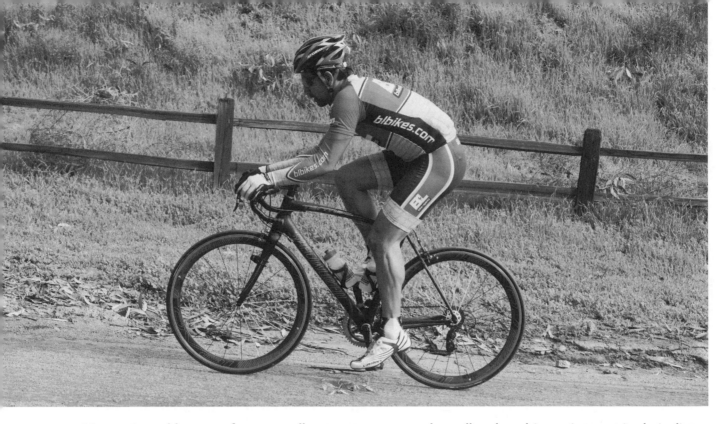

Vegetarian athletes perform as well as meat-eaters, and usually take a bigger interest in their diet.

and grain foods, while being lower in saturated fat and cholesterol. Let's take a look at each nutrient mentioned in the quote in association with the information on nutrition provided in chapters 1, 2 and 4 of this book.

Energy

Energy is the term given to kilojoules or calories. Some people become vegetarian to reduce their energy intake and lose weight. That is an admirable reason, but some take it too far by increasing the amount of training they do while following a rather spartan diet, or they find that they cannot eat enough food to match their training and experience unwanted weight loss. Too much weight loss in athletes becomes a problem because it affects their performance. This is more likely with a low-fat diet. Fruits and vegetables have a high water and fibre content so they are very filling while providing little energy. That's why they help people control their weight. The same holds true for legumes and whole-grain cereals—they're very filling.

If you are an endurance athlete training for 20 or more hours a week, you need to ingest some concentrated energy by doing things such as eating dried fruit, using extra oil in cooking or salad dressings, adding milk powder to yogurt or eating food bars. Fruit juice, nuts, tofu, cheese, peanut butter, tahini and avocados are other foods with a higher energy density. There are more ideas in chapter 12, which discusses muscle and weight gain.

If you are healthy and well and find that you are unintentionally losing weight, then you are not getting enough kilojoules to match your training and need to eat more energy-dense foods more frequently. (If you are unintentionally losing weight and not feeling well, then please see your doctor. Fit adults can still get medical conditions such as diabetes.)

Protein

First, let me make it clear that if you eat a well-balanced vegetarian diet, you are likely to be getting enough protein, even though it is thought that vegetarians need slightly more protein than meat eaters because plant protein is slightly less well digested than animal protein. Some plant protein doesn't get completely digested by the time it reaches the end of the small intestine, so it gets called 'resistant protein' meaning it is resistant to digestion. For this reason experts have recommended that highly trained vegetarian athletes eat 1.3 to 1.8 grams of protein per kilogram of body weight per day, slightly more than meat eaters. This is relatively easy to achieve by including milk, yogurt, cheese, soy foods, eggs and high-protein food bars.

In addition to eating adequate protein, vegetarians must also eat enough energy as carbohydrate and some fat to make sure the protein is performing its role of building and repairing muscle. If you begin to lose weight, then it is likely that your body is using some protein as an energy source and your muscles are beginning to break down.

Vegetarian protein alternatives based on soy protein are also very useful sources of protein (e.g., Sanitarium products and soy-based beverages). Table 10.2 lists some foods that are useful sources of protein in a vegetarian diet. Also use the protein guide in chapter 2 and the Nutrient Ready Reckoner in the appendix on page 215 to ensure that you are getting enough protein each day. If you weigh 80 kg (176 lb), then you need around 120 grams of protein each day.

It was long believed that vegetarians need to eat protein combinations (e.g., legumes with grains, such as baked beans on toast) in the same meal to meet all their amino acid needs. In chapter 2 you may recall that I said that was no longer the advice. As long as you eat a good range of protein sources each day, you will meet your amino acid needs.

TABLE 10.2 Sources of Protein for Vegetarians

Food	Protein (g)
Cheese, cheddar, 30 g	7.0
Milk, 200 mL	7.0
Soy milk, 200 mL	7.0
Yogurt, 200 mL, average per serve	10.0
Ice cream, 1 scoop	2.0
Egg, 1 whole, 50 g	7.0
Bread, 1 slice	3.0
Breakfast cereal, 1 serve, average	4.0
Weetabix, 2	5.0
Porridge, 1 cup	4.0
Vegetables, 1/2 cup, average	1.0
Peas, green, 1/2 cup	4.5
Sweet potato, cooked, 1/2 cup	2.0
Mushrooms, 1/2 cup	1.5
Potato, baked, 1	3.0
Kidney beans, lentils, chick peas, 1/2 cup	7.0
Fruit, 1 serve, average	1.0
Pasta, cooked, 1 cup	8.0
Pasta sauce, 1/2 cup, average	2.0
Rice, cooked, 1 cup	5.0
Fruit cake, 1 slice, 50 g	2.0
Muesli and nut bar, 40 g	3.5
Cereal bar, average	2.0
Protein sports bars, 60 g	18.0
Sustagen Sport, 1 flat tbsp, 15 g	3.0
Nuts, 30 g, average	4.0
Peanut butter, 1 tbsp (30 g)	7.0
Tahini, 30 g	6.0
Milk chocolate, 50 g	4.0
Popcorn, 1 cup	1.0

There are more protein figures in the Nutrient Ready Reckoner in the appendix at the end of the book.

Fat

Fat is included in the opening quote only because many vegetarian athletes also follow a low-fat diet. Although low-fat milk is a good choice because it often has more calcium than regular milk, the main concern is that vegetarians eating too little fat can have difficulty meeting the energy needs of a rigorous training schedule. As mentioned earlier in the chapter, if you find you are losing weight, or finding it very difficult to maintain weight and increase muscle mass, then you are probably getting too few kilojoules, or calories. One simple way to add extra energy to your diet is to include more polyunsaturated or monounsaturated oil and margarine in your cooking or on bread and toast. Nuts, seeds and avocados are also good sources of healthy fats.

Because vegetarians avoid fish, they could be getting insufficient omega-3 fats (fish oil). They have the option of taking fish oil as a supplement (1,000 mg of omega-3 fats) or including dietary sources of alpha-linolenic acid (ALA) such as flaxseed, walnuts, eggs, green leafy vegetables, canola oil and soy (National Heart Foundation of Australia 2009). The ALA can be converted to omega-3 fats in the body. Some foods have been fortified with fish oils (e.g., milk, food bars, bread and breakfast cereal), so consider including them in your diet if it suits your reason for being vegetarian.

Iron, Zinc and Vitamin B$_{12}$

Iron is very important for athletes because it is part of haemoglobin and myoglobin, critical molecules in the delivery of oxygen to active muscles. Low iron stores results in decreased sports endurance and performance.

Iron is often mentioned as a nutrient of concern in vegetarians for three reasons:

1. The iron in plant food is less easy to absorb from the gut than iron in animal foods; that is, the iron is less bioavailable.

2. Most vegetarians are young women who have the highest need for iron and are at the highest risk for too little iron.

3. Vegetarians generally have lower iron stores when compared to meat eaters, even if they have similar iron intakes.

Although there is plenty of iron in plant foods, the body is unable to absorb much of it because of the presence of compounds that can bind tightly to the iron so it cannot be absorbed (e.g., oxalates, phytates). Because spinach is high in oxalates, it is not a good source of iron, despite what you may have heard. Spinach is, however, a good source of beta-carotene and folate, so don't be thinking it has no place in your diet.

In addition to the lower bioavailability of iron from plant foods, the iron is present as non-heme iron, which first needs to be converted to heme iron before it can be absorbed. There is little you can do to make iron easier to absorb if it is bound to oxalate or phytate, but you can eat vitamin C–containing foods (e.g., salad vegetables, fruit and fruit juices) to help convert non-heme iron to heme iron.

Australia's National Health and Medical Research Council (NHMRC) states that: 'Absorption [of iron] is about 18% from a mixed western diet including animal foods and about 10% from a vegetarian diet; so vegetarians will need intakes about 80% higher' (NHMRC 2006, 189). That means that vegetarian athletes need to be extra vigilant in choosing high-iron foods. A vegetarian male athlete could need 14 milligrams of iron daily, and a female vegetarian athlete, up to 32 milligrams. Although male vegetarians can easily meet their iron needs through smart food choices, female vegetarian athletes may need the assistance of an iron supplement, because their iron needs are very high. I would strongly recommend that all athletes have their iron levels checked to determine whether they are truly low in iron before taking any iron supplementation. As I explained in chapter 4, around 1 in 250 people have a condition called hemochromatosis, in which their high levels of iron cause fatigue. Taking additional iron in this situation is very dangerous to health.

Many iron-fortified foods are on the market. A lot of breakfast cereals are now iron fortified, and a reasonable athlete-sized serve provides 6 milligrams of iron, about 20 per cent of the needs of a vegetarian woman aged 19 to 50, and about half of the needs of a vegetarian man. Powdered food drinks, Milo and soy drinks often have added iron. If you are constantly tired despite eating well, it is worthwhile getting your iron levels tested. If you are low in iron, you will require an iron supplement to quickly raise your iron stores, and you will need to modify your meals to include more iron-containing foods. See table 10.3 for non-meat sources of iron.

Because zinc is more common in, and more bioavailable from, animal flesh, and with vitamin B$_{12}$ coming mainly from animal foods

TABLE 10.3 Sources of Iron for Vegetarians

Food	Iron (mg)
Breakfast cereal, 45 g	2.0–3.0
Vegetable juice, 200 mL	2.0
Tofu, firm, 50 g	1.4
Bread, whole-grain, 1 slice	0.8
English muffin, 50 g	1.0
Muesli, natural, 1 cup	3.5
Porridge, 1 cup	1.8
Fresh fruit, average serve	0.3
Gnocchi, cooked, 1 cup	0.8
Pasta, cooked, 1 cup	0.6
Rice, cooked, 1 cup	0.6
Chocolate, dark, 50 g	2.2
Milk chocolate with nuts, 50 g	0.8
Licorice, 30 g	2.6
Fruit, fresh, average serve	0.3
Vegetables, cooked, 1/2 cup, average	0.5
Tofu, firm, 50 g	1.4
Egg, 50 g	1.0
Milo powder, 1 tbsp	3.0
Drinking chocolate, 200 mL	0.4
Baked beans, lentils, dal, 1 cup	2.5
Falafel, 3 pieces	1.8
Tabouleh, 1/2 cup	0.8
Tahini, 30 g	1.5
Sesame seeds, sunflower seeds, 30 g	1.3
Almonds, 30 g	1.2
Cashews, 30 g	1.5
Peanuts, 30 g	0.3
Peanut butter, 30 g	0.4
Muesli bar, 40 g, average	0.8
Broccoli, cooked, 1 cup	0.9
Asparagus, 4 spears	0.8
Avocado, 50 g	0.3
Mushroom, stir-fried, 100 g	0.5
Sustagen Sport, powder 15 g	3.2

Sources: Food Standards Agency (2002) McCance and Widdowson's The Composition of Food, Sixth summary edition. Cambridge: Royal Society of Chemistry. NUTTAB 2010 Online Searchable Database; Food Standards Australia New Zealand.

(mushrooms contain a modest amount), these two nutrients are listed as being at risk of being lacking in vegetarians. It is rare to see an obvious zinc deficiency in vegetarians. Zinc can be found in cheese (a lesser amount in milk and yogurt), eggs, grains, legumes, seeds, nuts, peanut butter, wheat germ, Vegemite, Marmite, dark chocolate and muesli bars. There is a small, but appreciable, amount in vegetables, especially green peas.

As with iron and calcium, compounds in plant food, such as phytates and oxalates, may inhibit the absorption of zinc from the diet. We are all encouraged to eat plenty of fibre, yet these same foods can also make it a bit harder to absorb iron and zinc, so ensure that you are eating plenty of zinc-containing foods. Men require about 14 milligrams a day of zinc; women, about 12 milligrams a day. Table 10.4 shows the zinc content of some vegetarian foods.

Vitamin B_{12}, vital for healthy blood, is found in all animal foods including dairy foods and eggs, and a few breakfast cereals and soy drinks are fortified with B_{12}. Fresh mushrooms also provide a modest amount. If a food is fortified with vitamin B_{12}, then the vitamin will be listed in the nutrition information panel. Vitamin B_{12} is also found in some spreads such as Marmite. People need around 2.4 micrograms of B_{12} each day, which can easily be achieved by consuming dairy and eggs. Table 10.5 (page 158) lists the vitamin B_{12} content of non-meat foods. Vitamin B_{12} deficiency is more likely in vegans and those on very restrictive vegetarian diets, such as fruitarians; these people should take a vitamin B_{12} supplement if they don't include foods fortified with vitamin B_{12} in their diets.

Iron is covered in more detail in chapter 4, and minerals and vitamins in general are covered in chapter 1.

Calcium, Vitamin D and Riboflavin

Calcium, vitamin D and riboflavin are more likely to be low in those following very restrictive vegetarian diets such as the vegan diet. Most vegetarians consuming dairy foods or calcium-fortified soy drinks, and getting enough sunshine, do fine on the calcium, riboflavin and vitamin D front. Those avoiding dairy foods find it very difficult to meet their calcium needs and may require a calcium supplement because few other foods provide a concentrated source of calcium unless they are calcium fortified, such as some soy beverages and breakfast cereals.

Calcium absorption (bioavailability) is lower from vegetable foods (including soy products) than it is from dairy foods. For example, spinach may appear to be a good source of calcium, but much of this calcium is bound to oxalate and is not bioavailable. Low-oxalate vegetables such as broccoli are better sources of calcium.

Calcium and vitamin D are particularly important for healthy bones. The generally higher fruit and vegetable intake of vegetarians tends to result in less calcium loss from bones, whereas a high salt intake increases bone loss. You may recall from chapter 4 that eating a high-salt diet increases the loss of calcium from the bones via losses in the urine. Calcium losses are also high in female athletes who have stopped menstruating as the result of an intense training program.

Look for foods that are calcium fortified to get your calcium needs. Many milks are calcium fortified; if you are not a milk drinker, then look to calcium-fortified soy drinks, calcium-set tofu, fruit juice and breakfast cereals. Refer to table 10.1 (page 151) for non-dairy sources of calcium (dairy sources are listed in table 4.2 on page 57).

Vitamin D greatly assists the body in the absorption of calcium from the intestines. If your training or work keeps you inside for most of the day, then you may not be getting enough sunlight to generate adequate vitamin D. In that case you must rely on dietary sources such as margarine, cheese and sunlight-exposed mushrooms, or a vitamin D supplement, for your daily vitamin D. Vitamin D supplements commonly provide 25 micrograms (1,000 IU) in a single capsule.

Riboflavin is abundant in milk, yogurt, eggs, breakfast cereals, yeast extracts, almonds and Brazil nuts, so most vegetarians find it easy to meet their riboflavin needs. Riboflavin may be lacking in those who follow the more strict versions of vegetarianism (e.g., fruitarians).

Calcium is covered in more detail in chapter 4, and vitamins in general are covered in chapter 1.

Supplements

Vegetarians are often told that they cannot get enough nutrition through a diet based on plant foods, dairy and eggs. You can see that with a judicious choice of foods, vegetarians can be just as well nourished as anyone else. You may want to take a multivitamin supplement, but if you do, choose one that provides 50 to 100 per cent of your daily needs in a tablet. You won't need any more than that, and probably only

TABLE 10.4 Sources of Zinc for Vegetarians

Food	Zinc (mg)
Drinking chocolate, cocoa, Milo, 200 mL	1.0
Soy milk, 200 mL	0.8
Tofu, firm, 50 g	0.8
Bread roll, whole-grain, 50 g	0.5
English fruit muffin, 50 g	0.5
Muesli, natural, 1 cup	1.3
Breakfast cereal, 50 g	0.7–2.0
Gnocchi, cooked, 1 cup	0.3
Pasta, cooked, 1 cup	0.5
Chocolate, dark, 50 g	0.5
Milk chocolate with nuts, 50 g	0.8
Cheddar cheese, 30 g	1.0
Milk, plain or flavoured, 240 mL	1.0
Yogurt, 200 mL	1.2
Egg, 1 whole, 50 g	0.6
Fresh fruit, average, 1 serve	0.2
Baked beans, lentils, dal, 1 cup	1.0
Falafel, 3	1.0
Tabouleh, hummus, 1/2 cup	0.3
Tahini, 30 g	1.5
Sesame seeds, sunflower seeds, 30 g	1.5
Almonds, 30 g	1.0
Cashews, 30 g	1.5
Peanuts, 30 g	0.8
Muesli bar, 40 g average	0.4
Broccoli, cooked, 1 cup	0.6
Green beans, green peas, 1/2 cup	0.8
Avocado, 50 g	0.3
Mushroom, stir-fried, 100 g	1.0
Sustagen Sport, powder, 15 g	2.2
Breakfast cereal, fortified, 50 g	1.8

Sources: Food Standards Agency (2002) McCance and Widdowson's The Composition of Food, Sixth summary edition. Cambridge: Royal Society of Chemistry. NUTTAB 2010 Online Searchable Database; Food Standards Australia New Zealand.

TABLE 10.5 Sources of Vitamin B$_{12}$ for Vegetarians

Food	Vitamin B$_{12}$ (mcg)
Egg, 1 whole, 50 g	0.6
Milk, average, 240 mL	2.0
Yogurt, average, 100	0.3
Cheese, cheddar, 30 g	0.7
Cheese, camembert, 30 g	0.3
Cottage cheese, 30 g	0.2
So Good soy milk, 240 mL	1.0
Up&Go, 240 mL	1.0
Bread, 2 slices, average	0.15
Milk chocolate with nuts, 50 g	0.2
Milk chocolate, 50 g	0.15
Licorice, 50 g	0.15
Mushroom, 100 g	0.01–0.1
Sustagen Sport, powder, 15 g	1.0
Vegemite, 2 tsp (Marmite)	1.0

Sources: Food Standards Agency (2002) McCance and Widdowson's The Composition of Food, Sixth summary edition. Cambridge: Royal Society of Chemistry. NUTTAB 2010 Online Searchable Database; Food Standards Australia New Zealand.

one every second day if it is a high-dose vitamin supplement. Seek advice from a sports dietitian to determine whether you need a mineral supplement as well, especially if you have a very restricted diet, because iron, calcium and zinc may be compromised.

If you have read chapter 9 on supplements for sports performance, you realise that both creatine and beta-alanine can offer benefits to athletes involved in sprint training or resistance exercise such as weightlifting. Both creatine and carnosine (made using beta-alanine) levels are lower in the muscles of vegetarians when compared to meat eaters, so taking them as a supplement for high-intensity exercise would likely be beneficial. Here is an important warn-ing: Sports supplements are generally expensive and are better suited to athletes who are trying to reach elite level rather than those exercising for fitness and health.

Performance

There is no evidence that a vegetarian athlete will perform better or worse than a meat-eating athlete, assuming they are both well nourished. Put another way, becoming vegetarian will not necessarily improve your performance. If your consumption of protein, carbohydrate, vitamins and minerals meets those recommended to athletes, then you will have the nutrition to perform at your best.

FINAL SCORE

- Most vegetarians easily meet their nutrition goals by consuming dairy foods, eggs, and calcium-fortified soy drinks.

- Because a vegetarian diet may provide less energy than a meat-rich diet, endurance vegetarian athletes may not consume adequate energy. They may need to increase the energy density of their meals and snacks.

- Protein needs should be easily met by vegetarian athletes who includes milk, yogurt, cheese, soy, eggs, legumes and grains in their diet.

- To get enough omega-3 fats, vegetarian athletes need to include foods fortified with fish oils and eat foods that contain the fat alpha-linolenic acid.

- Because the best sources of iron, zinc and vitamin B_{12} are of animal origin, the vegetarian athlete needs to make judicious food choices to get enough of these nutrients.

- Calcium, riboflavin and vitamin D needs should be easily met by consuming dairy foods and calcium-fortified soy drinks for calcium; dairy foods, eggs, meats, breads and breakfast cereals for riboflavin; and by eating vitamin D–fortified foods, eggs, margarine, oily fish and light-exposed mushrooms, as well as by getting adequate sun exposure, for vitamin D.

- Seek advice about the need to take a specific nutrient or nutritional supplements.

- Because creatine and carnosine levels are generally lower in the muscles of vegetarians compared with those of meat eaters, supplements of creatine and beta-alanine may benefit elite vegetarian athletes involved in sprint training and resistance exercise such as weight training.

Meal Tips for Restaurants and Road Trips

> When we went on the road, we ate as a team, so I had to eat the Japanese stuff. All kinds of stuff: moving stuff, live stuff, stinky stuff, ugly stuff. I talked to the interpreter to make sure they had some fried chicken or else I would have starved.
>
> *Brian Williams, Chicago Cubs baseball pitcher on his return from a season in Japan (2000)*

It is not always convenient to prepare all your own meals and snacks. Often you will have to eat on the road, at airport terminals or at restaurants. Sometimes, like Brian Williams, you may have to make arrangements to have your style of food available. It is still important that you keep to your nutrition goals for optimal performance. This chapter is a guide to making the best choices when you cannot prepare your own meals.

Snacks

Your mother was right—one of the best snack foods is a piece of fruit for its carbohydrate, vitamins, fibre and antioxidants, all at a very good price. The only thing going against fruit is that it doesn't always travel well on hot days and can be easily bruised. This can be overcome by storing it in a cooler bag. Another snack favourite with athletes is the food bar, and a great variety is available. Many food bars are low in total fat and saturated fat. If nuts or seeds are added, the fat is higher. Of course, nuts and seeds are healthy ingredients, and their fat is mainly unsaturated.

Some snacks have added sugar, possibly in the form of honey, to improve the taste, thus raising the carbohydrate content. This should not cause alarm because fit people can afford some kilojoules as sugar, and the extra carbohydrate will be burned during training and sport. Table 11.1 lists the highs and lows of various snacks' nutritional values.

Take-Aways

With some smart thinking you can choose a better class of take-away, which includes fast food and carry-out food. Some are not the perfect choice, but in a tight situation they can still keep you on track for a good dose of your daily carbohydrate and essential nutrient needs. Many franchised take-aways are now offering salad bars, fruit, vegetarian meals and a range of low-fat choices. Importantly, most of the franchised chains provide the nutrition profiles online or

TABLE 11.1 Snack Guide

Food	Higher nutritional value	Lower nutritional value
Fruit	• The fastest food around. Choose your favourite. Canned fruit and dried fruit are also good choices.	• Fruit juice because of minimal fibre (however, still a good source of carbohydrate and water).
Food bars	• There are low-fat versions of fruit bars, muesli bars, sports bars, and breakfast bars. Recommend less than 4 g fat and more than 20 g carbohydrate per food bar weighing 30–45 g.	• Coated food bars such as yogurt and chocolate coating because they usually have a high saturated fat coating (i.e., are not real yogurt or real chocolate; compound chocolate is less healthy than good-quality chocolate).
Milk	• Flavoured milk. (Most flavoured milks are based on reduced-fat milk. Sure, they have some sugar, but not enough to diminish the value of the milk nutrients.) • Reduced-fat and non-fat milk. Make a smoothie with fresh or canned fruit or flavouring for carbohydrate and taste.	• Full-cream milk (still nutritious, but higher in fat).
Bread and bread rolls	• Fruit bread rolls with dried fruit. • Whole-grain breads because they have fibre—they take longer to chew and are more filling. • Bread rolls, Lebanese bread, pita bread, Turkish bread.	• Rolls with cheese, bacon and other savoury flavourings. • White breads. • Croissants.
Muffins	• Plain English muffins to which you can add your own spread. • Sweet muffins.	• Savoury muffins with fatty ingredients.
Nuts	• Plain, unsalted.	• Roasted and salted.
Take-aways	• See Dining Out Guide (table 11.2) on page 164.	
Sandwiches	• See Dining Out Guide (table 11.2) on page 164.	

in-store for their entire menu. Check the profiles to identify the lower-fat and lower-salt choices. Check the energy (kJ or cal) content if you are watching your waistline. Here are some suggestions for healthier fast foods.

Still Number One   The most popular take-away of all time is the sandwich or bread roll. Ask for little or no margarine if you are watching your waist, and get them to reduce the fatty fillings such as cheese. Lean fillings with plenty of salad is the best way to go.

Fowled Out   Take a precooked chicken home, remove the skin and serve with micro-waved vegetables or salad and bread. The breast meat is lowest in fat. Finish with some canned fruit and a little ice cream. A dead-easy meal.

Rice Is Nice   Steamed rice is available from every Asian or Chinese take-away. To this carbohydrate source, add some lean meat or seafood for protein, and some vegetables. You can add a steamed spring roll for variety.

Veg Out   Any meal that is high in vegetables is likely to have less fat and more carbohydrate than a meat-dominated meal. Corn and peas are filling, low in fat and high in carbohydrate. Don't add butter or margarine if you need to restrict your fat intake. Ask for plenty of vegetables, or vegetable-based foods, when getting a take-away (but not just hot chips and fries!).

Pasta Lasta Longa   Pasta is always a favourite with athletes. Make sure you get a big serve if you are doing lots of training, and ask them to reduce the oil. The topping is crucial—a tomato- or seafood-based sauce has less fat than other sauces. Remember, only a sprinkle of cheese on top.

Pie-Eyed   Meat pies and pork pies are still popular in Australia and the UK. Fortunately, some lower-fat types are becoming available, and although lower in fat than in the past, they aren't a great source of carbohydrate. Athletes need to supplement a pie with fruit, fruit juice or a fruit bun. A vegetable pie or pastie can be a good choice because they are often lower in fat than meat pies.

Chewing Your Spud   The baked potato is making a comeback! Try toppings such as baked beans, coleslaw, salsa and creamed corn. Go light on the cheese topping. This makes a great, inexpensive meal.

Pizza Hit   The best pizza choices are those with a vegetarian, pineapple or seafood topping.

You could ask for less cheese to get the fat content even lower. Beware of fatty toppings such as cabanossi and other fatty meats. And remember that you can easily make your own pizza at home with frozen pizza base, pasta sauce and your favourite toppings.

Remove the Fat of the Land   Try removing the following from take-away foods:

- Skin from chicken
- Batter from fish
- Excess fat from meat

Tijuana Tucker   If you go Mexican, aim for a burrito or enchilada with salad, lean meat, chicken or beans. Corn chips with cheese and sour cream may taste great, but they have a lot more fat than carbohydrate.

Lebanese, Please   You might have to do some negotiating here. Kebabs, cabbage rolls, tabouleh, vegetarian kibbi and flat bread are the best choices. Beware of any dish that's fried or deep-fried. Often you can choose 'wet' dishes made from potatoes, beans, lentils or rice. Hummus and baba ghannouj are popular. Eat these with plenty of rice or bread.

Salad Days   The popularity of the salad bar is on the rise. The response to the obesity issue has meant that many take-away outlets now offer fresh fruit and a range of salads. Some offer a decent breakfast, too. Take advantage of this trend.

Have the Day Off!   There is no harm in eating the occasional fatty meal especially if you are more than a couple of days away from competition. Make sure your eating habits improve before the big event. The more often you stray from wholesome eating, the more likely you will be to deep-fry your chances of success. It's your decision.

Tips for Dining Out

More and more restaurants now offer lower-fat, 'light' meals to patrons, making it a little easier to eat well when away from home. Table 11.2 (page 164) is a guide to making dining out fit into your health and performance goals. Enjoy the experience.

Wait Staff Don't Bite!   Feel comfortable asking the wait staff for information about the menu. You can also ask them to make simple changes if possible: 'The grilled fish is fine, but

TABLE 11.2 Dining Out Guide

Food	Higher nutritional value	Lower nutritional value
Sandwiches and rolls	• Fillings: Lean meat, salmon, tuna, chicken breast, turkey, baked beans, banana, cottage cheese, ricotta, salad vegetables. • Go easy on the margarine or butter. • Whole-grain roll if possible.	• Fillings: luncheon meats (e.g., salami), hard cheese, cream cheese, sausages.
Chicken	• Remove skin and stuffing. Breast meat is lowest in fat.	• Deep fried, battered or crumbed pieces. • Chicken nuggets.
Burgers	• Hamburgers with grilled meat patty and lots of salad.	• Burgers with fried meat patties, cheese and bacon. • Battered and deep-fried fillings.
Chips, fries	• Smallest serve with large size chips/fries/wedges! (Large chips/fries/wedges have a lower fat content per weight compared to thin varieties.)	• Thin chips, fries, wedges. • Thin chips have more fat.
Pizza	• Vegetarian, lean meat or seafood topping; minimal cheese.	• Fatty toppings such as salami, bacon, cabanossi, cheese. • Garlic bread.
Pastries, pies	• Pasties, pies and shepherd's pies, and other pastries with less than 10% fat (10 g per 100 g).	• Pies, pasties, croissants, sausage rolls, hot dogs, and chips • Any deep-fried foods
Seafood	• Grilled fish, steamed shellfish and seafood.	• Battered fish. • Cream and fatty sauces.
Indian and Asian	• Steamed rice, vegetable-based dishes, lean meat, seafood, clear soups, noodles, steamed spring rolls and steamed dim sims, dal, lentils, curries (minimal fat), naan bread.	• Fried rice or fried noodles, deep-fried and battered dishes such as sweet and sour pork, duck. • Fried dim sims, excess satay sauce.
Lebanese	• Souvlakia, kebabs, flat bread, salad, cabbage roll, tabouleh, vegetarian kibbi, lady fingers.	• Felafel, fried kibbi, hummus and baba ghannouj (all nutritious but moderate fat). • Any fried or high-oil food.
Italian	• Pasta with tomato, seafood or pesto sauce—low oil, minestrone soup, plain bread, salad, pizza with minimal fat such as vegetarian or seafood	• Lasagne; cannelloni; cream, butter and cheese sauces such as alfredo; garlic bread; pizza with fatty meats and excess cheese.
Mexican	• Taco, burrito or enchilada with salad; fish, lean meat, chicken, beans; gazpacho; salsa.	• Dishes with cheese, sour cream or refried beans; nachos; corn chips.

Food	Higher nutritional value	Lower nutritional value
Salad bars	• All salads, vinaigrette dressing, fruit salad, whole-grain bread, baked potato, corn cobs.	• High-fat salad dressings and mayonnaise, cream, sour cream.
Potato	• Baked potato (minimum sour cream or cheese). • Toppings: baked beans, cottage cheese, coleslaw, avocado and tomato, creamed corn.	• Hot chips, french fries (wedges are a better choice). • Potato cakes, potato scallops.
Family restaurant	• See advice for above foods. • Most soups are also low in fat. • Fruit salad and fruit platter for dessert.	• See advice for above foods.
Drinks	• Water, mineral water and diet soft drinks are the best choices if you are controlling body fat.	• Regular soft drinks, fruit juice, sensible amounts of alcohol.
Dessert	• Low-fat frozen yogurt, fruit salad, low-fat ice cream.	• Sweet pastries, cakes, ice cream.

please leave off the butter sauce'. Beware of the grease factor. Cheese, cream and oil can add lots of fat to a meal.

Be Fruitful   Eat one or two pieces of fruit before you go out. Then you won't arrive at the restaurant so hungry that you forget all your good intentions.

Get Wet   Ask for a jug of water to quench your thirst before you order other drinks. Drink water, mineral water, juice or a soft drink between alcoholic drinks. Choose a broth or a clear soup if you need to boost your fluids after a solid day of training. Drink alcohol sparingly, especially when you are close to competition—remember that it's a dehydrating fluid.

Read That Menu   Descriptions that include the words *pan-fried, butter sauce, cream sauce, sautéed, fried, battered* and *creamed* are dead give-aways for a high-fat meal. It's easy to ask for the sauce to be left off.

Beware the Smorgasbord Monster!   A smorgasbord demands that you have a little bit of everything until your plate is so loaded you can't see the first three selections you made. This can easily lead to overeating. So, try three or four choices at first and go back for more later if you're still hungry. Here, I shall mention the Japanese expression *Hara hachi bu*. It translates to: 'Eat until you are 80 per cent full', meaning 'Don't eat until you are bloated just because

there is plenty of food available'. The key is self-control and self-respect.

Well Bread   Many athletes eat more food than sedentary people do. The bread roll is a useful adjunct to any athlete's meal. Ask for extra bread rolls if necessary, especially if the meal has been delayed and will be served well past your usual eating time. Bread can also supplement a low-carbohydrate meal.

Salacious Salads and Voracious Vegetables   Salad bars are usually inexpensive. Very active people can fill up on salads made from rice, pasta, potato or beans for a carbohydrate base. Order salads without oil and fatty dressings. Although side salads are very nutritious, they are generally low in carbohydrate. If the main course comes with vegetables, ask for extra potato, peas and corn to meet your carbohydrate needs.

Welcome Asia   Asian meals are always a good value for health. Get plenty of steamed rice, stir-fried vegetables, lean meat or seafood. Ask for extra steamed rice if you are hungry; don't fill up on greasy food.

What's Your Perspective?   If you have been eating plenty of carbohydrate at breakfast and lunch, then don't be fanatical about the carbohydrate in an occasional meal out. For example, a meal of grilled fish and salad is good nutrition and although it is low in carbohydrate, you may have made up for this earlier in the day. Life and sport are meant to be enjoyed. Just make sure that you eat plenty of carbohydrate at the next meal and in the two days before sports events.

On-the-Road Nutrition

Eating while on the road is a very personal affair, as demonstrated in the opening quote of the chapter. Travelling to compete in sport usually signals the culmination of all your training. Unfortunately, travel can often mean delays, different time zones, take-away or restaurant foods and uncomfortable beds. Whether you're travelling overseas or interstate, or spending a couple of hours in the car, your aim is to arrive as fresh as a gazelle ready to produce the performance of a lifetime. Following are some tips to maintain your nutrition goals when travelling. You may already be happy with what you arrange to eat. The following may help you refine your food choices to get the best out of your body while on your travels.

Plan Ahead   If possible, travel so that you can keep close to your normal routine and try to avoid travel that causes you to rise too early or stay up too late. This becomes more important when you're flying (see the section Minimise Jet Lag). If you are travelling somewhere with a restricted or unreliable range of foods, then it's worth taking a daily multivitamin supplement with you.

Take Your Own Feed Bag   You might decide to bring your own meals rather than rely on hotels and take-aways. Grab your own breakfast cereal and milk (there are reduced-fat versions of powdered milk and UHT milk—ideal if you don't have refrigeration). Breakfast bars, muesli bars, fruit bars, liquid meals (e.g., Up&Go), fresh fruit, dried fruit, nuts, canned fruit and fruit juice all travel well.

Minimise the Strain   Long hours of travel can upset your digestive system. Low-fibre meals, combined with being seated for long hours, can block your down-pipe. To minimise constipation, eat fibre-rich foods such as fresh fruit, fruit salad, whole-grain bread, breakfast cereals and vegetables.

Don't Starve   When travelling by car, bus or train, don't let yourself get too hungry or the first fast-food outlet you see might tempt you to make less-than-wise choices. Take some snacks with you such as fruit, sandwiches and low-fat muesli bars.

Don't Overeat   Because you are not active when you travel, you need less food than on training days. Don't confuse boredom with hunger or you will overeat—a big problem in sports with a weight limit. Some major event venues provide athletes with unlimited amounts of a big range of food, which makes it very easy to eat more than normal. You will need to consciously control your eating.

Feast Without Fear   You may have to eat lots of meals from restaurants and take-aways when on the road. Ask for plenty of steamed rice, pasta, bread or potatoes to provide enough carbohydrate, with vegetables and fruit for fibre. See table 11.2 for more ideas on the best choices when on the road. Contact the hotel at your destination a week or so before you travel to ensure that they have, or are willing to have, your favourite foods or meals. I used to deal with the catering managers of hotels around Australia to make sure they knew the key nutrition requirements of travelling athletes and teams.

This Is No Holiday   Travelling for competition can often take on a holiday atmosphere, especially for a new destination, pushing good nutrition to one side. Your goal is still to eat mainly wholesome, least-processed foods. Ask the people serving you for assistance when choosing from a menu. It's no problem for them to go light on the margarine or hold the cheese sauce.

Minimise Jet Lag

Airline travel can be arduous. On long trips that cross time zones, your 24-hour biological time clock, or circadian rhythm (from *circa diem*, Latin for 'about 24 hours'), becomes disrupted. This condition is called circadian dysrhythmia, or jet lag.

More than 300 bodily functions occur with a 24-hour rhythm. These functions normally have high and low points during the 24-hour period, corresponding to a sleep–wake cycle. For example, body temperature (which peaks at around 6 p.m.), heart rate (which is higher in the afternoon), and the stomach (which empties more quickly in the morning than in the evening) all have a circadian rhythm. Your performance can be affected by this sleep–wake cycle. Most people seem to be at their peak between 11 a.m. and 4 p.m., so it is no surprise that most world records are set in the afternoon.

Your circadian rhythm resynchronises at a rate of around 90 minutes a day after westward travel across time zones, and 60 minutes a day after eastward travel. This explain why jet lag seems more apparent after travelling east, when we 'lose time' and the body clock resynchronises more slowly, than it is after travelling west, when we 'gain time'.

Change Your Body Clock Time When travelling across time zones, some people adjust their body clocks to their destination time in the two or three days before departure. On arrival they can quickly adopt local times for eating and sleeping. This can be very effective when crossing one to four time zones. For example, if you are travelling east, gradually get up earlier each morning so that you are one or two hours closer to your destination time zone. Getting sunlight early in the morning also helps this transition. Do the reverse if you are travelling west. Adjust to getting up later before you leave and expose yourself to bright sunlight in the evening if possible so that your body feels like it is closer to your destination time zone.

Natural daylight is important for adjusting the body clock. Exposure to light early in the morning advances your body clock so it feels like it is farther east, hence the reason to get up earlier and get some early morning sun before you travel east. Light in the evening helps your body feel more like it is farther west (Reilly et al. 2007).

If you move into a different time zone for only a day or two, keep to your regular home time zone so you don't have to change your body clock twice in 48 hours.

When travelling to another country, the first thing to do on arrival is to forget what time it is in your home country. As soon as you get on the plane, set your watch for the time in the country of destination and start thinking like a local. Experiment with adjusting your body clock times and find out what is comfortable to you.

Be an Early Bird If possible, arrive at your destination well before the event to allow time for your body to adjust to the new time. As a guide, arrive one day early for every time zone crossed; that is, arrive three days early to adjust for a three-hour time difference. For international travel crossing six or more time zones, athletes seem to return to their peak within four to seven days of arrival, so allow a week in your new country before competition. Of course, not everyone has this luxury.

When travelling for events, devise an eating plan. You may need to bring some of your own snacks with you.

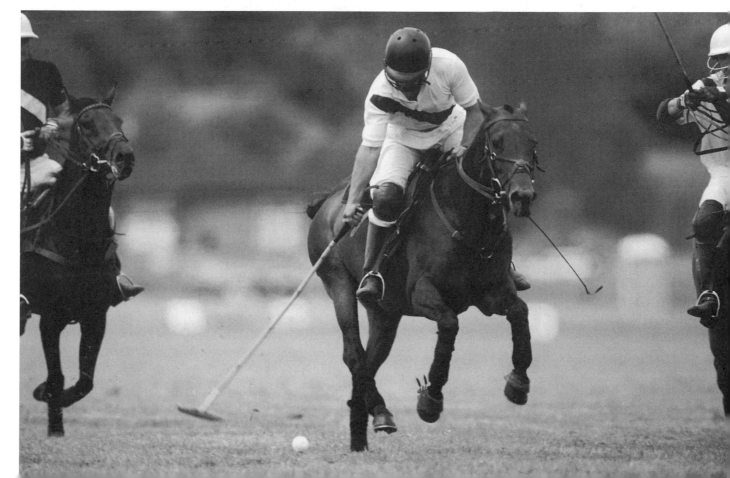

Acclimatise If you are travelling from a cool climate to a warm one, it can take 7 to 10 days for your body to acclimatise to the warmer weather. Your sweat and general cooling physiology take a little time to get used to the higher temperature. Sweat will have a higher sodium level initially; then the sodium levels drop to adjust to the warmer weather and the need to conserve sodium. To speed up the acclimatisation, exercise in warmer conditions before you leave home. Some athletes do this inside with the heater on or by wearing extra clothing during training.

Fly Well Fed Contact the airline at least two days before departure to see whether they can cater for special meals. Most airlines provide low-fat meals, possibly your best choice, or vegetarian meals. Both types of meals are likely to be higher in fibre to help keep you regular. Some airlines are so accustomed to working with sports teams and athletes that they even offer a high-carbohydrate athletes' meal. The bonus is that you tend to get served first! Some airlines are happy to provide extra bread and fruit for the hungry athlete. Teams can negotiate special arrangements with airlines.

Soak It Up Keep up the non-alcoholic fluids. The humidity in an aircraft is around 10 to 15 per cent, which means that moisture is lost from your body more quickly than normal, an estimated extra 20 millilitres an hour (Reilly et al. 2007). Some new aircraft have a higher humidity to counter the extra fluid loss. The extra humidity may also reduce jet lag symptoms. Drink mineral water, soft drinks or fruit juices when travelling by air. Bringing your own water bottle on long flights is a great idea. Tea and coffee can also be a part of your fluid intake; up to five cups in a flight hydrates the body equally as effectively as water. Just remember to minimise caffeinated drinks if they upset your sleeping. During long international flights you might need to get the best possible sleep, and both caffeine and alcohol can disrupt sleep cycles. Give alcohol a miss because it also dehydrates the body.

Stretch It Out While flying, occasionally get up and do some stretches, especially during flights that are longer than two hours. This also helps keep you alert and relieves the monotony. Airlines now advise stretching and wriggling your toes and feet to minimise the risk of deep vein thrombosis (DVT). You can also try walking up and down the aisles to improve the blood flow in your legs. A quick wash near the end of the flight can help you feel fresh.

Loosen Up Your feet tend to swell on long flights, so wear comfortable shoes that can be easily loosened or removed, such as runners. Wear loose clothing and avoid anything that digs into your body.

Zoom With a View I prefer a window seat. That way, no one has to climb over me if I'm having a snooze. Others prefer an aisle seat because they can stretch their legs and get up whenever they please. Nobody fancies a middle seat! Some airplanes have more leg room near the exit doors. If you are a frequent flyer, seating arrangements can be made to suit you.

Make It a Good Night Being on the road can play havoc with your sleeping habits. Changes in time zones, a different bed and pillow, unusual noises outside and different weather conditions all play their part in disrupting your sleep. To improve your chances of getting a good night's sleep, try these tips:

- Go for a light training session, or a good walk, about three hours before bedtime.
- Eat a high-carbohydrate snack before bedtime. It increases brain serotonin, which may help you to sleep.
- Keep the bedroom cool. Warm rooms can upset the sleep cycle. (I know, hotel room air conditioning can be tricky to get right.)
- Don't nap during the day; you may not get to bed tired enough to sleep.
- Regulate your sleeping habits to local time as soon as possible.

▶ Avoid Disease

Before travel, discuss your destinations with your doctor because they will be aware of any inoculations or vaccinations you require to minimise disease risk. Some disease outbreaks can occur even in other parts of your own country. Most governments have websites giving travel advice for other countries (e.g., Foreign and Commonwealth Office in the UK, Centers for Disease Control and Prevention in the USA, Safe Travel in New Zealand and Smartraveller in Australia).

▶ Avoiding Food Poisoning

When travelling for competition, you don't want to be laid low with a bout of food poisoning. Here are some important guidelines on food and drink safety to prevent travellers' diarrhea and food poisoning:

- If you are not sure of the quality of the local water supply, use well-sealed bottled, boiled or sterilised water for drinks and teeth brushing. Avoid ice, mixed drinks and foods washed in local water. Avoid tap water for brushing teeth.
- If you are not sure of food preparation cleanliness, avoid raw foods, including unpeeled fruits and vegetables, washed salads, shellfish and so forth.
- Avoid undercooked meat or unpasteurised milk products.
- Avoid buying foods from local stalls and markets, where hygiene may be poor.
- Look for food that is well cooked and served hot (not warm).
- Avoid food from buffets that is not served very hot or chilled, or that you suspect has been there for a long time at ambient temperature.
- Consider taking probiotic live cultures (acidophilus, bifidus) or cultured yogurt with you as a preventive measure. There is some evidence that taking probiotics (e.g., Yakult) for four weeks prior to travel reduces the risk of travellers' diarrhea. Take probiotics if you do get food poisoning because they will help your bowels restock with healthier bacteria.
- Wash your hands regularly, or use an alcohol-based hand sanitiser to clean your hands. Dry your hands with a clean towel or hand dryer.

Food Safety

When at home, you probably wash your hands before you prepare food, make sure all perishable foods are stored in the refrigerator and don't use foods past their use by dates. When you are away from home, you often have to trust that your meals have been made under hygienic conditions. Your trust is well placed in virtually all quality airlines, hotels and restaurants. In some countries and in some food outlets, however, it is wise to take precautionary measures to avoid food poisoning.

◯ FINAL SCORE

- Be prepared to ask questions about the choices at take-aways and restaurants. With more knowledge, you can make wiser decisions.
- Download nutrient profiles of menu items from franchise restaurants' websites so you can identify the best choices.
- Generally, the lower-fat, higher-carbohydrate, least-processed choices are the most nutritious and best suited to athletes' needs.
- Plan ahead for travel. The quicker you can adapt to local conditions, the quicker you will recover from the lethargy of travelling.
- Consider food safety when travelling to other countries to reduce any chance of food poisoning.
- The Australian Institute of Sport website has a number of fact sheets on travel nutrition. Their web address is listed in the resources section on page 241.

PART III

Weight Management for Athletes

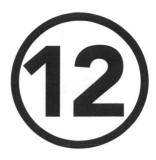

Muscle Building and Weight Gain Strategies

> So I started my final diet. On Sunday and Monday I ate the new diet, labored strenuously through my workouts, and slept like a baby. But by Tuesday, without adequate fuel, I began to lag. My two egg whites for breakfast were hardly enough. I worked out in the morning listlessly. . . . I was so weak that even when I halved the amount of weight I normally pushed, I barely got through the workout.
>
> *Sam Fussell (1991, 219)*

All elite athletes, and many recreational athletes, now weight train to increase muscle strength and muscle mass. Formerly the domain of male athletes, strength training is becoming a useful part of women's sport training. Good nutrition can help, but we have to look beyond the hype and find what is scientifically proven to help the strength athlete and those looking for greater muscle mass. Certainly, the spartan diet followed by bodybuilder Sam Fussell may have been high in protein, but it lacked the carbohydrate to fuel his workouts, hence his weakness. There is a smarter and healthier way to eat when trying to bulk up.

Formula for Strength and Muscle Bulk

To have the best chance to gain extra muscle, you need to have the basics in place first: the right genes, weight training, good nutrition and patience. These are discussed in the following sections.

The Right Genes

All athletes can increase their strength, but not all find it easy to naturally increase muscle bulk. Take a look at your blood relatives, especially those of the same gender as you. If they were skinny at a similar age, then you may find it a little tougher to gain muscle mass than if your immediate relatives were solidly built, in which case you would have a better chance of being able to pack on more muscle. The good news is that, independent of your genetics, you can always increase muscular strength with weight training even if the increase in muscle size is not spectacular.

Women have more difficulty gaining muscle mass than men do because of their lower levels of the hormone testosterone. Women notice a change in shape, definition, firmness and strength more than a change in muscle mass. Men have more testosterone and larger muscle fibres, a combination that gives them bigger muscles than women. Most women, with the exception of female bodybuilders, prefer muscle strength over bulk. They can achieve this by following the nutrition guidelines in this chapter and engaging a strength and conditioning coach.

Weight Training

Muscles get bigger and stronger only when you use them—muscle protein is manufactured in response to resistance exercise. Nothing else will make them bigger. Protein powders and amino acids won't make muscles bigger unless your muscles have been exercised. Resistance exercise such as swimming (for the upper body), cycling (for the legs) and weight training all stimulate muscle protein synthesis. Directly following exercise, some muscle breakdown occurs, but this is less than subsequent muscle synthesis providing there is good nutrition after a workout.

Good Nutrition

If you want to gain muscle, you have to eat good-quality food. You need adequate amounts of both protein and carbohydrate. The right amount of protein is quite easy to get. The average athlete already eats more protein than needed for weight training. (Protein needs are covered in chapter 2.) Your meals have to have a reasonable amount of carbohydrate to fuel the muscles so they can do a longer and more efficient workout to increase muscle mass. Otherwise, you will feel as tired as Sam Fussell, quoted at the beginning of the chapter.

When you put muscle under stress through weight training, long-distance running or sprint sessions, a small amount of muscle damage occurs naturally. This is not cause for alarm because with time and healthy eating, the body repairs the damage. If you can eat enough protein and carbohydrate to minimise muscle breakdown, then it makes sense that you can gain muscle

Weight training is a useful adjunct to women's sports to improve muscle strength.

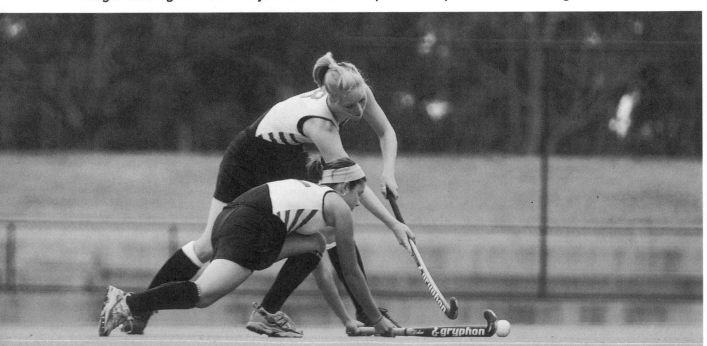

mass more quickly through training. Some supplements are thought to reduce muscle damage, thereby enhancing muscle gain. I mention some supplements later in this chapter. Supplements are covered in more detail in chapter 9.

Patience

Creating bigger muscle takes time and effort. Although it happens more quickly in some than in others, it's likely to take 6 to 12 months to achieve significant gains in muscle size, even if you work hard at it. Realistic gains will be between 0.2 and 1.0 kilogram (0.4 and 2.2 lb) per week. The rate of weight gain is usually faster in the first months and slows down thereafter.

An athlete might gain 3 kilograms (6.6 lb) in the first month of weight training, but gain only 1 kilogram (2.2 lb) in the fourth month. The remainder of the chapter focuses on nutrition and bulking up. I'll leave it to you to organise your own weight training program and to address the issue of patience. There's nothing you can do about your genes.

Who Can Benefit From Gains in Muscle and Weight?

Generally, five kinds of people want to increase their muscle mass for specific health or sports benefits.

- **Skinny people.** Some people are naturally lean and believe it is a disadvantage in sport and life. Gains in muscle mass may be slow, but gains in muscle strength can be significant. With a little extra muscle mass, they are likely to get more respect in sport and on the street.

- **Unintentional weight losers.** Some athletes find it hard to maintain their weight as a sporting season progresses. This is common in football and rowing, in which training demands are heavy and the kilojoules going in don't match those going out. Athletes in these situations need to eat more kilojoules to maintain their weight.

- **Set position athletes.** Some positions in team sports require strength and bulk, whereas others might rely on speed and additional muscle bulk slows them down. Those athletes who need extra muscle mass need to adjust their diet and put in some extra time at the gym.

- **Unfit and overweight people.** Increasingly, unfit people are turning to weight training as a means to lose body fat and increase bone density. As they lose weight, they can increase their level of aerobic training.

- **Older folk.** Older people now attend gyms because they know that weight training slows down osteoporosis and makes them less prone to falls, diabetes, heart disease and some types of arthritis. Rather than building muscle mass, their primary goals are increased muscle strength, bone density and fat burning.

Although people often ask me how they can gain weight, what they really want to know is how they can increase muscle mass without increasing body fat. This can be difficult, especially if genetics has designed someone to be very lean. Following are six nutrition tips that can help you increase muscle mass through weight training.

Nutrition for Bulking Up and Gaining Weight

Following the nutrition guidelines outlined in this section, in conjunction with a weight training program, will enable you to get maximal gains in muscle size. A summary of these guidelines is given in table 12.1. Based on all the scientific research, it is very unlikely that

TABLE 12.1 Nutrition for Increasing Muscle Mass

Nutrient	Amount each day (in g per kg of body weight)
Protein	• 1.5–1.7 for muscle growth in men • 1.3–1.5 for muscle growth in women • 1.0–1.2 to maintain muscle mass in men and women
Carbohydrate	• 4–5 for 30- to 60-minute workout/day • 6–8 for 60- to 90-minute workout/day
Fat	• 0.6–1.0
Supplements	• Creatine (see chapter 9) • Sports drinks (see chapter 5) • Hydroxy methylbutyrate (see chapter 9)

you will need more than 2 grams per kilogram of body weight of protein daily. If your training sessions are strenuous, you may need more than 8 grams of carbohydrate per kilogram of body weight. The fat guideline given in table 12.1 is more for general good health than for any training benefits. If you eat more fat than suggested, make sure it is mainly unsaturated fat. Nutritional supplements *may* help you, but you should read chapter 9 carefully before you spend any money on them.

Eat Adequate Protein

There is no doubt that athletes need greater amounts of protein than sedentary people do. Certainly, strength athletes and those doing resistance exercise need extra protein. However, it doesn't follow that they need a protein supplement. A high-quality diet with plenty of carbohydrate will almost always meet the protein needs of an athlete. (The protein needs of athletes are discussed in chapter 2.) It is not wise to eat most of your protein in one or two meals because the protein will be used for energy; it is best to spread your protein intake over the day to stimulate muscle development, and include some protein in the meal or snack you eat in the two hours after a workout.

Athletes doing weight training often find that protein supplements increase muscle mass. Usually, they could have taken extra carbohydrate and achieved the same result. Why? Because the extra protein in the supplement is not necessarily being converted to muscle—if the protein is in excess of needs, then it is being converted to muscle fuel (glucose), allowing a longer workout, which in turn is increasing muscle mass, just as carbohydrate would have done.

The International Olympic Committee Consensus Statement on Sports Nutrition (2010) states: 'Foods or snacks that contain high-quality proteins should be consumed regularly throughout the day as part of the day's total protein intake, and in particular soon after exercise, in quantities sufficient to maximise the synthesis of proteins, to aid in long-term maintenance or gain of muscle and bone and in the repair of damaged tissues. Ingestion of foods or drinks providing 15-25 g of such protein after each training session will maximise the synthesis of proteins that underpins these goals'.

That amount of protein (15 to 25 g) is easily met through good nutrition (e.g., a ham sandwich). If you eat 1.5 to 1.7 grams of protein per kilogram of body weight per day (men) or 1.3 to 1.5 grams per kilogram of body weight per day (women) early in a weight training program, you will be getting enough protein for muscle growth. That's about 125 to 145 grams of protein for an 85-kilogram (187 lb) man, or 90 to 105 grams of protein for a 70-kilogram (154 lb) woman. This can be readily achieved by eating a normal diet (see chapter 2 on protein).

Eat Plenty of Carbohydrate

Muscles get bigger and stronger with resistance training, such as weight training. It makes sense to feed the muscles high-carbohydrate food so they have the fuel to get them through a tough training session. You will need a minimum of 3 grams of carbohydrate per kilogram of body weight to fuel a single tough workout, possibly more if your training is heavy or intense. You are likely to need at least 6 grams of carbohydrate per kilogram body weight each day to cover your needs (see chapter 3 on carbohydrate for more information). The trick is to eat extra good-quality food to fuel both the workout and the gain in muscle mass, without putting on extra weight as fat. That might mean an extra 2,100 to 4,200 kilojoules (500 to 1,000 cal) a day.

There is good evidence that eating a mix of protein and carbohydrate before and after a workout promotes muscle repair or, at least, minimises muscle breakdown after exercise. Having an adequate amount of carbohydrate before a workout will make you less likely to use muscle protein as a fuel, and eating a mix of protein and carbohydrate after training reduces the amount of muscle breakdown. A snack or meal with both protein and carbohydrate also promotes muscle protein synthesis. The carbohydrate stimulates insulin production, and the insulin reduces protein breakdown and promotes protein uptake by the muscles. It is not clear what the best mix of protein and carbohydrate is, but the evidence suggests that the meals need to be more carbohydrate than protein, meaning that flavoured milk, bread, rice, pasta, granola bars and muesli bars can be part of an ideal muscle-building diet. (See chapter 8 for more advice on what to eat after sport.)

Men and women differ in their nutritional needs in several ways, in addition to those mentioned earlier. It seems that women burn less glycogen than men do when weight training (Volek, Forsythe and Kraemer 2006). Women appear to burn less of both glycogen and protein as fuel, while making up the difference with a greater use of fat as an energy source. Carbohydrate is still important to maintain glycogen stores, but women strength athletes probably don't need as much as male athletes do. Equally, women still need good-quality protein sources in their diet, although at a slightly lower level per kilogram body weight than do men.

Eat Frequently

Athletes need to eat frequently, especially if they are doing a lot of training. That means three meals and three or more snacks a day. If you eat too little, you will not have enough fuel to train efficiently. Some people like to follow a set plan (e.g., eating every two hours); what you do is up to you. I think you can be less regimented and still achieve your goals.

Don't skimp on an eating opportunity. Eat something before going to bed. Supper provides an extra nutrition boost and is useful for topping up your glycogen stores before an early morning training session. If it's high in carbohydrate and low in fat, and you are an active person, it won't turn to body fat.

Concentrate on the Kilojoules

Without enough kilojoules, your body won't have the means to create extra muscle mass. One very effective way of getting more nutrition is to make your meals and snacks energy dense—that is, more concentrated in kilojoules. This is an important technique for the athlete who is unintentionally losing weight or having difficulty gaining weight. Eating more food may not be

a practical option. By fitting more kilojoules into the same amount of food, you don't end up eating a mountain of food. There are simple ways of getting more nutrition into food (e.g., adding non-fat milk powder and table margarine to mashed potatoes).

Try some extra nutritious foods that are high in carbohydrate and low in fat but simple to eat in addition to your normal meals. Aim to get another 100 or more grams of carbohydrate into your diet to support the energy needs of your training program and encourage weight gain. You could possibly fit in more bread, rice, pasta, flavoured yogurt, breakfast cereal, dried fruit, fruit juice, flavoured milk or food bars (see table 12.2). For extra kilojoules with healthy fat, eat more nuts, peanut butter and avocados, and use olive oil and other unsaturated oils in salad dressing and cooking.

Drink Plenty of Nutritious Fluids

Fluids provide a simple way of getting extra kilojoules. Drinks such as reduced-fat milk, milkshakes and smoothies (preferably made with reduced-fat milk or soy drinks) are very nutritious. You can add extra non-fat milk powder to milk for extra carbohydrate and protein. Commercial liquid meals such as Sustagen Sport are usually based on milk powder. You might also try plain fruit juices or add some yogurt to the juice.

Many protein supplemental drinks are on the market. Although many of them are nutritious, they are usually expensive. You can make your own at a fraction of the cost. Try some of the great body boost drink ideas on page 178 or

TABLE 12.2 Examples of Nutritious, Energy-Dense Foods

Food	Kilojoules per serve	Calories per serve
Dried fruit, 1/2 cup	528	125
Nuts, 25 g (0.9 oz)	600	143
Peanut butter, 1 tbsp	720	170
Avocado, 1/2 medium	1,000	238
Unsaturated margarine, 1 tbsp	600	143
Unsaturated oil, 1 tsp	190	45
Milo, Ovaltine, 2 tbsp in 200 mL (7 oz) reduced-fat milk	760	180
Milk chocolate, 50 g (1.8 oz)	1,040	248
Muesli bar, 1	500	120

▶ Body Boost Drinks

Use these drinks to supplement your regular well-chosen diet. They are simple to make and inexpensive, and they provide a good balance of protein and carbohydrate without excess fat. They are ideal after a workout to replenish glycogen and stimulate muscle repair and growth. Nearly all of them are good sources of calcium, and four provide a modest amount of iron, both essential minerals, especially for athletes.

TRIPLE G (GLENN'S GARGANTUAN GAINER)

Ingredients

240 mL (8 oz) non-fat or reduced-fat milk

3 tbsp (30 g) non-fat milk powder

1 scoop ice cream

2 tsp Milo, AktaVite, Ovaltine, Nesquik or Horlicks

Method

Blend all ingredients together until smooth.

Nutrition Analysis

Kilojoules: 1,425	Calories: 340	Protein: 26 g
Fat: 7 g	Carbohydrate: 47 g	
Calcium: 880 mg	Iron: 2.5 mg	

BANANA POWERSHAKE

Ingredients

240 mL (8 oz) non-fat or reduced-fat milk

1 banana

1 scoop ice cream

1.5 tbsp glucose powder or sugar

pinch nutmeg

Method

Blend all ingredients together until smooth. Sprinkle nutmeg on top. Serve chilled.

Nutrition Analysis

Kilojoules : 1,715–1,820	Calories: 410–435	Protein: 14 g
Fat: 6 g (non-fat milk)	Carbohydrate: 75 g	
Calcium: 430 mg	Iron: negligible	

FRUIT SURGE

Ingredients

240 mL (8 oz) non-fat or reduced-fat milk

1 cup canned fruit

3 tbsp (30 g) non-fat milk powder

1 scoop ice cream

1 tbsp glucose powder or sugar

Method

Blend all ingredients and serve.

Nutrition Analysis

Kilojoules: 1,885–1,990	Calories: 450–475	Protein: 26 g
Fat: 5.5 g (non-fat milk)	Carbohydrate: 76 g	
Calcium: 850 mg	Iron: 1.0 mg	

SUSTAGOGO

Ingredients

200 mL (7 oz) reduced-fat milk

3 tbsp Sustagen Sport powder

Method

Blend together and serve hot or cold.

Nutrition Analysis

Kilojoules: 920	Calories: 220	Protein: 16 g
Fat: 4 g	Carbohydrate: 32 g	
Calcium: 500 mg	Iron: 3.1 mg	

YOJUICE

Ingredients

200 mL (7 oz) fruit juice

3 tbsp low-fat flavoured yogurt

Method

Blend ingredients and serve cold.

Nutrition Analysis

Kilojoules: 500	Calories: 120	Protein: 4.2 g
Fat: 0.2 g	Carbohydrate: 25 g	
Calcium: 120 mg	Iron: 0 mg	

▶ Can Muscle Turn to Fat?

No, not if you mean a direct conversion from one to the other. If you don't use a muscle group, it will get smaller (atrophy). If, at the same time, your exercise levels drop or you start eating too much food, then the excess kilojoules will be stored as body fat. It just appears that muscle is becoming fat. On the other hand, many people want to gain muscle mass while losing body fat and that can be tricky because muscle gain requires adequate kilojoules, whereas body fat loss requires a deficit of kilojoules. It is easier to increase muscle mass first and then work out often enough to maintain the muscle mass, while slightly cutting back on food so that you are losing 0.5 kilogram (1 lb) per week. The extra muscle produced by resistance training will really help your weight control. More muscle results in an increase in basal metabolic rate, which burns more kilojoules at rest. Kilojoules burned are kilojoules *not* stored as body fat.

make up the protein powder recipe (Glennergy) provided in chapter 2. I've named the first one Glenn's Gargantuan Gainer tongue in cheek, because many commercial products use titles to suggest rapid and massive muscle gain. Of course, muscle gain is gradual.

Nutritional Supplements

Many nutritional supplements are promoted as enhancing muscle growth. Unfortunately, the

Hours in heavy equipment can promote greater fluid loss and a need for greater strength.

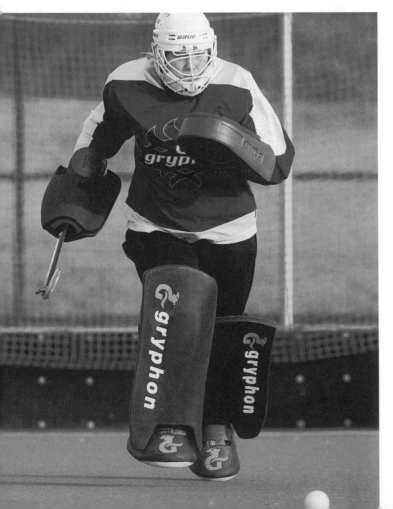

scientific studies do not justify the hype surrounding many of them. In this section I briefly describe the supplements that may be of some value for increasing muscle. For more details on each one, see chapter 9.

Creatine certainly increases weight gain in many athletes, with an initial gain in the region of 1 kilogram (2.2 lb), most of which is likely to be fluid, not muscle. Any subsequent and sustained weight gain is likely to be extra muscle mass providing you are also doing a regular weight training program. Creatine allows you to do extra repetitions, leading to muscle growth.

Hydroxy methylbutyrate (HMB) studies suggest that it can reduce muscle damage during resistance exercise and increase muscle mass. Any benefit is most likely to be in elite athletes and very serious recreational athletes because they usually work their muscles hard. Fitness enthusiasts may get little benefit because they usually suffer less muscle damage after exercise.

Other supplements promoted as helping muscle gain in the past, such as chromium picolinate (see chapter 9 for more detail), vanadyl sulphate and boron, do not seem to provide any benefit to weight training athletes in either muscle strength or muscle mass. Their hype was way in advance of the research.

Cutting Up

In the month before competition, bodybuilders go through the process of 'cutting up' to enhance muscle definition. They consume a very low fat diet to reduce subcutaneous fat. Bodybuilders who dramatically restrict their food intake before competition run the risk of losing muscle mass. That's because when there is too little food, the body breaks down muscle for fuel.

That makes all the hard work in the gym a waste. Ensure that you consume enough carbohydrate to spare your muscle stores from degradation.

Some believe that carbohydrate loading at this stage can increase muscle girth. For every extra gram of glycogen stored, an extra 2.4 to 4.0 grams of water are stored, which is believed to plump up the muscle size. However, one well-controlled study was unable to find any muscle definition difference between bodybuilders who carbohydrate-loaded and those who ate a regular diet before competition (Balon, Horowitz and Fitzsimmons 1992).

Some bodybuilders dehydrate in the 24 hours before competition to make the skin 'tighter' to improve muscle definition. Unfortunately, dehydration can cause fatigue, headaches and faintness, which is not the best way to feel just before the competition starts. So-called fat mobilisers are also popular during the cutting-up phase, even though they do not help with loss of body fat at all. Read the section on fat mobilisers in chapter 9. It could save you a pile of money.

Building muscle takes a lot of resistance training. Good eating provides the fuel, the nutrients and the extra protein needed to increase muscle mass. Progress will be slow and steady. Don't expect a supplement promoted as a muscle mass booster to be any more helpful than good nutrition.

FINAL SCORE

- Increasing muscle mass requires a combination of the right genes, resistance training, good nutrition and patience.
- Nutrition for increasing muscle mass includes adequate carbohydrate for training and adequate protein and kilojoules for muscle growth.
- You will likely need 5 to 6 grams of carbohydrate per kilogram of body weight each day to fuel weight training workouts. It is also likely that you will need around 1.5 grams of protein per kilogram of body weight daily while you are increasing muscle mass.
- Eat a meal or snack with a mix of protein and carbohydrate soon after a workout to replenish muscle glycogen stores and repair muscle protein damage.
- Many nutritional supplements promoting muscle growth are not well researched, or the research suggests little or no value. Creatine is a supplement that may assist muscle growth in those doing adequate resistance exercise.

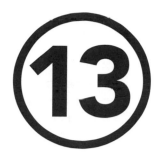

Fat Burning and Weight Loss Strategies

Laffit Pincay Jr. is a jockey of legendary status in U.S. racing. In a career encompassing over 35 years, he rode over 9,500 winners, the most of any rider before he retired in 2003. A story is told of Pincay, who, while on a plane flight, took a single peanut from the packet, broke it in half and ate the first portion, saving the second half to eat later in the flight!

Be assured, you will not have to go to the lengths Laffit Pincay went to, to control your own body fat. Active people are normally lean, but plenty of fit people still have difficulty shedding very small amounts of weight. This chapter details the best eating strategy for long-term success in losing body fat, or not gaining any, and keeping lean. If you are looking for a quick fix, a magic diet or a rapid weight loss program, you will not find it here because they rarely work, are generally unhealthy and certainly won't help you stay fit. They work only for as long as you can handle plain starvation.

Questions Athletes Ask

If you are carrying a little too much body fat, then your first step is to set yourself a realistic goal. Your goal may not even be a set weight. Your goal could rightfully be just to feel a lot better and fitter than you do now. Be warned, before you go any further, that this is not a food-obsessed chapter that will ask you to measure everything you eat and delete every taste pleasure you ever pursued. If you want that, buy the latest diet book. This chapter is about eating to successfully control your weight while including such foods as wine, chocolate, pizza or ice cream on occasions. Successful people don't 'diet'. Success depends more on what goes on inside your head than on what goes on your plate. That is, your attitude will determine your success. Let me answer five common questions before I explain further.

'**N**o pizzas, toasted cheese sandwiches, hot chips, potato chips, sausage rolls, vanilla slices—there's not much left for me except for cereal and some baked beans', revealed Australian cricketer Shane Warne in a 2002 press briefing during a tour in South Africa. 'I haven't eaten pizzas or drunk beers for the last couple of weeks. I've dropped about eight kilos' (Crutcher 2002).

http://www.espncricinfo.com/wc-timeline/content/story/114575.html

1. Why Do I Put on Body Fat?

Please appreciate that you are designed to gain body fat. Humans evolved to gain body fat easily when food was abundant; that extra stored body fat acted as an energy reserve during food shortages. Those who put on body fat easily were better able to survive the rigours of human survival. If you gain body fat easily, you are normal. If it is difficult to lose body fat, you are normal. To lose body fat, or not gain it, you must treat your body as it was designed. That often means eating more vegetables and fruit, eating less treat foods, drinking less alcohol and sugared drinks and doing more activity even if you are already fit.

As we age, our body weight tends to increase and our body shapes change. One contributing factor is that our metabolic rate decreases with age, but the more common reason is that we do less activity as we age without eating less food (and often eating more). Regular exercise and weight training to increase muscle mass will keep your metabolic rate elevated and slow any age-related weight gain.

▶ What Causes Athletes to Gain Weight?

- **Off-season.** Less training and more time for partying can be a simple recipe for gaining extra body fat. This is common in athletes involved in team sports that often have a two-month break after the season has ended.

- **Injury.** Again, a lower training level is the key reason for weight gain. Being injured can also mean feeling depressed because you can't compete, possibly turning you to food for solace. A sports psychologist can help you with your thinking.

- **Alcohol.** Alcoholic drinks are strongly associated with male team sports. Alcohol is also strongly associated with dehydration, poor sports performance, poor recovery from injury and increases in body fat. Alcohol needs to be treated with respect. Excess alcohol does not mix well with sport or life.

- **Grease.** Too much fat in foods, and a reliance on take-away foods, can easily make your navel move farther from your spine. Take-aways are often chosen for convenience, especially by athletes who have just left home and don't have any cooking skills. Choosing less energy-dense foods and drinks will help control body weight (see chapter 11 for ideas for healthy take-away choices).

2. Am I Too Fat?

Scientists use all types of formulae to judge whether someone is too fat. One is the waist circumference (see figure 13.1). Ideally, for good health, your waist circumference should be 80 centimetres (31.5 in.) or less for women and 94 centimetres (37 in.) or less for men. Having a waist circumference above 88 cm (35 in) for women and above 102 cm (40 in) for men is linked to a much greater risk of problems such as heart disease. Health authorities say that above those waist measurements you are likely to have stored excess fat around the pancreas, liver, kidneys and heart, which is not good news for your health. The waist circumference measurement should be done in line with the belly button for men and at the narrowest part of the waist, just above the hips, for women.

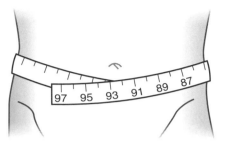

FIGURE 13.1 Waist measurement (at the level of the belly button) should be less than 88 centimetres (35 in.) for women and 102 centimetres (40 in.) for men. More than this can contribute to poor health due to being overweight.

Why measure here? The fat around your middle is the most dangerous to your health. Once that gets above the recommended circumference, your health can decline. Fat here will raise blood cholesterol and blood pressure, while dramatically increasing your risk of diabetes. Get a tape measure and find the circumference of your middle. If you are overfat, change your eating and exercise habits such that your belt goes in a notch every few weeks or so. If your waist is normal, then eat sensibly and remain active to ensure that it stays that way.

You can also determine your body mass index (BMI), a common indicator of fatness based on your height and weight using the following equation:

$$BMI = \frac{Weight\ (kg)}{Height\ (m)^2}$$

For example, if you weigh 80 kilograms (176 lb) and you are 180 centimetres (1.8 m; 5 ft 9 in.) tall, then your BMI is 24.7:

$$\frac{80}{1.8 \times 1.8} = \frac{80}{3.24} = 24.7$$

A BMI between 20 and 25 is considered a healthy weight. A person with a BMI over 25 is considered overweight, whereas someone with a BMI over 30 is considered obese. The BMI is not always the best measurement of overweight in athletes because it doesn't account for muscle mass. A well-muscled athlete is likely to have a BMI higher than 25, yet can still have a low body fat level. In these circumstances, your waist measurement is a better gauge of fatness.

A common way to determine the fat levels of athletes is to measure their skinfolds. This should be done by a trained kinanthropometrist using a set of skinfold callipers to determine the levels of body fat just below the skin. Various sites can be measured, but the most common are the biceps, triceps, subscapula (just beneath the shoulder blade) and abdomen (just beneath the rib cage). A sum of the measurements gives an indication of the level of fatness. The same person should do the measurements with the same callipers on the same sites to ensure consistency. The measurements are commonly done on elite athletes to find the measurements that provide the best performance and to give some extra incentive to lose fat. Recreational athletes probably need no more than a waist measurement to determine whether they need to lose body fat.

Please be aware that not all athletes want to be superlean. Obviously, some sports require bulk rather than speed, in which case a little extra body fat is acceptable. Yes, sumo wrestlers are an obvious example, but consider long-distance open-water swimmers. They often swim in cold waters, and extra body fat provides insulation against the cold as well as some buoyancy.

3. Can I Lose Weight Fast?

The answer is no—well, not if you want to remain healthy and sane. It is easy to believe that we have become fat really fast and that Christmas, Easter or the annual holiday is to blame for the excess weight. This is very unlikely. Most athletes remain at a steady weight over their competitive lifetimes. Any weight is likely to be slow and gradual over a period of months

▶ The Cathy Freeman Weight Loss Program

'Fruit, vegetables, water, skin off the chicken, no McDonalds, no alcohol—oh, maybe one or two glasses of red wine—but training hard is the thing', is the secret of Cathy Freeman, 400-metre Olympic gold medalist, Sydney 2000. In 2002 she had gone from 65 kilograms (143 lb) to 54 kilograms (119 lb) in ten weeks. 'It's no big deal', she said as she closed in on her 52-kilogram (114 lb) 'fighting weight'.

or years. Sometimes, body weight can fluctuate significantly. During a lay-off as a result of injury or the end-of-season break, an athlete could gain 2 to 5 kilograms (4 to 11 lb). This process needs to be reversed gradually and permanently, ideally at a rate of 0.5 kilogram (1 lb) per week. It may sound frustratingly slow, but a faster rate could result in a loss of muscle.

Some simple changes to your diet could be all you need. For example, if you changed from drinking 600 millilitres (20 oz) of full-cream milk a day to a reduced-fat milk, you would save 150,000 kilojoules (35,800 cal) a year. Potentially that's a loss of 5 kilograms (11 lb) per year. Instead of two cream biscuits for morning tea, eat a piece of fruit instead to save well over 200,000 kilojoules (47,800 cal) a year, a potential loss of 6.5 kilograms (14 lb). Simple changes to your eating can make a big difference—over time. (Note: I say a *potential* loss of a certain weight because that is what the math suggests. In reality, the body adjusts as weight is lost and fewer kilojoules are burned because the body is carrying around less weight; as a result, actual weight loss is less than potential weight loss.)

If you are a jockey, boxer, lightweight rower, bodybuilder, wrestler, diver, synchronised swimmer, figure skater or gymnast, you are probably under pressure to be a certain weight or shape. Being 2 or 3 kilograms (4.4 to 6.6 lb) over your

Some athletes in weight restricted sports dehydrate to meet their weight class, yet this will cause fatigue and affect performance.

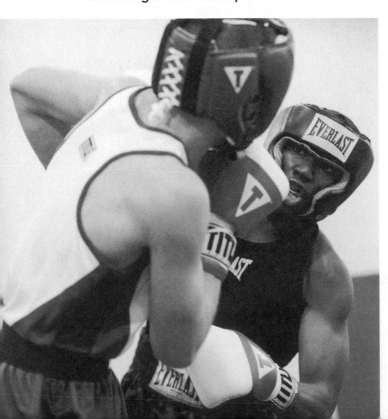

'fighting weight' can come as a shock, so you want to get it off fast.

The first problem with this issue is the term *fast*. Fast means that you will have to do just that: fast . . . as in *go without food*. Without food, or following a very restricted diet, your body runs out of glycogen and dumps the water needed to store that glycogen. In other words, you run out of energy and lose weight mainly as water.

Rapid weight loss, especially by dehydration, will torpedo your endurance as well as your sprinting or intense training programs. Rapid weight loss can also affect your thinking and concentration—and feeling tired and irritable is not the best way to go into an event.

You may need to ask yourself, 'Am I competing in the right weight class for my natural weight and health?' There is little point in becoming weak and wasted just to make a lower weight class and risk injury for not being at your optimal weight, too. A thin athlete is not always a fast athlete, and a hungry athlete is a weak athlete. You would be smart to plan weeks, not days, ahead and get that extra weight off slowly and permanently. That way you retain your health, strength and ability, both physical and mental.

4. Will Exercise Affect My Appetite?

Yes. When you do no exercise at all, it is easy to overeat—that is, eat more than you need, which leads to weight gain. A moderate amount of exercise, around one hour a day, tends to return appetite to normal. The result is that kilojoules in equal kilojoules out, and your weight remains steady. As exercise levels increase, so might your appetite to meet your increased needs. When training sessions becomes intense and last many hours, you may find that you can't eat enough food and your weight begins to inadvertently decline. In that case, refer to the tips for increasing your energy intake from chapter 12.

5. How Can I Raise My Metabolism?

You may already know that your basal metabolic rate (BMR) burns quite a few kilojoules each day. Your BMR is the energy burned to keep you alive—that is, to keep your heart beating; lungs breathing; and liver, kidneys and brain functioning. You can estimate your BMR using the following equations:

Male

> 63 × body weight (in kg) + 3,000 = kJ

> 15 × body weight (in kg) + 716 = cal

Female

> 50 × body weight (in kg) + 3,000 = kJ

> 12 × body weight (in kg) + 716 = cal

Adjustments for Age

30–35 years	reduce BMR by 5%
36–50 years	reduce BMR by 10%
51–69 years	reduce BMR by 15%
70+ years	reduce BMR by 20%

Reprinted from *Nutrition Research*, 19(7), A. Movahedi, "Simple formula for calculating basal energy expenditure," 989-995, copyright 1999, with permission from Elsevier.

When you do the calculations, there is a good chance you will have a figure of 5,000 to 6,700 kilojoules (1,200 to 1,600 cal) for women and 5,800 to 8,400 kilojoules (1,400 to 2,000 cal) for men. For example, if you are a 32-year-old 65-kilogram (143 lb) woman, your BMR will be about 6,250 kilojoules (50 × 65, then add 3,000, then take off 5%) or 1,420 calories. A healthy adult is very unlikely to have a BMR less than 4,200 kilojoules (1,000 cal), when measured accurately. Remember, these figures are just for your BMR. You will need more than this to cover your daily activities and training. Fit people need to multiply these figures by 1.5 to 2.0 to get an indication of their total daily energy needs.

A common question is, 'How can I raise my metabolism?' People hope to be able to help the body burn fat while they are at their desk or sleeping. The answer is, 'Yes, you can raise your metabolism, but there is not an easy method.' The three most effective ways to raise your basal metabolic rate are as follows:

- **Exercise.** This is by far the best method. Exercise burns kilojoules and generally increases your muscle mass depending on the exercise. Swimming increases upper body muscle, and running increases lower body muscle. I suspect that you already have this method as part of your life.

- **Weight training.** Muscles have a higher metabolic rate than body fat has. Weight training is the most effective way of increasing muscle mass, but don't rely on it as the sole method of losing body fat. Aerobic exercise usually burns up fat stores at a faster rate. You could, of course, do light weights as part of a general fitness program.

- **Small, frequent meals.** Some research has suggested that dividing your food into five or six smaller meals helps raise metabolic rate compared to eating just one or two big meals a day.

Often, you will hear stories that certain foods will raise your metabolic rate above what it is normally. You may hear, for example, that chilli, green tea and caffeine raise metabolic rate. This is true, but it is unlikely that you can eat enough chilli or drink enough cups of green tea at every meal, day after day, to make a big difference to your metabolic rate. You might burn an extra 200 kilojoules (50 cal) per day, but that doesn't hold a candle to the 1,250 kilojoules (300 cal) burned in a 45-minute walk or the 820 kilojoules (200 cal) saved by cutting out the two cream biscuits at coffee break. Eat sensibly, rather than hoping a certain food (or supplement) will be helpful in weight loss.

Body Shape

There is a great deal of pressure to conform to cultural ideals of the ideal body shape. Providing that your waist circumference is within the guides given earlier in the chapter, then your shape may not be easy to change. Compare the body shapes of the athletes in figure 13.2 (page 188). They are all lean athletes, but they have

 ## The Lauren Burns Weight Loss Program

For the 2000 Sydney Olympics, the taekwondo gold medallist Lauren Burns had to work hard to compete in the under-49-kilogram (108 lb) division. 'It took me three months, because under 49 kg is way too light for me. I had the help of the Victorian Institute of Sport and its dietitians', said Lauren, who now weighs 54 kilograms (119 lb). 'That's my natural weight', she said.

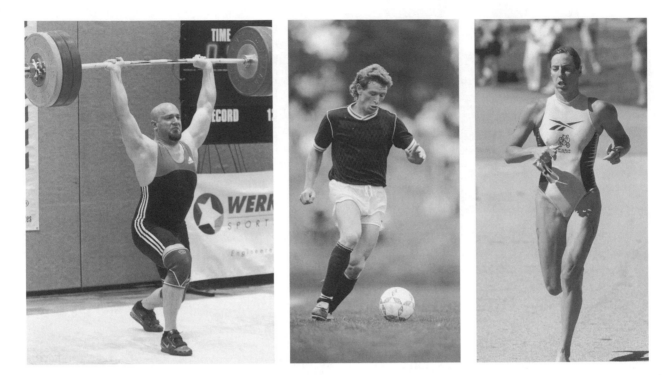

FIGURE 13.2 Lean bodies can come in a variety of shapes.

different body shapes. Sure, exercise or weight training will improve your musculature, but beyond that you are better off accepting your shape than trying mythical ways to sculpt your body to some ideal shape. For example, it is well established that you cannot spot reduce. Doing abdominal exercises will improve the strength of the abdominal muscles, but it won't magically get rid of abdominal fat. The only way you can do that is to eat less energy than you burn.

> It is an amazing paradox that our culture, with its great flexibility and liberal ideas, attempts to superimpose one form of body build on those whom nature has endowed differently.
>
> *Hilde Bruch, 1957 (Seid 1989, 133)*

If your waist circumference does not fall within the guidelines given earlier in this chapter, then you may want to evaluate whether your body shape is normal and healthy. The pear body shape is generally a female shape with fat deposits on the hips, thighs and buttocks (see figure 13.3). This is normal for women. Human survival relied on women having fat in this part of the body so that in the case of a food shortage, they had fat reserves to ensure that pregnancies

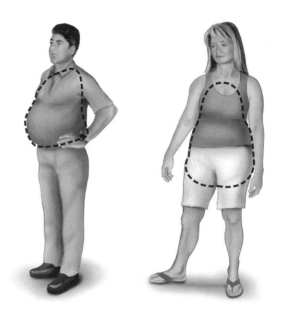

FIGURE 13.3 The apple shape occurs when abdominal fat increases, which in turn increases the chance of heart disease, diabetes and other medical problems. The pear shape is commonly found in women and is not linked to any health problems.

went to term and that they could also breastfeed the infant. Because the Western diet hasn't had a food shortage in the last 60 years, we haven't had to rely on fat stores for survival.

The apple shape is associated with excess body fat in men and women. Excess body fat around the abdomen is a long-term health risk because it can raise blood cholesterol, blood pressure and blood glucose levels, leading to a higher risk of heart disease, stroke and diabetes. Apple-shaped people also have a greater chance of back pain and breast and bowel cancer. In short, pear shape is healthy, and apple shape is unhealthy, although no one should gain excess weight, no matter their shape.

Weight Loss Quackery

Before you think about changing your food choices, you first need to ignore the distractions of weight loss charlatans promoting fad diets and slimming products. History has taught us that there has never been a weight loss breakthrough. It is reasonable to suggest that there is unlikely to ever be a healthy, simple new idea or product that will make body fat loss easy. You can buy diet books, fat loss products (fat metabolisers, tablets, meal replacement drinks), weight loss machinery (especially those advertised on TV), weight loss tablets, diet soups or cellulite creams, but all these will prove disappointing because you are really buying hope, not success. Why don't they work? Let's take a brief look at some of them.

Diet Books

Every diet book is written to a formula. They are all prescriptive and restrictive. That is, they dictate what you eat and they cut out a huge range of foods, including all your favourite foods. If you don't follow their exact program, you probably won't lose weight. For a diet book to work, it must control your actions and decisions. Take a diet book, any diet book, and this is what you will be told:

- You can't eat pastries, take-aways, snack food, soft drinks, confectionery (candy), biscuits, cookies, cakes, fatty foods, butter and margarine or any treat you might enjoy.
- You can eat vegetables, legumes, lean meats, low-fat dairy foods, fruits and whole-grain cereals (unless it is a low-carbohydrate book, in which cereals and some fruits and vegetables are deleted).

Over the years, the low-carbohydrate diet has been promoted to athletes and the public alike. It is interesting to note that low-carbohydrate diets have been popular since the 1950s. (The first one was published by William Banting in 1864, about 150 years ago, so it is not a new idea.) In 2003 researchers from Stanford University checked all the research on low-carbohydrate diets and concluded that they work only because they are low-kilojoule diets (Bravata et al.).

A low-carbohydrate diet book often mentions that you can eat all the fat you like. That sounds great until you realise that there aren't any potatoes for the sour cream, no bread for the butter, no pasta or rice for the oil, no fruit for the cream. Ever tried eating fat on its own? Of course not. By deleting the carbohydrate, you also end up eating less fat and therefore fewer kilojoules.

When you limit food intake to low-carbohydrate foods such as salad vegetables, lean meats, cheese, yogurt and a small number of fruits, it becomes very difficult to overeat. Of course, when you limit food to fruits, vegetables, oats, pasta, rice, bread, lean meats, low-fat dairy foods and the occasional treat, it is also difficult to overeat. The latter style is called healthy eating, a concept too difficult to embrace by pop nutritionists.

Do low-carbohydrate diets work? Yes, in the short term; no, in the long term. The low-carbohydrate diet can produce greater weight loss over three to six months, but there is little difference between low-carbohydrate eating and low-kilojoule eating after 12 months. It is also important to note that there is a very high drop-out level for both types of diets, which should remind us all that any weight loss diet is hard to stick to.

If foods high in carbohydrate were implicated in weight gain, why have we conveniently forgotten the Pritikin Diet, the wonder diet of the 1970s and 1980s? It was a very high carbohydrate, low-fat diet that trimmed the body fat off millions. Clearly, carbohydrate wasn't fattening itself. The Pritikin Diet was so extreme in its avoidance of fat that most people returned to their old style of eating very quickly and replaced any lost weight.

All the emphasis on reducing carbohydrate has forgotten that athletes and other active people need carbohydrate for muscle fuel. Depriving endurance athletes of their carbohydrate will reduce their endurance capacity. As a result, they will tire quickly and not meet their performance goals.

The 2010 Dietary Guidelines for Americans, sums up the situation:

There is strong and consistent evidence that when calorie intake is controlled,

189

macronutrient proportion of the diet is not related to losing weight. A moderate body of evidence provides no data to suggest that any one macronutrient is more effective than any other for avoiding weight regain in weight reduced persons. A moderate body of evidence demonstrates that diets with less than 45% of calories as carbohydrates are not more successful for long-term weight loss (12 months). There is also some evidence that they may be less safe. In shorter-term studies, low calorie, high protein diets may result in greater weight loss, but these differences are not sustained over time. A moderate amount of evidence demonstrates that intake of dietary patterns with less than 45% calories from carbohydrate or more than 35% calories from protein are not more effective than other diets for weight loss or weight maintenance, are difficult to maintain over the long term, and may be less safe.

http://tinyurl.com/7ulnd4m

Put simply, the guidelines are saying that, to lose or maintain weight, there is no advantage of one diet over another; don't follow extreme diets, such as low carbohydrate, because they may be unhealthy. For athletes, it means: Eat well and don't over-restrict carbohydrate foods.

Magic Products

So-called fat metabolisers or mobilisers are touted as weight loss agents, especially to bodybuilders and personal trainers. Common claims are that they convert fat to body fuel and improve muscle definition, making them attractive to anyone trying to lose body fat. The brochures imply that they will melt away the excess fat, turning you into a chiselled beefcake or beach babe in no time. However, they work only in conjunction with a calorie-controlled diet, which is their way of saying, 'If you want to lose weight, eat fewer kilojoules or calories, but please buy our supplement so you get the impression the supplement also played a role'.

The most common ingredients of fat metabolisers are the compounds carnitine, inositol and choline. Other ingredients include lecithin, methionine, herbs and vitamins. There is no scientific evidence that any of these ingredients cause fat loss or help to control your appetite.

Another favourite claim is that certain products stop you from digesting fat or carbohydrate.

The fact is that undigested fat or carbohydrate would pass into your large intestine, causing abdominal pain, gas and diarrhea. The manufacturer of the product chitosan claimed that it binds to fat in the gut and passes undigested into the stool. In 2003, University of California researchers revealed that a full daily dose of chitosan saved 42 kilojoules (10 cal), the amount of energy burned in a two-minute walk (Gades and Stern 2003)! Other research shows that chitosan did not assist in the loss of body fat (Ni Mhurchu et al. 2004). (Chitosan is not to be confused with the drug Xenical, which does reduce fat digestion and absorption, but you have to be on a low-fat diet in the first place so that you don't get diarrhea.)

Some products are plain ridiculous, such as slimming soap, which supposedly dissolves fat from your thighs and waist as you wash. This is a rip-off at the criminal end of the scale. Yes, people do buy this stuff . . . but only once. In summary, don't waste your time or money on weight loss diets or gimmicks. To lose excess body fat, you must eat less energy (kilojoules or calories) than you burn up each day. Why? Because that is the first law of thermodynamics—it's been in place since the beginning of time. To lose excess body fat, you must be prepared to do extra training or modify your eating, which is discussed later in this chapter.

Facts About Cellulite

Cellulite seems to be an exclusively female concern, despite the fact that cellulite is not linked to any health condition. Even if you are fit and eat well, and your waist measurement is normal, you may still have cellulite. What is cellulite? According to *Taber's Cyclopedic Medical Dictionary* (2009), cellulite is a 'colloquial term for subcutaneous deposits of fat with dimpling of the skin, especially in the buttocks and thighs'. Put simply, cellulite is round, fatty lumps just under the skin and features, to some degree, in 85 to 98 per cent of women (Khan 2010a). Having cellulite does not mean that you have excess fat. Cellulite can be present in lean, healthy women.

Cellulite fat stores and regular fat stores appear to differ structurally. In cellulite, fibrous connective tissue separates the fat cells into clusters (see figure 13.4). Much of the connective tissue is collagen, a protein. With age, extra collagen is formed to change the structural geography of the stored fat. Evidence suggests

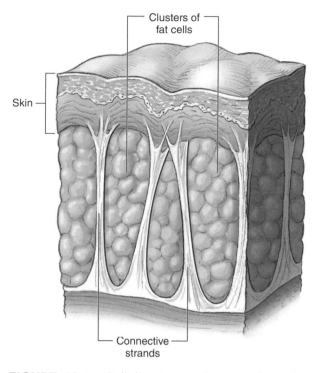

Skin

Clusters of
fat cells

Connective
strands

FIGURE 13.4 Cellulite is just clusters of regular fat cells beneath the skin, giving a dimpled effect.

The cellulite effect may become more obvious in the following cases:

- In overweight women as fat cells enlarge and the fat begins to bulge from the fat cell compartments to accentuate the cellulite appearance. Fat cells can only enlarge to a certain size. If more fat is stored, the body must produce new fat cells. It follows that cellulite can diminish with weight loss in overweight women, but this doesn't happen for everyone.

- With high-salt diets because the sodium may cause more fluid retention. Just deleting salt at the dinner table may not help because about 80 per cent of all salt in the diet is added by food manufacturers. A better choice is to eat reduced-salt foods, preferably with sodium levels under 120 milligrams per 100 grams listed on the label.

- During the week pre-menses with fluid retention.

Unfortunately, once a fat cell has been created, it stays forever. It can be reduced in size, but it won't go away. Cellulite is more common in women because their skin is thinner and their fat compartments are larger and more rounded than men's. The result is a dimpling appearance on the surface of the skin. It can occur in overweight and normal weight women. If a woman has cellulite, then her daughters are more likely to have cellulite. Genetics can be a nuisance sometimes.

Cellulite is not a build-up of toxic waste or undigested food, and it is not caused by faulty circulation, as some have claimed in the past. Cellulite creams are not a solution. The creams seemed to work because gentle massaging of the skin temporarily flattens some of the bumpy areas. In other words, you can rub whatever you like into the cellulite area and the skin will

that blood flow in the cellulitic areas is slower, but the role this plays is unclear.

These changes encourage a mild edema in the area, with the extra water giving rise to the orange peel look. Further pronouncement of the cellulite occurs if the fat cells enlarge and the skin loses elasticity with time. Certainly, a greater amount of fluid appears to be associated with cellulite areas when compared to other areas of body fat. One theory is that cellulite has a higher level of proteoglycans, molecules of proteins and sugars combined, which have high water-attracting properties.

Cellulite often increases with age, possibly compounded by female sex hormones and extra weight. Cellulite is more common in white women than in black or Asian women.

The Dean Lukin 'Yeah, Did That Years Ago' Weight Loss Program

Los Angeles Olympics gold medal super-heavyweight weightlifter, Dean Lukin, went from 145 kilograms (319 lb) in 1984 to a lean 95 kilograms (209 lb) eight years later. He revealed all in the *Dean Lukin Diet* (1993). In the book he described being a big lad and going to his girlfriend's house for dinner. He sat on the toilet and crushed the porcelain bowl, breaking it into jagged pieces. 'I have never been so thankful for the invention of toilet seats', said Lukin. Dean does hand out lots of sensible nutrition advice in the book. Guess that's why it wasn't a best-seller.

become smoother for a short time. There is no single treatment of cellulite that is completely effective (Khan 2010b). See your dermatologist if you believe that your life would improve without cellulite; just don't expect a magic solution. The good news is that new therapies are being trialed, and one may just provide the answer many women have waited for.

Wise Food Choices

No matter how you look at it, gaining body fat is due to eating more kilojoules than you burn through activity each day. This may be only a small discrepancy, with an average body fat gain of 1 to 3 grams a day (30 to 90 kJ [7 to 21 cal]) a day. That's around 1 to 3 kilograms (2.2 to 6.6 lb) every three years. (Note: Although food fat is 37 kJ [9 cal] per gram, body fat is 29 kJ [7 cal] per gram because some water is integrated with body fat.)

Fat loss is the opposite: You need to eat fewer kilojoules than you use each day so that you are forced to burn a little extra body fat each day. For some athletes, this is not easy. You may not succeed the first time around. Don't despair. This may take more than one attempt. Indeed, most successful people will tell you that they made more than one attempt to achieve their fat loss goals. A few food tricks can help put the odds in your favour, but don't for a moment expect this to be easy.

In 1980, Coca-Cola began to design a new diet drink. The can itself went through 150 designs, and over 10,000 consumers had taste-tested Diet Coke before its release in July 1982 using saccharin as the sweetener. By the end of 1983, Diet Coke was sweetened with the intense sweeteners saccharin and aspartame, before it eventually dispensed with saccharin (which, by the way, was cleared of all links with human cancer in May 2000). Unfortunately, the whole concept of sugar substitutes gave the impression that sugar was fattening and that the elimination of sugar was the road to salvation. Not so. Let me explain some nutrition points and link them to weight loss.

First, we must understand the origin of energy (kilojoules and calories). Only four components of the diet contribute energy: protein, fat, carbohydrate and alcohol. Fat and alcohol, when compared gram for gram, have around twice the kilojoules as protein or carbohydrate (see table 13.1). Therefore, it makes sense to limit the

TABLE 13.1 Energy Value of Food Components

Food component	Kilojoules per gram	Calories per gram
Protein	17	4
Fat	37	9
Carbohydrate	16	4
Alcohol	29	7

amount of fat and alcohol you consume if you want to lose excess body fat. Indeed, the scientific evidence supports this as the best decision.

Eat for Fat Loss

The dietary basics for losing body fat are to eat less fat and alcohol, and possibly eat more good-quality carbohydrate foods, such as fruit, and protein foods such as meat or legumes. This is the current, universally accepted style of eating for health and shedding body fat. Most adults gain weight because they eat too much fat, drink too much alcohol and do not eat enough staple foods such as fruits, vegetables and whole-grain cereals.

It is now well established that the fat in food is quite easy to convert to body fat. If you eat an extra 100 kilojoules as fat, 97 of them will go straight onto your waist. Carbohydrate and excess protein are generally used for energy production and are unlikely to be converted to body fat. Here, it must be noted that carbohydrate foods include sugars and starches; therefore, sugar in modest amounts is unlikely to be fattening. Protein and carbohydrate intakes are tightly regulated, and any excess consumption is burned up by the body rather than being stored as fat, although there is evidence that fat people are capable of converting some carbohydrate to body fat.

The body will preferentially convert food carbohydrate to blood glucose and glycogen stored in muscle and in the liver. Glucose is your primary muscle and brain fuel. Without carbohydrate you will have to convert muscle or food proteins to glucose, because fat is very poorly and inefficiently converted to glucose. Although it is possible to eat excess carbohydrate, in real life this is difficult if those carbohydrate foods are fruits, vegetables and whole-grain cereals. It is rare to find anyone who eats too many fruits and vegetables; indeed, 9 out of 10 adults eat too few.

Fat also has a poor feedback mechanism on appetite so it is easy to overconsume fatty foods before they satisfy the appetite. Both low GI carbohydrate and protein are much more efficient at telling the body when it is full so they tend not to be overconsumed. Beyond this, there is good evidence that foods with a high water content have a strong ability to satisfy the appetite for a relatively few kilojoules. Table 13.2 summarises the effects of the various food components on appetite and their ability to become excess body fat.

In a series of experiments, University of Sydney researchers showed that different foods with equal amounts of kilojoules had widely differing abilities to satisfy the appetite (Holt et al. 1995). For example, for the same number of kilojoules, boiled potatoes were six times more filling than a croissant. The upshot of this work was that foods with a high water content and a low fat content such as fruits and vegetables were far more satisfying than foods with a low water content and a high fat content such as cakes and pastries.

The University of Sydney study also revealed that high-protein, low-fat foods such as lean meat and fish had a high level of satiety (appetite suppression). You can see why a meal of meat and vegetables or salad is very satisfying. (Of course, this natural appetite-suppressing effect can be overridden at all-you-can-eat smorgasbord meals, Christmas dinner and other special events.)

We are conditioned to eat the same amount of food each day. I don't mean the same amount of kilojoules, but the same volume of food. Dr. Barbara Rolls' research at Pennsylvania State University, USA, revealed that we eat roughly the same weight or volume of food each day (Rolls and Bell 1999). Think about it. No matter what you do, you probably eat the same breakfast five or six days a week. You probably also expect the same amount of food on your dinner plate. If it is true that we eat the same volume of food each day, then it makes sense to eat foods with a low energy density—that is, low-fat, high-water, moderate-protein type foods (e.g., fruits and vegetables are around 90 per cent water and only 1 to 3 kilojoules per gram). Eating too much high-energy-density foods could be contributing to the midriff overhang. Table 13.3 shows the range of energy densities found in food.

Keep a Check on Fat

Fat is very energy dense; that is, it has a lot of kilojoules per gram compared to other food components. As table 13.1 shows, fat and alcohol have the most energy (in kilojoules or calories) per gram, making them the most energy dense components of food. This is why there is such a concern with the fat content of foods and why dietary fat has such a bad image.

I mentioned in chapter 1 that some diet advisers recommend that you count the fat in your diet, limiting it to 20 to 30 grams per day. That's a huge and dramatic drop when you consider that many people eat 80 to 100 grams of fat a day (probably more for lovers of fries, pizza and cheesecake). Of course, if you want palatable and enjoyable meals, I suggest you don't go any lower than 40 grams per day for women, and 50 to 60 grams for men, who are active each day. Count fat grams if you wish, but don't become fat obsessed because the food may start to control you rather than vice versa. The most dangerous fat, of course, is saturated fat. You can use the Nutrient

TABLE 13.2 Influence of Various Food Components on Body Fat

Food component	Energy content	Effect on your satiety	Ability to convert excess to body fat	Ability to make you fat
Fat	High	Moderate	Easy	High
Protein	Low	Good	Hard	Low
Carbohydrate (especially low GI)	Low	Good	Hard	Low
Alcohol	Moderate	Moderate	Hard	Moderate
Water	Nil	Good	Nil	Nil

TABLE 13.3 Energy Density of Selected Foods

Food	Kilojoules per 100 g	Calories per 100 g
Mushroom	98	23
Broccoli	125	30
Apple	180	45
Banana	358	85
Green peas	275	65
Potato, boiled	290	70
Milk, full cream	280	67
Milk, skim	146	35
Baked beans	395	90
Rice, steamed	490	115
Pasta, boiled	630	150
Meat, lean	730	175
Bread	925	220
Pizza	1,000	240
Muesli bar	1,680	400
Croissant	1,340	320
Meat pie	1,065	255
Potato crisps	2,100	500
Soft drink	170	40
Beer	170	40
Wine	315	75

Ready Reckoner on page 215 to get an idea of the fat content of foods. Don't forget that some fat-containing foods such as the avocados, nuts, peanut butter, seeds and cheese are very nutritious and should still have a place in your diet.

Drink Less Alcohol

Although small amounts of alcohol may be protective against heart disease, alcohol is high in energy and can also contribute to your waistline. Alcohol is dealt with as a toxic substance by the body, so it must be metabolised preferentially ahead of other nutrients. As soon as the body absorbs alcohol, it starts to metabolise it at around 10 grams (one standard drink) each hour. Each gram of alcohol is 29 kilojoules (7 cal). If these kilojoules aren't burned up through activity, more food fat will be converted into body fat. Put another way, alcohol isn't converted to body fat, but it will 'push' more food fat into becoming body fat.

The figures for alcohol given in table 13.3 suggest that soft drinks, beer and wine are not very energy dense. Be aware, however, that most people easily drink much more soft drink, beer and wine than they do, say, skim milk. Three cans of beer provide 1,890 kilojoules (450 cal), whereas a glass of skim milk provides 335 kilojoules (80 cal).

Can You Eat as Much Carbohydrate as You Like?

Carbohydrate is very efficiently stored as glycogen, but on the rare occasion that liver and muscle glycogen stores are full, carbohydrate can be converted to body fat. Yet even when large amounts of carbohydrate are eaten, its conversion to fat is slow and inefficient. The body's major adaptation is to increase the amount of carbohydrate used as a fuel source and store any excess dietary fat as body fat. It is possible to eat too much carbohydrate (more than 800 g [28 oz] daily), but I have never seen a fit and healthy person eat good-quality carbohydrate to excess. Fat, yes; carbohydrate, no. Don't think that eating lots of cakes, biscuits and pastries is a carbohydrate problem. Most of their kilojoules come from fat. (Half the kilojoules in a cream biscuit come from fat.)

Following is the view of the World Health Organisation (2003, 80) on what you should be eating to help control your weight:

The fat and water content of foods are the main determinants of the energy density of the diet. A lower consumption of energy-dense (i.e., high-fat, high-sugar and high-starch) foods and energy-dense (i.e., high free sugars) drinks contributes to a reduction in total energy intake. Conversely, a higher intake of energy-dilute foods (i.e., vegetables and fruits) and foods high in fibre (i.e., wholegrain cereals) contributes to a reduction in total energy intake and an improvement in micronutrient intake. It should be noted, however, that very active groups who have diets high in vegetables, legumes, fruits and wholegrain cereals, may sustain a total fat intake of up to 35% without the risk of unhealthy weight gain.

▶ Fat, Carbohydrate and Protein

Following are some reasons for reducing fat intake:

- Fat is energy dense, having twice the kilojoules as carbohydrate or protein.
- Excess fat is relatively easy to convert to body fat.
- Fat is less satisfying to the appetite compared to carbohydrate and protein. As a result, it is easier to overeat (think chocolate biscuits and pizza).
- Fatty foods (e.g., pastries, cakes, cookies) generally have low water content and a high energy density, which means they take longer to suppress the appetite. High-water-content foods seem to have a greater ability to satisfy the appetite than do high-fat, low-water foods.
- Keeping the fat, especially saturated fat, intake low may be the best nutrition strategy for long-term body fat loss and health.
- Many high-fat foods, such as crisps, pizza and snack foods, also have a high salt content.

Following are benefits of eating more carbohydrate and having a moderate protein intake:

- Unrefined carbohydrate foods such as fruits, vegetables and legumes are very filling, making them difficult to overconsume. These foods are generally low glycemic index.
- Lean protein foods such as lean meats and fish have a good ability to control appetite. Including a protein food at each meal can help to satisfy your appetite throughout the day.
- Fruits, vegetables and legumes have a high water content, which makes them quite filling.
- High-carbohydrate and moderate-protein foods such as breads, cereals and legumes provide essential nutrients and fibre.
- Carbohydrate foods are your only source of fibre. Adequate fibre will keep you regular, whereas too little could clog your down-pipe.
- Fruits, vegetables, nuts, seeds and cereals are your major source of antioxidants, which are linked to a reduced risk of heart disease and cancer.
- Protein foods offer a range of minerals, with calcium (milk, yogurt, cheese), iron and zinc (meats) being the minerals of most importance.
- Including some foods with 'natural' fat such as nuts, seeds, avocados and vegetable oils will enhance healthy eating, while still leaving some room for your favourite treats.

That quote is the conclusion of the of the WHO Technical Report on Diet, Nutrition and the Prevention of Chronic Diseases. Note that it says that very active people can have a bit more freedom with their fat intake if they are pretty lean already. A lower-fat, higher-carbohydrate diet is probably the best food balance to *minimise* body fat stores. There is no need to cut out all sources of fat.

Successful and Permanent Weight Loss

Because you are likely to be a fit and active person, then you are probably burning quite a few kilojoules each day. By focusing more on the energy consumed, you should achieve a steady rate of fat loss with some simple changes to your diet. I have given you what I think is the basis of successful fat loss. This is not just personal opinion. U.S. researchers have tracked 3,000 people who have lost at least 10 per cent of their body weight and kept that excess off for a year or more (Wing and Hill 2001). On average, the participants in this project lost 30 kilograms (66 lb) over five years. The researchers found that these successful weight maintainers had a lot in common. The most important factors in their success were as follows:

- They ate a healthy, low-fat diet (not a low-carbohydrate diet).
- They ate smaller portion sizes and rarely overate.

- They ate breakfast regularly.
- They allowed themselves the occasional treat without concern.
- They exercised, or were active, for at least one hour each day (and often had a friend exercise with them).
- They kept tabs on their weight, but weren't obsessive about it. They quickly changed their food and exercise habits if their weight began to creep up.

More recently, the same research group found other characteristics of those who successfully controlled their weight (Phelan et al. 2009):

- They ate less restaurant and take-away foods.
- They watched less TV and had fewer TVs in the house.

As you can see, success means a high level of self-management; that is, success is up to you and no one, and nothing, else.

Relationship Between Food and Exercise

You have probably heard a few people say that exercise intensity and time of day are very important as to how much fat you burn up. Well, it doesn't really matter. The biggest factor for burning up body fat is whether you do the activity in the first place. It may be interesting to speculate whether you burn more fat in certain circumstances, but here is a general guide:

- To burn fat, you have to be active. The fitter you are, the better your body is at burning fat. To get a reasonable level of fitness, you need to get up and move your body for three to five hours a week.
- It doesn't really matter whether you exercise in the morning or afternoon, or whether you exercise before breakfast or after breakfast. People will tell you that you are a better fat burner at certain times of the day, but this is without substantiation. If you exercise primarily for weight control, and your body burns more kilojoules than you consume in your diet, then you will be a fat burner, independent of when you exercise.
- It doesn't really matter whether you walk or jog. You will burn up more fat by jogging for 30 minutes than you will by walking for 30 minutes. On the other hand, you will burn up more fat by walking for 60 minutes than you will by jogging for 30 minutes.
- The amount of incidental activity you perform during the day will potentially burn more fat and kilojoules than a jog. Getting up from your chair, having a stretch or a quick walk around the office, taking the stairs up to the next floor, hand watering the garden, and so on, can burn more body fat through the day than a 30-minute walk. So, don't assume that 30 minutes of exercise a day is all you need to do for fat burning.
- Weight-bearing exercises such as walking, aerobics and jogging are better at burning up fat stores than are weight-supported exercise such as swimming and cycling over the same amount of time. However, it is better to do something you enjoy than to analyse its fat burning capabilities. Refer back to the first point.

Your Eating Habits

Sometimes, just the way people eat makes it very difficult to lose weight. Let me give you some examples.

- **Speed eaters.** Life is busy—so much to do, so little time. If you always eat your meals quickly, then you will likely eat more kilojoules than you need before your appetite is satisfied. Slow down your meals. Take time to chew your food. This will allow time for your body chemistry to assess when you have truly had enough to eat. The signal will come from a feeling of fullness.
- **Plate cleaners.** In my experience, almost half of adults feel compelled to eat everything on their plates, mainly because this was how they were brought up. Being a plate cleaner means you are responding to a visual cue rather than an internal hunger cue before you stop eating. If you have been given a large serve, then you will eat it all and likely overshoot your needs. The extra kilojoules are stored as fat.
- **Hara hachi bu.** Stop eating before you are full, and feel comfortable leaving food on your plate. *Hara hachi bu* is a Japanese expression meaning 'Eat until your stomach is 80 per cent full'. That means eating until

you are no longer hungry, rather than eating until you can't fit anything more in.

- **TV munchers.** Some people eat many of their meals in front of the TV or always like to nibble on a snack when watching their favourite programs. In this situation, you virtually have little knowledge of what, or how much, you eat. You have become distanced from the eating experience. Try eating your meals slowly at the dinner table. Eat with other people if possible, so that the table conversation helps slow down the rate at which you eat. If you do nibble while watching TV, make sure they are smart food choices such as fresh fruit, a whole-grain sandwich or roasted peanuts in the shell.

Food–Exercise Diary and Pedometers

Many health advisers suggest keeping a record of everything you eat and drink and all the exercise you do. This can be very useful way of reminding you of your habits and whether you are on target for your goals. Sometimes it is really easy to forget the last time you went for a walk or to the gym. The diary can serve as a useful reminder. There are a number of apps that track your movements via GPS on your phone to tell you how far you have travelled while walking, running or on your bike. There are also food diary and calorie counter apps suited to your phone or tablet PC. Check the descriptions and user evaluations for the best one for your purposes.

Wearing a pedometer can also be very handy. This neat and inexpensive monitor can be worn on the belt and measures the number of steps taken each day. The aim for previously sedentary people is 7,000 steps daily, although this will need to increase to 10,000 to 12,000 steps for effective body fat loss and maintaining that loss. A pedometer will give you a good indication of how much incidental activity you are doing. Again, a number of pedometer phone apps are available, either free or low cost.

Eating Disorders

Despite the impression that athletes are superhealthy, the eating disorders anorexia nervosa and bulimia are common among athletes, especially females, who make up 90 per cent of those afflicted. It occurs mostly in women under pressure to be the perfect weight and shape in sports such as diving, gymnastics, distance running and synchronised swimming. Men who have to keep within a set weight or need to look very lean are also prone to eating disorders (e.g., wrestlers, boxers, gymnasts and bodybuilders).

Eating habits can stray from normal long before athletes get stamped as having an eating disorder. They may start cutting back on fatty take-aways and snacks, but when they start cutting back on healthy food such as whole-grain bread, milk and starchy vegetables to lose weight or become a certain shape, then it could be a warning sign of an eating disorder. Occasional purging and other unhealthy habits to achieve weight loss may not be witnessed, although an obsession with the scales and skinfold callipers are likely to be obvious, especially if an athlete wants to be weighed and measured for skinfolds on a daily basis.

It isn't the purpose of this book to discuss how to prevent eating disorders, or how to solve them. All I can do is acknowledge their existence and point out some characteristics of eating disorders. If you suspect that you or someone you know has an eating disorder, I strongly recommend that you seek professional help or talk to an eating disorder support group.

Warning to Parents and Coaches

Parents and coaches can have a great impact on how athletes see themselves. Telling young athletes that they're fat, putting them on strict diets or demanding rapid weight loss can lead to obsessive eating behaviour and eating disorders. Instead, suggest they see a sports dietitian who will give them the knowledge and guidance to make changes that reduce body fat without reducing performance. Early education about

Athletes at greatest risk for poor micronutrient status are those that restrict energy intake or have severe weight loss practices, who eliminate one or more of the food groups from their diet, or who consume unbalanced and low micronutrient-dense diets.

Position of the American Dietetic Association, Dietitians of Canada and the American College of Sports Medicine: Nutrition and Athletic Performance (2009, 515)

healthy eating is more helpful than expecting quick changes in weight that encourages unhealthy weight loss ideas. Rapid weight loss will include muscle loss and make training much less effective.

Anorexia Nervosa

Anorexia means 'without appetite'. This condition comes from not eating as a result of listening to outside sources that stress the importance of keeping a lean shape. It starts with dieting and becoming preoccupied with food, body weight and body shape. It is then followed by an enjoyment of dieting, periods of starvation and possibly a very high level of exercise to help weight loss. Sometimes the exercise is a form of punishment for eating too much.

Anorexic athletes can progress to being on a permanent diet and always thinking about food.

Female athletes are most prone to eating disorders, especially in sports where weight and shape are important.

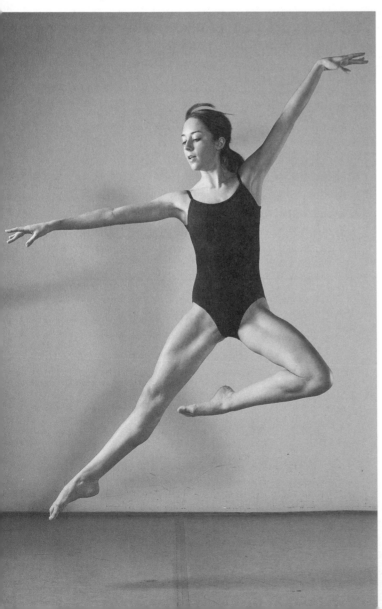

They feel fat when they are actually thin. The body becomes emaciated and skinfold measurements are low. Often they become constipated as a result of low fibre and food intake. The lack of food causes women to stop menstruating, increasing their risk of bone loss and stress fractures (see chapter 4). Dehydration can occur if they start to use diuretics, laxatives or fluid restriction to control their weight. Of course, all the food and fluid restrictions they impose on themselves means they won't be getting all the nutrition required for effective training. By this time they know the kilojoule content of every food in the supermarket. They may wear baggy clothes or multiple layers of clothing to hide their thinness and stay warm (they have too little insulating body fat to keep in the warmth).

Bulimia

People with bulimia are often on a strict diet, during which they sometimes eat lots and lots of food (binge eating), followed by purging through self-induced vomiting, laxatives or diuretics. People with bulimia usually eat very little in public, while tending to be closet eaters at home. They tend to visit the bathroom straight after eating. They may also engage in frequent vigorous exercise.

If vomiting is frequent, teeth repeatedly come into contact with stomach acids, causing erosion of the tooth enamel and eventual tooth decay. Often the family dentist is the first to suspect bulimia when an athlete comes in complaining of very sensitive teeth and the enamel on the inside of the teeth has suffered acid erosion.

If you are preoccupied with food and constantly worrying about your weight, maybe it's time to call for help. To read more on this topic, download the free fact sheet 'Eating Disorders in Athletes' from www.sportsdietitians. com.au/content/2583/EatingDisorders. Other resources include www.anad.org or the eating disorder group in your country, such as http:// au.reachout.com/find/articles/anorexia-nervosa in Australia.

Female Athlete Triad

Given the pressure many female athletes and dancers feel to maintain a very petite shape, they may become mindful of everything they eat or drink. This can lead to food obsessions, strict dieting, inadequate intake of essential nutrients such as calcium and disordered eating. With very little food, the body reacts by ceasing menstrual loss (amenorrhea). The combination of too little food (too few kilojoules or calories), amenorrhea or menstrual irregularity, and the subsequent loss of bone density is called the female athlete triad.

Amenorrhea is not a normal and healthy response to training. The loss of periods results in a drop in estrogen and progesterone levels, infertility and often a loss of bone density. Estrogen and progesterone are hormones that protect against bone loss. Their levels drop to those of postmenopausal women during amenorrhea. If amenorrhea continues for many months, bone density may never return to normal.

A loss of bone density increases the risk of bone stress fractures and the early onset of osteoporosis (brittle bones) later in life. Exercise and an adequate consumption of calcium in the diet can help offset bone loss in this situation, but it is unlikely to stop it altogether.

The athlete with female athlete triad should see both a sports physician and a sports dietitian and be properly assessed. The long-term consequences of this condition are severe and can lead to irreversible bone damage and possibly death in extreme situations. The earlier the intervention, the better for the health of the athlete.

FINAL SCORE

- Your level of body fat can be assessed in a number of ways. Waist circumference, body mass index and skinfold measurements are the most common methods. Measuring waist circumference is the easiest method for most athletes. Skinfold measurements should be done by a trained practitioner.

- Your metabolic rate will increase with extra training, an increase in muscle mass and possibly through dividing your meals into small, frequent snacks. Individual foods such as chilli, caffeine and green tea will have only a minor effect on metabolic rate or weight control.

- Diet books, diet plans, weight loss powders and pills, fat melters, exercise machines and any products promising quick weight loss are very unlikely to work in the long term.

- Sensible eating is the best route to long-term weight loss. It means eating less saturated fat–containing foods, less alcohol and more fruits, vegetables and whole-grain cereal foods.

- Choosing foods that have a low energy density (i.e., with the least amount of kilojoules or calories per 100 g) should be the basis of a fat loss eating plan.

- Be wary of over-restricting your food intake to meet a specified weight or shape. This could lead to disordered eating, inadequate nutrition and, for young women, female athlete triad.

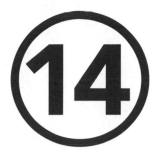

Nutrition for Selected Sports

Athletes will benefit from the guidance of qualified sports nutrition professionals who can advise on their individual energy, nutrient and fluid needs and help develop sport-specific nutritional strategies for training, competition and recovery.

International Olympic Committee Consensus Statement on Sports Nutrition (2010)

Sports nutrition has changed greatly over the last 30 years. Back in 1980 it was a novelty, dabbled in by long-distance runners, triathletes and football teams with money. Now, just about every elite athlete has access to a sports dietitian, or has at least attended courses put on by sports dietitians. The information that the elite athlete has been hearing has filtered down even to junior ranks, which is great news. Although no one is suggesting that an eight-year-old netballer needs to carbohydrate-load or that there should be sports drinks at a primary school sporting event, teenagers and adults can benefit from making smart nutrition decisions in all sports and activities. Some of these are covered in this chapter.

If your sport is not listed in this chapter, choose one that is similar. For example, the guidelines for volleyball would be similar to those for basketball and netball; baseball advice is similar to cricket advice; and triathletes will benefit from the advice to swimmers, cyclists and endurance runners. I suggest that you read the rest of the book first, before reading this section because it assumes that you have all the basic knowledge of sports nutrition. If specific advice is given, such as eating good sources of iron or protein, then refer to the chapter that covers the subject in more depth. Very little will be said about

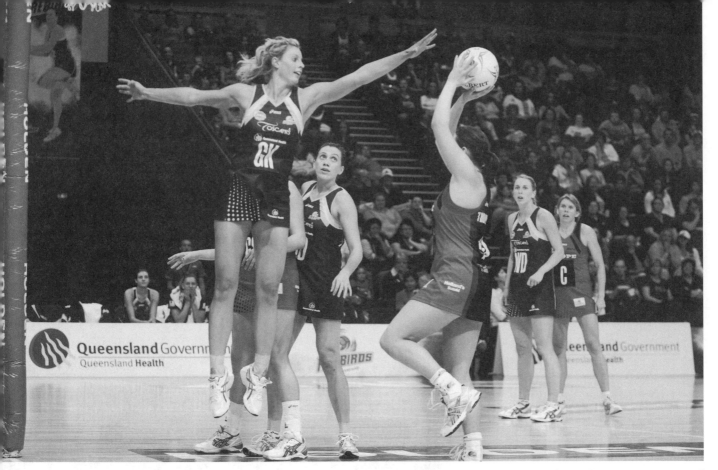

Young female athletes are at a greater risk than males of low iron stores and need to eat a range of foods high in iron.

supplements. Read chapter 9 to see if a supplement may benefit you in your sport.

Your sport's controlling body may also have food and nutrition tips on its website. Sports nutrition experts also provide nutrition advice for specific sports. Use the terms *sports dietitian* or *institute of sport* and the name of your sport in your search engine to find more help on eating for specific sports.

Basketball and Netball

Both basketball and netball are very popular in New Zealand, Australia, South Africa and the UK. Because many women's teams now wear Lycra bodysuits, there can be an emphasis on body shape and a desire to lose body fat (even though this may not improve performance). If you are trying to lose weight, please do it sensibly with the help of a sports dietitian. The common dietary method of cutting back on carbohydrate foods is not recommended because it may lead to low glycogen levels and tiredness. Any body fat loss needs to be gradual without interfering with training and performance. Weight gain is more likely during the off-season and when injured. These are special times to be more vigilant with food choices and also the best times to lose excess body fat.

Females are at a greater risk of low iron stores than males are because they lose more iron in sweat, have monthly blood loss and as a result of foot-strike hemolysis during training and games. Young women need a lot more iron each day than men and need to ensure that they eat a range of high-iron foods such as iron-fortified breakfast cereals and drinks and red meat. They should also boost their iron absorption by consuming vitamin C–containing foods at each meal and snack (e.g., fruit juice, salads and fresh fruit). Male basketballers, especially fit men, find it much easier to meet their iron needs than women do. They are more likely to feel tired from too little carbohydrate or constant mild dehydration during times of intense training.

Before Competition

Eat a main meal two to three hours before a game; allow longer if you get particularly nervous before a game. If you have to be at the venue a couple of hours before the game begins for ankle tape strapping or media commitments, take a carbohydrate snack with you. A banana or a food bar may be necessary to keep hunger pangs away. Make sure you are passing clear urine in the hour before the game or training. This is a reasonable indication that you are hydrated. You may not need to drink again until 10 to 15 minutes before the start. Drinking 200 to 300 millilitres then will ensure there is fluid in your stomach waiting to pass into the small intestine to be absorbed just as you start to sweat.

During Competition

Players are often not able to replace all their fluid losses during a game. Commonly, only half of sweat losses are replaced during a team game such as basketball or netball. Moreover, players vary greatly in their need for fluid: some sweat heavily and others, only lightly under the same conditions. Fluid needs may be lower in court games in which players spend some time on the bench and in enclosed air-conditioned areas. If you do have some bench time, take the opportunity to sip at a drink bottle. There is no need to drink huge volumes, just enough to have some fluid in the stomach and minimise dehydration during a game. Similarly, use time-outs and quarter-time breaks as opportunities to drink. Dehydrated players experience a decline in their passing and shooting skills.

After Competition

Your key postgame strategy is to replace any fluid losses accumulated during the game. That won't be a problem if you had only a short amount of court time. It will be necessary if you spent most of the second half on the court. Because you may have had less than an hour of activity during a game, you may not be hungry. It is still smart to eat some carbohydrate in the one to two hours after a game to initiate the glycogen replacement process, and then to have a larger meal later. If you had an evening or night game, eat a reasonably sized meal before going to bed so your meal can be digested and absorbed overnight (and, no, food eaten after 8 p.m. doesn't go straight onto your buttocks; it is used just as it normally would be, to replenish and repair the body).

Summary

Basketball and netball are sprint and precision-based sports that often involve some strength training as well. Because nutrition influences both endurance and skill, it is important to be well hydrated and well fuelled before and during games. Low glycogen stores near the end of a game can affect passing and shooting.

Cricket

Modern cricketers have to be moderately lean, strong, flexible and very fit. They are under pressure to be in control of their weight while also being involved in fitness, strength and skills training to improve their fielding, bowling and batting. The most common problems they face are dehydration and hunger because games can be held in very hot weather and over a number of hours. A fielding team in a cricket match can be out on the oval for six hours in very warm weather.

Before Competition

Be well hydrated before you start the game. Passing almost-clear urine about an hour before the game starts indicates that you are well hydrated. It is wise to eat about two hours before the game so very little food remains in your stomach and you do not feel hungry. If you end up being 12th man in cricket or not batting for a while, you can enjoy snacks and drink fluids while waiting your turn to be on the field, although you should still eat wisely and avoid fatty cakes and biscuits. In a professional cricket game that is played over four or five days, lunch and afternoon tea are provided. If you are batting, bowling or likely to bat or bowl in the hour following lunch, then do not eat too much food. If you do eat in a break, eat until you are not hungry, not until you feel full. You don't want to suddenly find yourself batting or bowling and feeling uncomfortable or at risk of heartburn, with food in your stomach coming up into your throat.

During Competition

Bowlers who find themselves bowling throughout the day will need to regularly consume fluids and high-carbohydrate foods and snacks. A regular bowler is likely to benefit from a sports drink, especially in hot weather. I remember Australian fast bowler Brett Lee saying that he would get cramps in the last session of a game if he bowled all day, until he started taking a sports drink that contained sugars and sodium. The sports drinks hydrated him, and the sodium reduced the chance of cramps.

Elite cricketers have access to cool fluids all through the day with drink bottles on the boundary and drink breaks every hour (every 40 minutes in very hot weather). Even club cricketers have a cool box with drinks on the boundary so that a bowler or fielder can take a drink between overs. If it is hot, ask the umpires to schedule extra drink breaks so everyone has a better opportunity to take on fluid.

A fielder may cover 5 to 10 kilometres (3 to 6 miles) during a day of fielding, so it is important to keep up fluids. During hot weather your body may use up glycogen at a faster rate than normal; a sports drink will be a useful source of glucose in this case.

The advice for batsmen depends on how long you bat for. On a bad day, it is a stroll out to the middle and back. On a good day, you might be batting for many hours, which means there will be much greater demands on your body and a greater demand for nutrients and fluids. Certainly, take every opportunity to drink fluids to replace sweat losses. Ideally, you should drink enough to match your losses. If you lose more than 2 per cent of your body weight during an innings, you are likely to be slower between wickets, think slower and have slower reactions to the bowling.

Longer breaks in play (e.g., a lunch break) offer an opportunity to eat solid foods. Whatever you eat will empty from your stomach over the next couple of hours, but you don't want to feel uncomfortable. I recommend that you don't eat so much that you feel full, especially if you are waiting to bat and don't really know when that will be. Liquid foods empty quicker from the stomach than solid foods do, so a smoothie made with low-fat milk or a soy drink would be a good choice. Otherwise, choose low-fat carbohydrate snacks such as fruit, cereal bars, yogurt, sports bars and even the good old sandwich, a banana or a pasta salad. If you know you won't be batting for a while, you can have a more substantial meal. Make sure you replace your fluid losses during this time and take a pee break before you go back on the field.

After Competition

Based on your activity and game involvement during the day, you will now have a better gauge as to how much, and what type, of food and fluid you need to replace what you have used. If you have played a lot during the day, you will need carbohydrate to replenish glycogen stores (e.g., fruit salad, pasta, sushi, bread rolls filled with meat and salad) and protein foods (e.g., yogurt, milkshake, meat, chicken, quiche) to help repair any minor muscle damage. Rely on non-alcoholic fluids to get yourself properly hydrated. Fluids after a game can include cordial, fruit juice and even tea and coffee on cooler days in addition to water and sports drinks.

In the last century, alcohol was strongly associated with the celebration and relaxation after a day's play. Now, elite cricketers realise that alcohol compromises injury recovery, rehydra-

tion and subsequent playing ability, especially in games lasting more than one day. If you, or your team, normally have a beer or other alcoholic drink after a game, then drink smart—that is, don't drink alcohol until you're well hydrated; then, drink only sensible amounts, and don't drink if you have been injured, to facilitate healing. I don't recommend that you drink alcohol at all if you are injured or if you have to play again the next day.

Summary

The characteristics of a cricket game can be very predictable if there are a limited number of overs; this makes planning your nutrition easy. In games in which you aren't sure how long you might be batting, fielding or bowling, you will have to give a little more thought to planning your food and drink intake before the game starts. Assume the best if you are batting; assume the worst if you are fielding. That is, expect to bat for a long time and be prepared to field or bowl for a long time.

Cycling

The nutrition advice for cycling depends on whether it is a single-day event or a multi-day event. If the event is just on one day, what is the duration? Is it over in an hour, or could it take six hours? The longer the event, the more you will have to plan to eat on your bike. Because much of the food and drink eaten on the bike can be low in essential nutrients, you need to eat particularly well at mealtimes to make sure essential nutrients such as iron and calcium feature in your diet. That means eating meat, whole-grain cereals and fortified breakfast cereals for iron, and yogurt, milk, cheese and fortified soy milk for calcium.

Some formulated sports bars, although expensive, are fortified with essential nutrients such as iron and calcium. Be wary that food bars and constant snacking on the bike can lead to gradual weight gain if you ride slowly and don't burn many kilojoules. If you have to cut back on training because of extended bad weather or injury, be sure not to overeat and gain weight.

Before Competition

Naturally, use your training sessions to get used to what suits you during a ride. Some cyclists need to eat something within the first hour of a ride; others can wait until later or find that a sports drink is enough in rides of two to three hours. Most recreational riders have to carry all their food and drinks with them, possibly stopping at water fountains or shops to restock food and fluids. Some cyclists prefer to eat a large meal two or three hours before cycling and then snack thereafter, with the idea that they can eat less food on the bike. Others prefer a light meal before cycling and then frequently snack during the ride.

Whatever technique you choose, it is likely that in long rides you will need to snack every 30 minutes or so. Just prior to a long ride, especially if it is warm, drink 200 to 300 millilitres of fluid so you have that fluid on board to be absorbed into the blood as soon as you begin to sweat.

During Competition

In shorter rides of less than two hours, you may get by with just water. On longer rides, you really do need the help of sports drinks and foods. All-time favourites of cyclists are ripe bananas (the riper they are, the softer and sweeter and quicker to digest they are), dried fruit bars, food bars and jelly confectionery such as jelly beans. They like these kinds of snacks because they can keep them in the pouches of their tops or, in the case of jelly snakes, wrapped around their handlebars so they can pull off small amounts to eat when needed. Some cyclists travel with carbohydrate gels as well. The emphasis is on carbohydrate foods because each leg muscle

contraction is burning carbohydrate. Getting too little carbohydrate will make your legs heavy due to glycogen depletion.

You will need sports drinks for longer training rides. Don't try to get by on one bidon (600 mL water bottle) in rides over an hour. You might make it to the end, but you will then spend the rest of the day tired while you make up the fluid deficit. You are better off having two or three bidons on the bike, possibly making an allowance for a drink stop during the ride to refill the bidons with water or a sports drink. Drink early and drink frequently to avoid dehydrating early.

One problem is that the rapid air movement across your skin while cycling causes sweat evaporation so you may not be aware of heavy sweat loss. This is especially common in warm weather. Hourly sweat losses can be as low as 300 millilitres on a cool day and up to 1,500 millilitres on a warm day.

Some cyclists ingest gels with caffeine because they allow them to ride for longer at a higher intensity. Experiment with caffeine gels during training rides to see if they make your longer rides easier. Make sure you wash gels down with extra water because they are a concentrated source of carbohydrate.

After Competition

Because you are likely on your bike every day (serious recreational cyclists often ride 300 to 400 kilometres, or 186 to 249 miles, a week),

Endurance cyclists will need plenty of fluids and snacks like gels, food bars and jelly confectionery to fuel a long ride.

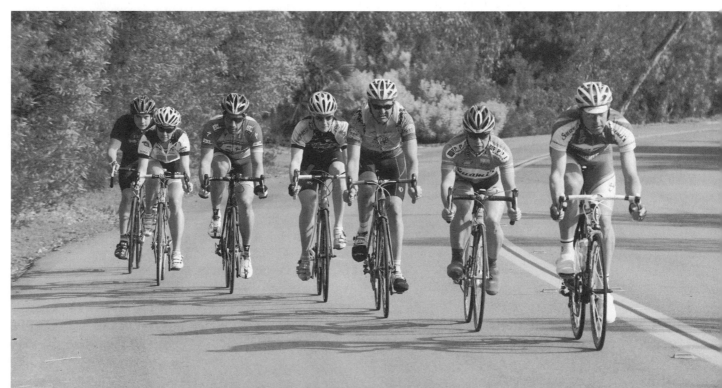

you need to listen to your body. On occasion, weigh yourself before and after a ride to gauge how much fluid you are replacing during a ride. Weigh yourself regularly during the week, especially after a big ride, because weight loss over a short time is likely to be fluid loss and an indication of dehydration. Once you are off the bike, it is time to refuel and replenish lost fluid. Although an obvious food choice would be a sandwich, and an obvious drink, water, high-water foods can also be helpful in replacing fluids (e.g., apples, oranges, steamed rice, yogurt) as can fluids such as fruit juice, milk, tea and coffee.

Summary

Cycling is a sport that involves a lot of training (i.e., a lot of kilometres and often on successive days). This makes nutrition and fluid replacement critical for your performance. It is not always easy to gauge sweat loss in the rain or if the wind current evaporates sweat as soon as it appears on the skin surface. Occasionally weighing yourself before and after a ride will give you a good indication of your fluid losses. You are likely to need to snack during long rides, so experiment to see what works best for you. You are the best person to tailor your own fluid and foods needs.

Football (Soccer, Australian Rules)

It seems prudent to recommend that football players training and or playing in the heat consider the benefits of limiting their body mass loss due to water loss during both training sessions and matches to less than about 2%.

S.M. Shirreffs 2010, 92

Players of all codes of football require high-level skills, speed (for intermittent bursts of sprinting), strength and endurance to get through 90 to 120 minutes of a game. During a game, players may cover 10 to 18 kilometres (6 to 11 miles), much of this at a dead run or sprint, and they do this while rapidly changing direction and duties (e.g., tackling, jumping, running backwards, passing). Therefore, players need both aerobic and anaerobic fitness.

Training during the preseason and season usually includes four to eight training sessions a week, including a recovery session after a game, flexibility and strength training sessions, skill sessions and endurance training sessions. This intensity of training mandates that footballers make judicious food and drink choices every day.

Once the off-season starts (which may be only six to eight weeks long for elite footballers), players have more time to enjoy restaurants, take-aways and time with friends and family; as a result, body fat levels begin to increase. Some highly paid footballers give their code a bad name by going off the rails and indulging in excess alcohol and illicit drugs. Fortunately, the majority of footballers know that limiting their alcohol consumption and eating well will extend their playing career and help them to control their weight.

Before Competition

Because a football season is so demanding, you need to eat enough carbohydrate each day to keep your muscles well fuelled. This is likely to be 5 to 8 grams of carbohydrate per kilogram of body weight. If you do not take in sufficient carbohydrate, you will quickly tire during training and games. It is important that you weigh yourself during the week, including before and after training. If you are losing weight or cannot gain weight through strength training, you may not be eating enough food. Rather than trying to eat more, you are better off trying to concentrate the kilojoules by adding milk powder or commercial food powders to milk and yogurt, and using other ideas found in chapter 12. Food bars taken to training are a convenient way to add energy-dense foods to the diet after training and before eating a meal. Weight loss during a training session will be mainly fluid and needs to be replaced, preferably before leaving the training ground. The best choices are water, sports drinks, fruit juice or even low-fat milk, the latter providing protein as well as carbohydrate and fluid.

If the game is not until the afternoon, then there is plenty of time to ensure good hydration and eat enough carbohydrate and protein at breakfast and lunch. Often, footballers have a larger meal about four hours before kick-off, followed by a smaller snack about two hours later. This ensures that they start the game with an empty stomach but not hungry. Studies of footballers indicate that those who don't eat enough carbohydrate before the game are slower, cover less ground, do less sprint work and experience

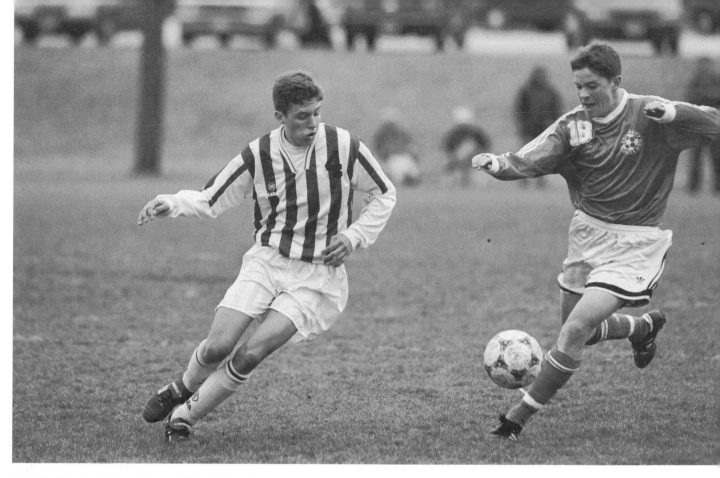

Footballers need to be well-hydrated and fueled so that their skills, thinking and endurance don't decline in the second half.

a drop in skills compared to their well-fuelled teammates (Currell, Conway and Jeukendrup 2009; Kirkendall 1993). Now, sports dietitians encourage footballers to drink water or a sports drink in the 10 minutes before the game starts, to get some reserve fluid on board before the sweating starts.

I once analysed the timing of goals scored in the top two divisions of English football; 23 per cent of all goals were scored in the last 15 minutes, compared to 8.5 per cent in the first 15 minutes. Do attackers get better as the game progresses, or do defenders become tired and dehydrated and make mistakes near the end of the game? You decide.

During Competition

Years ago, the only time a footballer could get fluid during a game was at the quarter-time and half-time breaks. Footballers can now also take advantage of any breaks in play (e.g., injury time, kicking penalties) to drink. Footballers who drink small amounts frequently report that they don't suffer gut bloating as much as those trying to meet their fluid needs just at the scheduled breaks. At the designated breaks (e.g., halftime) a footballer should nurse a drink bottle (i.e., take regular sips).

Generally, footballers drink only half their requirements during a game. In hot weather many are dehydrated by halftime and never are as good as they could be in the second half. On the other hand, during a cold winter's night game with plenty of stoppages, players can overdrink. This is why it is a good idea to know your rate of sweat loss in cool temperatures. If you lose only 600 millilitres per hour, then you need only 500 to 600 millilitres per hour as a replacement. Drinking a litre is counterproductive and may cause stomach upsets and the stitch.

After Competition

It goes without saying that you should drink to replace your sweat losses. Drinks can include tea and coffee, as well as cordials, soft drinks, water and sports drinks. For elite players, sports drinks are likely the best choice. Because football is usually played in the winter months, you may want cool drinks only when you are hot. Once you have cooled down and showered, you may prefer hot drinks. A cup of tea, coffee, milkshake and hot chocolate can all be part of fluid replacement.

In Australia and New Zealand, elite-level soccer is played in the summer months to coincide with the northern hemisphere winter season. Although games are played in the evening or at night, the temperature is likely to be high, making hydration a priority. If it's going to be some time before you get home or to the team hotel, you should have some food available after the game (e.g., sandwiches, a fruit platter, fruit juice, food bars or sushi).

Players continue to be fascinated with protein and the need to protect or build muscle mass. Although you will need protein in the postgame meal to repair any muscle damage, you don't need much. Just 100 grams of meat, fish or chicken will provide enough protein to cover any extra needs. Because you likely have a good appetite anyway, your protein needs are probably covered by normal eating. You can try powdered protein formulas if you wish (they are a convenient way to drink protein), but you probably won't need any more than one protein formula drink a day.

Summary

Many team sports such as football are played at a frenetic pace during the first half. The difference in teams can be seen in the second half. The team whose players are fitter, better fuelled (i.e., have more muscle glycogen) and better hydrated always perform better in the second half. That is the essence of team sports nutrition: eat well before the game and drink well during the game and you will have a better chance against the opposition.

Marathon and Endurance Running

The meaning of the term *long-distance running* depends on people's level of fitness and speed. For some people, *long distance* describes a 10K fun run that they hope to complete in an hour; others define it as a half marathon (21.1 km, or 13 miles) that they can finish in 75 minutes, a marathon (42.2 km, or 26 miles), or even an 80-kilometre (50-mile) or 24-hour ultra-long-distance event. You can finish a 10K run on a good regular diet and smart drinking during the event. When you start competing in events that take you an hour or much more, you need to give serious thought to nutrition. Distance running training can range from 30 minutes to three hours.

A note to women: Long-distance female runners are at a higher risk of low iron stores and anaemia, due to iron losses in sweat, foot-strike haemolysis, possibly blood loss from the gastrointestinal tract and, of course, menses. Read chapter 4 on getting plenty of iron in your diet, especially if you are vegetarian (in which case, read chapter 10 as well). If you eat well yet still feel tired, see your doctor and ask about getting a blood test for iron stores. You've heard it before, but I'll say it again: Don't go taking iron supplements unless you have a confirmed iron deficiency.

Before Competition

If you are training twice a day on most days and running 120 to 200 kilometres (75 to 124 miles) each week, you need to be serious about your nutrition and hydration. You can easily become slightly dehydrated from day to day if you don't make the effort to drink enough fluids between training sessions and in the evenings before retiring. Tiredness and headaches can indicate low-grade dehydration. Practise your eating and drinking tactics during your long runs. Plan long runs that enable you to take in regular fluids. If you are a recreational athlete, this may mean knowing where all the public drinking fountains are on the route.

Endurance runners need plenty of fuel in the form of carbohydrate. Knowing how to prepare a variety of simple high-carbohydrate meals (or knowing someone who will make them for you) will be an advantage. Long training sessions are tiring, and relying on a take-away outlet for your meals is convenient, but these come with a lot of fat and salt.

Many runners get up early and run before they have to start work. It is not practical to eat a meal at, say, 4 a.m. for a 6 a.m. run. The evening meal and any snack eaten before bed needs to provide sufficient carbohydrate to fuel the morning run. You might benefit from a carbohydrate drink before you start, such as fruit juice, although I suggest that you dilute it by at least a third so that it is quicker to absorb from the intestines. If your early morning run is long, and you know your guts can handle it, then a little bit of solid food such as a low-fat yogurt, a glass of low-fat milk or a banana will help top up your glycogen stores.

During Competition

You should drink 200 to 300 millilitres of fluid in the 10 minutes or so before you start a long run so that you are absorbing water the moment you start sweating. You will feel most comfortable if your previous meal has emptied from your stomach, which means you will need to have eaten your last meal at least two hours before your run. Food remaining in your stomach can bounce around and find its way into your throat—not pleasant. For a short run, you need only water to get you through. With runs of an hour or longer, you will benefit from the sugar and water of a sports drink for hydration and feeding the muscles. In most runs you need to be drinking every 15 minutes, possibly more frequently in warm conditions. Consider also taking a gel with you on very long runs because it will provide extra carbohydrate to improve endurance. Some gels have caffeine, which can reduce the feeling of tiredness in the second half of a run.

On rare occasions, runners in long-distance events overdo the hydration thing and drink more than they sweat to the extent that they suffer from hyponatremia (see chapter 5 on fluids for more on this potentially dangerous problem). Drinking more fluid than you lose through sweat usually occurs only if you run relatively slowly in cool weather for three hours or more. When this happens, your body accumulates too much water. This is why I keep emphasising the value of weighing yourself before and after endurance events—doing so gives you a good idea of how much fluid you lose in various weather conditions.

After Competition

Endurance running burns up a lot of kilojoules and depletes glycogen stores, so start replacing glycogen with carbohydrate snacks and foods soon after you finish a race to take advantage of the elevated levels of enzymes designed to quickly replenish glycogen. You will have some minor muscle fibre damage, too, which means you will need some protein as well. This normally comes naturally in your meal selection (e.g., milk, cereal and a banana after a morning run or pasta, meat and cheese after an evening run).

Naturally, replace any lost fluids as soon as you can. Keep drinking until you have had one or two pees to ensure that you are fully hydrated.

If you are running twice a day, or swimming or cycling in the morning and running in the afternoon as a part of triathlon training, then topping up your fluids and glycogen between training sessions is even more important.

Summary

Endurance running, and endurance sport in general, takes a lot out of the body. For this reason, a constant consumption of good-quality carbohydrate, protein and fluid is needed every day so you can train and compete at your best.

For runs less than an hour, you need only drink water. If you are fit, healthy and eat well, you probably need only water in sessions less than two hours long. Beyond that, you will need the help of sports drinks and possibly gels.

If you do engage in ultra-endurance events, I highly recommend that you consult a sports dietitian because you are likely to need a lot of food and need to understand the best way to get it. There is a limit to how much total food you can eat. You can't just keep eating more pasta to train for events that take several hours or days. A high-kilojoule diet will require extra fat and therefore extra oil in cooking; you may even want to make your own cakes and biscuits with flour, oats, dried fruit and oil. That way, you will need to eat only six times a day to get all your needs.

Orienteering, Rogaining and Bushwalking

Although the competitive versions of these sports, or activities, may entail running and sprinting between checkpoints, many people prefer the more relaxing walk. Orienteering events can be eight hours long, and some rogaining events are 24 hours long. Even a four-hour bushwalk can take a lot out of you.

Before Competition

You need to consider how far you are going and for how long. For a walk of less than two hours, you probably need only a water bottle or two to cover your sweat losses. If you will be out for more than two hours, you need to consider whether to carry any food or whether there are places on your route where you can get fluid and food. Some organised events have a central point where food is available, or food and drink stations occur throughout the course.

During Competition

Fluid is your most important consideration. Make sure you take plenty with you. Allow 600 millilitres per hour (more if the weather is warm). In sports such as rogaining there may be allocated drinks drops, but be aware that these may not be evenly spread through the course, and the water may not be cool. Take powdered sports drink to mix with the water if you plan to cover a long distance. The backpack-style hydration packs can be very handy because they are a lot easier to walk with than water bottles in a backpack or on your belt.

Some events provide catering and food stations, or hash houses. This is not the case for bushwalking and longer events, so if you will be away from food for some hours, have snacks with you. The banana is always a favourite. Make sure it is unlikely to get squashed during the event. Food bars, jelly confectionery, gels, trail mix and dried fruit are popular. Even chocolate can be a great pick-me-up when the weather is cool (or if you can keep it cool) during long events.

During long events you may start to lose your appetite for food because you are beginning to tire or you are not enjoying the repetition of your snacks (be sure to include a variety). Even if you aren't hungry, it is smart to snack on something every hour.

After Competition

As always, get yourself rehydrated as soon as possible after the event. You are likely to need a meal after longer events. This is sometimes provided by caterers, and orienteering and rogaining clubs have a good idea of what participants need. They often provide potato, pasta and rice dishes, both vegetarian and with meat, along with bread, fruit and a dessert. Other foods, such as yogurt and ice cream, are available depending on budget and refrigeration capabilities. Bushwalkers have to be prepared to cook their own meals or get to a suitable restaurant or café for a meal, although some bushwalking clubs provide catering for organised events.

Summary

If you are enjoying a two-hour walk, then a water bottle is all you need. Once you become involved in longer events up to 24 hours, you need to plan ahead. If you are new to orienteering or rogaining, talk to those who are experienced for practical advice on food, fluids and the best way to transport them. With good planning you will enjoy your event or your walk without going hungry or becoming dehydrated.

Rugby

Although Rugby Union and Rugby League have seasons, usually in the colder months, many professional rugby players play almost the entire year and may get only four to six-week breaks from the sport. During that time they are still expected to remain fit, lose very little strength and endurance, and not gain too much fat. Some players need to be swift and very athletic, whereas other players need to be heavy (not fat) and strong to hold up a scrum in Rugby Union. Training involves skill training, speed and interval training, strength training and some endurance work.

Usually, rugby teams play once per week, often alternating between a home game and an away game, so they need to consider pregame nutrition, fluids during a game and postgame recovery. If travel involves a long bus trip or flights, then tactics for eating on the road need to be considered (see chapter 11). During the week there are likely to be two or three strength training sessions and three to five team training sessions. Injured players have rehabilitation sessions that may involve swimming, jogging and weight training.

Before Competition

Strength is critical for all rugby players, which explains the emphasis on strength training. To develop and keep muscle mass, players need to eat sufficient protein and carbohydrate. A forward in Rugby Union can weigh 90 to 120 kilograms (198 to 265 lb) and must have a high food intake to maintain this weight and have sufficient energy for training. The backs are lighter and more agile and may weigh 80 to 95 kilograms (176 to 209 lb). They should emphasise carbohydrate for endurance because they cover greater distances on the field. Just because players burn a lot of energy doesn't mean they can eat just about anything; a diet of pizza and cake (and beer) can quickly result in weight gain from the high fat content of take-aways.

Many professional rugby players are encouraged to consume protein powders and creatine to assist in building muscle and strength training. Although protein needs can be met through a prudent diet, some players like the security of including a protein drink or protein food bar in their diets. To get enough carbohydrate and kilojoules each day, they need to eat at least five times a day, possibly up to eight times a day.

Eat a meal at least a couple of hours before you start playing rugby. Having food in your stomach when tackling or being tackled will not feel comfortable, and it will put you in danger of heartburn. Remember that pre-season training is during the warmer summer months. Make sure you are passing light-coloured urine an hour or so before playing. That is a simple indication that you are well hydrated.

During Competition

The game of rugby is played in two 40-minute halves. Players cover around 5 to 8 kilometres (3 to 5 miles) in a game, which is less than what many players in soccer or Australian Rules football run, but rugby players often run at a higher intensity. The running backs cover more distance that the heavier, stronger forwards. During the game a number of stoppages can a occur as a result of injuries, kicking penalties and conversions, and for scrums and line-outs. Players may also find themselves substituted or sin-binned. These are all great opportunities to get a drink and, of course, reflect on your behaviour if you got binned! Drinking is critical if you sweat a lot or are playing in warm weather.

If you know that you tire near the end of a game, taking a sports drink during the game and the half-time break is a smart move; taking in some more carbohydrate as a gel or jelly confectionery can be very useful, too. First experiment with taking a gel during longer team training sessions to make sure it suits you because gels don't agree with everyone.

After Competition

Professional rugby teams often have breakfast, snacks or milkshakes provided after training or a game. Most players, though, won't be that lucky. If you can make it home soon after a game or training session, then eat a meal comprising protein and carbohydrate to help replace glycogen stores and repair any muscle damage. If you won't be home for a while, take food with you, such as bananas, food bars, gels, yogurt, sandwiches or milk-based drinks, or purchase wisely from a take-away venue (see chapter 11).

Because rugby is a contact sport, there is a good chance you have been bruised or even injured during the game. Drinking alcohol afterwards will promote the bruising and delay repair. Even if you have had stoppage time for drinks during the game, you will probably be mildly dehydrated afterwards, so drink non-alcoholic fluids such as water, sports drinks and fruit juice. Remember that straight after training or a game, your body is geared up to replace fluids and glycogen and build and repair muscle, so eat and drink within an hour or so after finishing.

Summary

Rugby is a very demanding sport. Taking advantage of breaks in the game to drink will minimise the risk of becoming dehydrated. Even mild dehydration can slow you down. Because strength training is important at the elite level, eat protein foods at each meal; carbohydrate foods are necessary for fuelling all training sessions and games. As you hear me say repeatedly, start training well hydrated, and make sure to rehydrate as soon as you can after training and games.

Swimming

Because it isn't evident, many people wonder whether swimmers sweat. The answer is yes. Swimmers generally sweat less than land-based athletes, partly because they are swimming in a cooling medium that surrounds the body, whereas most land athletes have to rely on air currents to evaporate sweat (which is difficult in still conditions and when playing in high

Swimmers and water polo players lose less fluid than running-sport athletes, although their food needs can be very high.

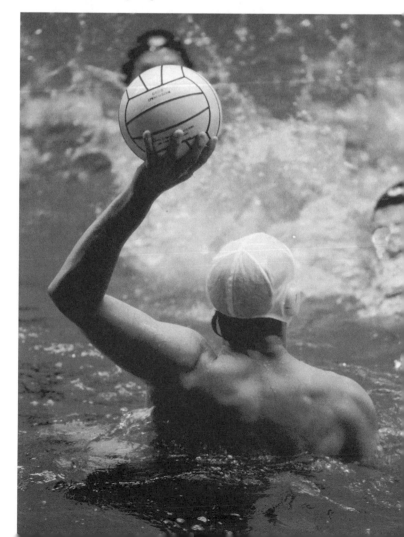

humidity). It is a good idea to weigh yourself before and after a swimming training session of two hours or more. This will give you a good idea of how much fluid (sweat) you have not been able to replace by drinking.

A study of elite swimmers found that males lost 330 millilitres of sweat per hour and females lost 300 millilitres per hour during intense training (Maughan et al. 2009). They were able to replace most of this during the session. Indeed, some swimmers actually gained weight during the session indicating that they drank more fluid than they lost. The Australian Institute of Sport states that elite swimmers lose an average of 125 millilitres of sweat per kilometre swum. During sprint training, sweat losses were around 170 millilitres per kilometre swum. Your sweat levels may differ depending on your level of fitness (higher if you are unfit) and training intensity (higher if you train at a high intensity).

Elite swimmers usually train twice a day for four to six hours. Triathletes might train for 60 to 90 minutes in the morning and go for a run or a bike ride in the evening. In these heavy training situations, it is critically important that you not miss an opportunity to eat well and rehydrate fully, especially if you have to squeeze school, university or a paid job into your day.

Before Competition

Swimmers can generally get away with eating closer to training and event time without having the feeling of a bloated stomach. If you experience heartburn or regurgitation of food during training, give yourself more time between eating and training. If you are training twice a day and for long periods, have some carbohydrate snacks on hand, such as fruit, muesli bars, fruit bars, sports bars, flavoured yogurt or a commercial liquid meal. These come in handy for when you travel from the pool to home or work.

Long training sessions require that you eat plenty of carbohydrate foods beforehand to pump up your glycogen stores. You need to eat only until you are comfortably full. If you have a big training session in the morning, you may need both a high-carbohydrate meal and a snack before going to bed, something like fruit toast with sliced banana or fruit salad and yogurt.

During Competition

During training it is easy and convenient to have one or more drink bottles at the end of the lane. Although you may sweat less than you

do running or cycling, it is still important to be well hydrated during long training sessions. You should be able to just about match your sweat losses with fluid consumed during training. Use sports drinks for long sessions. If the training sessions are particularly long, such as is the case for long-distance open-water swimming in which you may swim 10 kilometres (6.2 miles) in a session, then consider having gels, dried apricot or sugar confectionery available at the end of the lane or from your support crew. Obviously, it is not necessary to drink during events of 50 to 1,500 metres.

Taking on fluid and food is more important for long-distance swimming; in these situations, you will need a support crew to give you food and fluids at predetermined times. If you are training for an open water swim competition, practise eating and drinking the same food and fluids as you are likely to consume during an event.

After Competition

Following your swimming event, solid food may be more important than liquids because you may be only mildly dehydrated yet exceptionally hungry and needing to replace glycogen stores. Eating a food bar or fruit bar straight after swimming may give you enough energy to get back to home base. Now you can rely on the usual fare of high-carbohydrate foods and protein foods. If you have another training session that day, you will need to refuel during the day with foods such as fruit, sandwiches, pasta salad and fruit yogurt. If you are working or studying , make sure you take food with you unless you have access to good-quality food at your workplace, school or university.

Summary

Swimmers burn a lot of kilojoules during intense training sessions. Fluid replacement is relatively easy because swimmers lose less sweat per hour than runners or cyclists do. Energy replacement requires a little more thought, especially if you are training two or three times a day. In that case, every meal and snack needs to provide carbohydrate and protein.

Sprints and Power Sports

Although sprints and power sports such as the 100-metre sprint and powerlifting don't involve a lot of aerobic exercise, they can involve long and gruelling training sessions. A focus on protein to the exclusion of carbohydrate could make those training sessions very tiring. Weightlifters and bodybuilders commonly choose a low-carbohydrate diet in the belief that this will help them get stronger quicker and avoid weight gain. A far better choice is to eat a healthy diet that is relatively low in fat and provides good-quality carbohydrate in the form of fruit, vegetables and whole-grain cereals, and good-quality protein sources such as lean meat, skin-free chicken, fish, eggs and low-fat dairy foods.

In this section, I am assuming that you are trying to increase strength, and possibly muscle size, naturally and not with the aid of drugs or mail-order supplements from countries with lax regulations on what can be added to supplements.

Before Competition

For sprints and power sports, you need the classic healthy diet, but you need more of it than the average person. Your protein needs will be 1.5 to 1.7 grams per kilogram body weight each day, which can easily be met with a healthy diet. If, after reading chapter 2, you believe that you need extra protein, buy something reasonably priced in the form of skim milk powder, protein bars or meal replacement powders. Remember that protein in excess of your needs will be converted to glucose, a carbohydrate, which may be used for muscle contraction. Excess protein is not stored as muscle. You need 5 to 7 grams per kilogram body weight of carbohydrate to fuel two to three hours of training a day. Chapter 3 shows you how to achieve that.

Strength and sprint training athletes can benefit from creatine supplementation (see chapter 9). Check with your sporting body for the supplements they allow. Some supplements for strength training have been found to be tainted with banned or illegal substances. You need to be wary if you get randomly tested for banned substances in your sport.

If you are cutting up for bodybuilding, then make sure your weight loss is gradual. Rapid weight loss will definitely include muscle loss. Make sure you meet your protein needs to maintain muscle mass and still eat enough carbohydrate to get through a training session without tiredness. Be very wary of limiting your fluids to try to make your skin tighter. Dehydration will affect your training and your thinking.

During Competition

In a training session of two hours, you will need to replace fluid lost as sweat. Water is probably all you need, unless you are a heavy sweater and prone to cramping; in that case, a sports drink will be helpful with its extra sodium. A sports drink will also help keep up blood glucose during really tough training sessions. Sweat loss may not be a lot in an air-conditioned gym; it could be 1,000 millilitres an hour, though, if you are training outside in the heat. Because most training sessions are likely to be less than three hours long, there is no need for snacks during training.

After Competition

Eat a meal that focuses upon carbohydrate to replace glycogen stores used in muscle contraction, and protein to help repair the small amount of muscle damage caused during strength training. You may even find a protein drink useful if it is going to be over an hour before you can get a meal. Naturally, also replace fluid losses with water or other non-alcoholic drinks such as tea, coffee, low-fat milk or a soft drink (low joule if you are trying to control your weight). As mentioned earlier, you could take a sports drink if your training session was particularly strenuous. If you are still hungry after a meal, eat fruit, fruit salad and low-fat yogurt, chicken and salad, open sandwiches with lean meat, or sardines on toast. These choices are usually more nutritious and cheaper than the expensive protein supplements marketed to strength athletes.

Summary

Strength and sprint training does require a little more protein than the average person eats. Wise food choices can usually provide all the protein and carbohydrate you need. Be wary of the many supplements that are marketed to strength athletes and bodybuilders. Most are of no value, promising a lot and delivering little.

Considering the characteristics of your sport will guide you towards the best nutrition strategies. You need to eat for good health because no supplement will counter the problems of unhealthy eating. Make sure you are well hydrated because your body cannot adapt to dehydration and poor drinking habits. The timing of snacks, meals and fluid intake is critical to your success. I recommend that you read the nutrition information provided by your professional sports body, institutes of sport and well-respected websites such as the Australian Institute of Sport and Sports Dietitians Australia. This nutrition advice comes from experienced professionals you can trust. If you are getting serious about your sport and plan to enter into the elite category, get personal advice from sport dietitians, sports physicians and exercise physiologists, along with a sports psychologist to get mentally prepared. Some nutritional supplements can help, but don't expect them to elevate you into the elite level. Good luck!

Nutrient Ready Reckoner

This chart provides a list of common foods with their protein, fat, carbohydrate and energy content. The alcohol content of common drinks is also included. Follow this list of foods as you record all that you eat and drink for a day, and gauge your protein, carbohydrate, fat and alcohol intake. I suggest you do this for three consecutive days and take a daily average. Because new foods are constantly being released onto the market and other foods may be reformulated, you also need to check labels for nutrient profiles. Fast-food chains regularly add new products, delete others, and change the recipe and serve sizes of their items. Check their websites for the latest nutrition profiles because most of them happily declare the protein, total fat, saturated fat, total carbohydrate, sugar and sodium content of their foods. If you want to know the fat and kilojoule content of foods not listed, check the websites given at the end of this appendix, or go to the food company website—many now provide the nutrition information of all of their products. There are phone apps that scan the bar code and give you a nutrition summary of the food. These can be helpful when shopping.

Notes:

- All protein, fat and carbohydrate figures are in grams.
- All measurements are metric (metric cups and spoons are available from supermarkets at little cost).
- Spoon measurements are level (flat).
- Numbers given are rounded numbers and in many cases can only be approximate values because the nutrition profile varies depending on cooking method, processing method and brand name.

Food	Protein	Fat	Carbohydrate	Calories	Kilojoules
FRUIT—FRESH, CANNED, DRIED, JUICES					
Apple, canned, 1 cup	1	0	22	92	385
Apple, 1 med.	0	0	14	56	235
Apple juice, 200 mL	0	0	21	84	350
Apricot, canned, 1 cup	2	0	21	92	385
Apricot, dried, 1/2 cup	3	0	30	132	550
Apricot, 1 med.	0	0	4	16	65
Avocado, 1/2 med.	2	27	0	250	1,050
Banana, 1 med., peeled	2	0	22	96	400
Blackberry, canned, 1 cup	2	0	36	152	635
Blueberry, canned, 1 cup	2	0	41	172	720
Cherry, 10 (40 g)	0	0	5	20	85
Fig, dried, 2 pieces (30 g)	1	0	16	68	285
Fig, 1 med.	0	0	3	12	50
Fruit juice, av., 200 mL	0	0	20	80	335
Fruit juice drink, 200 mL	0	0	20	80	335
Fruit salad, canned, 1 cup	1	0	24	100	420
Fruit salad, fresh, 1 cup	2	0	31	132	550
Grapes, 1 cup	1	0	25	104	435
Grapefruit, 1/2	1	0	5	24	100
Grapefruit juice, 200 mL	1	0	12	52	215
Honeydew, no skin, 1 cup	1	0	11	48	200
Kiwi fruit, 1 med.	1	0	8	36	150
Lychees, canned, 1/2 cup	1	0	20	84	350
Mandarin, 1 med.	1	0	6	28	115
Mango, 1 med.	1	0	19	80	335
Mixed fruit, dried, 1 cup	3	1	98	413	1,730
Nectarine, 1 med.	1	0	6	28	115
Nectarine, canned, 1 cup	2	0	15	68	285
Orange, 1 med.	2	0	12	56	235
Orange juice, 200 mL	0	0	17	68	285
Paw paw, no skin, 1 cup	1	0	10	44	185
Peach, 1 med.	1	0	6	28	115
Peach, canned, 1 cup	2	0	19	84	350
Pear, 1 med.	0	0	18	72	300

Food	Protein	Fat	Carbohydrate	Calories	Kilojoules
Pear, canned, 1 half	0	0	6	24	100
Pineapple, canned, 1 ring	0	0	4	16	65
Pineapple, fresh, 1 slice	1	0	9	40	165
Plum, 1 med.	0	0	6	24	100
Plum, canned, 1/2 cup	0	0	25	100	420
Prune, 10	2	0	35	148	620
Raspberry, canned, 1/2 cup	1	0	18	76	320
Rockmelon, 1 cup	1	0	8	36	150
Strawberry, 1 cup	2	0	4	24	100
Sultanas, 1/4 cup	1	0	35	144	600
Tangerine, 1 med.	1	0	6	28	115
Watermelon, 1 cup	1	0	10	44	185

BREAKFAST CEREALS

Food	Protein	Fat	Carbohydrate	Calories	Kilojoules
Allbran, 1 cup	9	3	27	171	715
Branflakes, 1 cup	6	1	28	145	605
Breakfast bars—see snack foods					
Cornflakes, 1 cup	2	0	25	108	450
Fibre Plus, 1 cup	4	1	30	145	605
Fruity Bix, 10	3	1	29	137	575
Good Start, 2	5	3	32	175	730
Healthwise, 45 g	4	1	23	117	490
Just Right, 1 cup	4	1	36	169	705
Mini Wheats, 20 (40 g)	4	0	32	144	605
Muesli, Swiss style, 1 cup	15	12	65	428	1,790
Muesli, toasted, 1 cup	9	15	50	371	1,555
Muesli, untoasted, 1 cup	7	7	45	271	1,135
Nutrigrain, 1 cup	6	0	22	112	470
Nut Feast, 45 g	4	4	26	156	655
Oat bran, 1 tbsp	2	1	6	41	170
Porridge, 1 cup	4	3	20	123	515
Puffed Wheat, 1 cup	3	0	14	68	285
Rice Bubbles, 1 cup	1	0	18	76	320
Rolled oats, 1/2 cup	5	4	31	180	755
Shredded Wheat, 2	5	0	42	188	785
Special K, 1 cup	8	0	29	148	620

▶ continued

▶ *continued*

Food	Protein	Fat	Carbohydrate	Calories	Kilojoules
BREAKFAST CEREALS (CONTINUED)					
Sports Plus, 1 cup	4	1	32	153	640
Sustain, 1 cup	6	2	50	242	1,015
Weet-Bix, Vita Brits, 2	4	1	20	105	440
Weetabix, 2	5	1	27	134	570
Weeties, 1 cup	12	2	65	326	1,365
Wheat germ, 20 g	4.5	1.5	6	60	255
Wheat bran, unproc., 1 tbsp	1	0	1	8	35
LEGUMES AND GRAINS					
Baked beans, canned, 1 cup	10	1	25	149	625
Chickpeas, cooked, 1 cup	13	4	26	192	805
Flour, 1 cup, av.	16	2	85	422	1,765
Kidney beans, canned, 1 cup	15	1	30	189	790
Lentils, boiled, 1 cup	14	1	19	141	590
Lentils, canned, 1/2 cup	7.5	1	24	139	580
Millet, 100 g	11	4	63	355	1,490
Quinoa, 100 g	12	7	62	375	1,570
Refried beans, canned, 1/2 cup	5.5	0.5	11	82	345
Soybeans, canned, 1 cup	19	12	4	200	840
Three-bean mix, canned, 1 cup	14	1	30	185	775
VEGETABLES					
Asparagus, 3 spears	0.5	0	2	10	42
Beans, green, 1/2 cup	0.5	0	2	10	42
Beetroot, 2 slices av., 60 g	1	0	5	24	100
Broccoli, 2 florets	1.5	0	1	10	42
Cabbage, 1/2 cup	0.5	0	1.5	8	35
Capsicum, 1/2 cup, chopped	1	0	1.5	10	42
Carrot, 1 cup	1	0	8	36	150
Cauliflower, 1/2 cup	2	0	2	16	70
Champignons, 1/2 cup	1	0	2	12	50
Cucumber, 4 slices, 30 g	0	0	1	4	17
Eggplant, 2 slices, 60 g	0.5	0	1.5	8	35
French fries, 100 g	4	15	20	231	965
Lettuce, 1 cup, shredded	0.5	0	0.5	4	17
Mushrooms, 1/2 cup	1.5	0	1	10	42

Food	Protein	Fat	Carbohydrate	Calories	Kilojoules
Mushrooms, canned, butter sauce, 100 g	1.5	1	5	35	145
Peas, green, cooked, 1 cup	9	1	9	81	340
Parsnip, cooked, 1/2 cup	1	0	7	32	135
Potato, boiled, 1 med. (120 g)	3	0	16	76	320
Potato, baked, 1 med.	3	8	16	148	620
Potato, mashed, 1 cup	6	1	30	153	640
Potato chips, 100 g	4	7	20	159	665
Potato chips, 10 oven fries	3	4	24	144	605
Potato wedges, 100 g	4	9	20	177	740
Pumpkin, boiled, 1 cup	6	2	18	114	475
Pumpkin, baked, 100 g	7	7	22	179	750
Sweet potato, cooked, 1 cup	4	0	40	176	735
Sweet corn, kernels, 1 cup	5	2	30	158	660
Tomato, 1 med. (100 g)	1	0	2	12	50
Zucchini, 100 g	1	0	2	12	50

RICE AND PASTA

Food	Protein	Fat	Carbohydrate	Calories	Kilojoules
Continental Rice meal, av., 1 cup	7	5	52	281	1,175
Pasta, boiled, 1 cup	8	1	50	241	1,010
Rice, steamed, 1 cup	5	1	50	229	960
Spaghetti, canned, 1 cup	5	1	30	149	625
Tortellini, cheese and spinach, 1 cup	16	8	58	368	1,540
Rice cakes, 1	1	0	10	44	185

RICE AND PASTA SAUCES

Food	Protein	Fat	Carbohydrate	Calories	Kilojoules
Chicken Tonight, 1/2 cup, av.	2	5	10	93	390
Coconut milk, lite, 50 mL	0	7	2	71	295
Coconut cream, 50 mL	0.8	9.5	2	96	400
Dolmio, chunky, 1/2 cup, av.	2	0	14	64	270
Dolmio, heat and serve, 1/2 cup, av.	2	2	10	66	275
Leggo's, stir through, av. serve	2	8	8	96	400

BREADS, BISCUITS AND CAKES

Breads

Food	Protein	Fat	Carbohydrate	Calories	Kilojoules
Bread, 1 slice, (30 g)	3	1	15	81	340
Bread roll, 1 med. (60 g)	6	1	27	141	590
Crumpet, 1	3	0	20	92	385

▶ continued

► *continued*

Food	Protein	Fat	Carbohydrate	Calories	Kilojoules
Breads (continued)					
Fruit bun, 1 med. (80 g)	7	3	40	215	900
Fruit bread, 1 slice (30 g)	2	1	15	77	320
Garlic bread, 2 slices	6	10	32	242	1,015
Lebanese bread, 1 circle	10	3	57	295	1,235
Muffin, 1 English style (80 g)	7	1	28	149	625
Scone, av. (50 g)	4	5	25	161	675
Cakes					
Black forest cake, 100 g	4	19	40	347	1,450
Cheesecake, large slice (120 g)	5	23	42	395	1,655
Fruit cake, 1 slice (50 g)	2	5	28	165	690
Lamington, 1 (75 g)	4	9	36	205	860
Mudcake, 100 g	3	16	38	308	1,290
Rock cake, av. (50 g)	3	8	29	200	835
Swiss roll, 1 slice (30 g)	1	2	19	98	410
Vanilla slice, 130 g	4	15	35	291	1,220
Biscuits, crackers					
Biscuit, ginger, 1	0	1	7	37	155
Biscuit, plain, sweet, 1	1	2	7	50	210
Biscuit, chocolate chip, 1	1	4	9.5	78	325
Biscuit, choc. coated, 1	1.2	5	12	95	400
Crispbread, 2 av.	1	0	8	36	150
Digestive biscuit, 20 g	1	4	14	87	365
Pretzels, 20 sticks	1	1	8	45	190
Rice crackers, 10	1	0	14	60	250
Ryvita, 2	2	0	13	60	250
Water crackers, 4 av.	2	2	12	114	475
Pastry, pies					
Apple pie, 150 g	4	15	40	311	1,300
Croissant, 65 g	7	15	23	255	1,065
Danish pastry, 1	8	16	36	320	1,340
Doughnut, 50 g	3	10	20	182	760
DAIRY FOODS, SOY MILK, TOFU					
Brie, Camembert, 30 g	6	8	0	96	400
Cheese, hard, av., 30 g	7	9	0	109	455

Food	Protein	Fat	Carbohydrate	Calories	Kilojoules
Cottage cheese, 30 g	4	2	0	34	140
Cream cheese, 30 g	3	10	1	114	475
Feta, 30 g	5	7	0	83	345
Ice cream, 1 scoop	2	5	10	93	390
Milk, skim/non-fat, 200 mL	8	0	12	80	335
Milk, reduced-fat, 200 mL	8	4	12	116	485
Milk, whole, 200 mL	7	8	9	136	570
Milk, evaporated, 200 mL	16	16	23	300	1,255
Milk, evaporated skim, 200 mL	16	1	23	165	690
Milk, flavoured, 300 mL, av.	12	6	25	202	845
Milk powder, whole, 3 tbsp	8	8	11	148	620
Milk powder, skim, 3 tbsp	11	0	15	104	435
Parmesan, 30 g	11	9	0	125	525
Processed cheese, av., 30 g	6	8	0	96	400
Ricotta, quark, 30 g	3	3	1	43	180
Yogurt, skim, plain, 200 mL	14	0	12	104	435
Yogurt, skim, flavoured, 200 mL	10	0	26	144	605
Yogurt, reg., plain, 200 mL	12	9	9	165	690
Yogurt, reg., flavoured, 200 mL	9	4	25	172	720

SOY PRODUCTS

Food	Protein	Fat	Carbohydrate	Calories	Kilojoules
So Good, 200 mL	7	7	9	137	575
So Good Lite, 200 mL	7	1	12	85	355
So Good, flavoured, 200 mL	7	6	14	138	580
Tofu, firm, 100 g	5	2	6	62	260
Tofu, Thai style, 100 g	18	9	5	173	1,725

DRINKS

Food	Protein	Fat	Carbohydrate	Calories	Kilojoules
Cordial (1:4 dilute), 200 mL	0	0	15	60	250
Drinking chocolate powder, 25 g	1	1.5	20	98	410
Dry ginger ale, 200 mL	0	0	17	68	285
Energy drinks, 240 mL	0	0	27	108	450
Flavoured milk, 300 mL	12	6	25	202	845
Fruit juice, av., 240 mL	0	0	30	120	500
Fruit juice drinks, 240 mL	0	0	30	120	500
Gatorade, 500 mL	0	0	30	120	500
Horlicks powder, 25 g	2.5	1	20	99	415

▶ continued

▶ *continued*

Food	Protein	Fat	Carbohydrate	Calories	Kilojoules
DRINKS (CONTINUED)					
Lucozade Sport, 500 mL	0	0	32	128	530
Milo, AktaVite, Ovaltine, av., 1 tbsp, 10 g	1	1	6	33	140
Mineral water, flavoured, 375 mL	0	0	42	168	705
Powerade, 500 mL	0	0	40	160	670
Soft drink, diet, 375 mL	0	0	0	0	0
Sports water, 240 mL	0	0	6	24	100
Sports water, low joule, 240 mL	0	0	0	0	0
Soda water, 200 mL	0	0	0	0	0
Soft drink, av., 375 mL	0	0	40	160	670
Sports drink, av., 500 mL	0	0	30	120	500
Staminade, 240 mL	0	0	18	72	300
Sustagen Sport, 1 flat tbsp, 15 g	3	0	11	58	244
Sustagen Sport, 240 mL	18	0	49	268	1,120
Up&Go, 250 mL	9	6	36	178	740
Tonic water, 200 mL	0	0	17	68	285
Hot chocolate, powder, 20 g	2.5	2.5	12	79	335
Water, plain mineral	0	0	0	0	0
SNACK FOODS					
Solid snacks					
Apricots, 5, dried	1	0	15	64	270
Breakfast bar, av.	2	3	28	147	615
Cereal bar, av.	2	0.5	27	120	500
Fresh fruit, av.	1	0	15	64	270
Muesli and nut bar, 40 g, av.	3.5	7.5	20	162	680
Fruit bars, 50 g, av.	1	0	30	124	520
Fruit strap, 1 strap, 15 g	0.5	0	11	50	210
Fruit bun, 1 med.	7	3	40	215	900
Jelly beans, 10	0	0	30	120	500
Marathon bar, 55 g, av.	11	7	54	323	1,350
Potato crisps, 50 g	3	16	24	252	1,055
Power bar, 55 g	10	2	42	226	945
Raisin bread, 1 slice	2	1	15	77	320
Rice crackers, 1	1	0	10	44	185
Sultanas, 1/4 cup	1	0	35	144	605

Food	Protein	Fat	Carbohydrate	Calories	Kilojoules
Oven baked fruit bar, av.	1	1	29	129	540
Uncle Tobys muesli bar, av.	2	3	22	123	515
Uncle Tobys Twist bar, av.	2	1	30	137	575
DESSERTS AND YOGURTS					
Frûche, 1 carton, 130 g	10	4	19	152	635
Frûche Lite, 1 carton, 130 g	8	1	18	105	440
Fromais, reg., 175 g	6	10	33	246	1,030
Fromais, light 175 g	8	2	26	154	645
Crème caramel, 150 g	6	6.5	29	198	830
Ice cream, 2 scoops	4	10	20	186	780
Ski Double UP, 200 g	8	1.5	36	189	790
Yogurt, reg., 200 g	10	6	32	222	930
Yogurt, low-fat, 200 g	10	0	36	184	770
Yogurt, diet, 200 g	10	0	14	96	400
Yoplait, reg., 200 g	9	2	16	118	495
Yoplait, light, 200 g	10	0	16	104	435
Yogurt, non-fat, flavoured, 200 mL	10	0	26	144	605
JAM, MARMALADE, JELLY					
Glucodin, 1 tbsp	0	0	16	64	270
Honey, 1 tbsp	0	0	22	88	370
Jelly, reg., 1/2 cup	2	0	19	84	350
Jelly, low-joule, 1/2 cup	2	0	0	8	33
Marmalade, jam, 1 tbsp	0	0	14	56	235
Mayonnaise, 1 tbsp	0	6	4	70	295
Popcorn, 1 cup	1	2	4	28	115
Sugar, glucose, 1 tsp	0	0	4	16	65
Vegemite, 1 tsp	1	0	0	4	17
FAT AND OILS					
Butter, 1 tbsp	0	16	0	144	600
Copha, 1 tbsp	0	20	0	180	755
Margarine, reg., 1 tbsp	0	16	0	144	600
Margarine, reduced-fat, 1 tbsp	0	8	0	72	300
Oils, 1 tbsp	0	20	0	180	755
NUTS AND SEEDS					
Almonds, 25 g	4	13	1	137	575

▶ continued

▶ continued

Food	Protein	Fat	Carbohydrate	Calories	Kilojoules
NUTS AND SEEDS (CONTINUED)					
Brazil nuts, walnuts, 25 g	3	17	0	165	690
Cashews, 25 g	4	13	4	149	625
Peanut butter, 1 tbsp (30 g)	7	15	3	175	735
Peanuts, 25 g	6	12	3	144	605
Sesame seeds, 30 g	6	15	0	159	665
Sunflower seeds, 30 g	7	14	0	154	645
Tahini, 30 g	6	18	0	186	780
EGGS, MEAT, CHICKEN AND SEAFOOD					
Black pudding, 100 g	10	22	17	300	1,255
Chicken, leg, lean, 100 g	27	10	0	198	830
Chicken breast, lean, 100 g	28	5	0	157	655
Crab, 100 g	12	1	0	57	240
Egg, 1 whole, 50 g	7	6	0	82	345
Egg white, from 1 egg, 40 g	4	0	0	16	67
Egg yolk, from 1 egg, 20 g	3	6	0	66	276
Fish, av., cooked, 100 g	22	5	0	133	555
Fish, canned, brine, 100 g	22	5	0	133	555
Fish, canned, oil, 100 g	22	15	0	223	935
Ham, canned/cured, 30 g	5	2	0	38	160
Lobster, prawn, 100 g	22	1	0	97	405
Luncheon meats, av., 30 g	4	10	0	106	445
Meat, lean, av., cooked, 100 g	27	8	0	180	755
Mussels, 12 boiled	20	2	0	98	410
Oysters, 6 raw	6	1	0	33	140
Paté, 1 tbsp (20 g)	4	5	0	61	255
Pork pie, 100 g	11	26	24	365	1,520
Sausage, 100 g	15	20	5	260	1,090
Scallops, 6 steamed	13	1	0	61	255
Scotch egg, 1 whole, 100 g	12	16	13	240	1,005
Tuna, canned, salsa, 100 g	19	5	3	133	555
Tuna, canned, Thai, 100 g	18	11	5	191	800
SAUCES, GRAVY					
Barbeque sauce, 1 tbsp	0	0	9	36	150
Chilli sauce, 1 tbsp	0	0	4	16	65

Food	Protein	Fat	Carbohydrate	Calories	Kilojoules
Gravy, commercial, 1 tbsp	1	2	2	30	125
Soy sauce, 1 tbsp	1	0	0.5	6	25
Tomato sauce, 1 tbsp	0	0	5	20	85
Tartare sauce, 30 mL	0	8	4	88	370
Worcestershire sauce, 1 tbsp	0	0	4	16	65

TAKE-AWAYS

Subway Australia and United Kingdom

Food	Protein	Fat	Carbohydrate	Calories	Kilojoules
Chicken salad	17	2.7	7.4	126	526
Chicken teriyaki, 6 in.	23	4.5	42	306	1,280
Italian BTM, 6 in.	20.5	15	37	323	1,560
Subway Melt	22	11	38	349	1,470
Subway Club, 6 in.	17.4	4.8	37	269	1,130
Turkey wrap	12.5	6	39	283	1,180
Roast beef, 6 in.	17	4	37	260	1,190
Veggie Delite, 6 in.	9	2.5	35	205	859

Hungry Jacks Australia

Food	Protein	Fat	Carbohydrate	Calories	Kilojoules
Chicken nuggets, 6	14	11.5	18.5	232	974
Chicken wrap	14.5	28	40	472	1,977
Fries, reg.	5	16	42	336	1,409
Fries, large	6	19	51	409	1,713
Hashbrowns	1.6	8	17	160	673
Shake, strawberry, med.	12.4	10.7	69	424	1,776
Whopper	30	40	49	688	2,882

Red Rooster Australia

Food	Protein	Fat	Carbohydrate	Calories	Kilojoules
Peri peri wrap	24.5	11.5	46	394	1,650
Chicken roll	35	21	54	650	2,722
Fish burger	15	13.5	32.5	320	1,340
Burger, fries and Coke	20	30	68	939	3,930
Chicken, bacon and egg wrap	25	20	33	418	1,750

Chicken Treat Australia

Food	Protein	Fat	Carbohydrate	Calories	Kilojoules
1/2 chicken and chips	67	53	14	1,113	4,660
Chicken cheese burger	21	21	46	440	1,842
Hot chicken roll	37.5	24.5	56.5	612	2,565
Roast potato, 100 g	4.5	2.5	10.5	87	365
Chicken nuggets, 6	16.5	15.5	21	286	1,200

▶ continued

▶ *continued*

Food	Protein	Fat	Carbohydrate	Calories	Kilojoules
Taco Bell					
Beef enchirito	13	21	31	360	1,505
Chalupa supreme beef	14	24	31	370	1,550
Chicken burrito supreme	21	12	51	400	1,675
Chilli cheese burrito	16	18	40	390	1,630
Double Decker taco supreme	14	15	40	350	1,465
Gordita supreme steak	14	11	29	270	1,130
Nachos	4	20	31	330	1,380
Soft taco, beef	10	10	21	210	880
McDonald's Australia					
Bacon and Egg McMuffin	16.5	13.5	26	297	1,240
Big Mac	25	27	35	493	2,060
Cheeseburger	15	12.5	26.5	284	1,190
Double cheeseburger	26	23	27.5	430	1,800
Seared chicken Caesar wrap	28	23	40	397	1,660
Filet-o-fish	13.5	13	31.5	303	1,270
French fries, small	2.5	13.5	28.5	303	1,070
French fries, medium	4	20	41.5	255	1,540
French fries, large	5	24.5	51	368	1,900
Garden salad	1.2	0	1.5	453	64
McFlurry, double choc. fudge	8	15	74	15	1,960
McNuggets, 6	16	18	13.5	468	1,160
Milkshake, choc., med.	12	10	67.5	415	1,740
Quarter Pounder	33.5	30	33.5	549	2,300
Sausage McMuffin	15	12	25.5	277	1,160
KFC Australia and New Zealand					
Original recipe chicken, 2 pieces	33.7	29	13	449	1,880
Zinger burger	27.5	18	45.5	460	1,930
Original burger	27	14.5	42	412	1,724
Chicken nuggets, 6	17	15.5	13	260	1,090
Fries/chips, large	8.5	25	74	573	2,400
Mashed potato and gravy, reg.	1.7	3.2	10	79	329
Wicked wing, 3 pieces	20	28	16.5	395	1,657

Food	Protein	Fat	Carbohydrate	Calories	Kilojoules
PIZZA HUT AUSTRALIA AND NEW ZEALAND					
Deep pan pizza					
Cheese, 1 slice	10.5	10.5	25	243	1,017
Hawaiian, 1 slice	10	8.5	24.5	217	907
Super supreme, 1 slice	10.7	15	35	227	949
Veggie supreme, 1 slice	8	7	25.5	203	850
Thin 'n crispy pizza					
BBQ chicken, 1 slice	9	6	19.5	169	708
Pepperoni, 1 slice	7.5	7.5	15.5	145	608
Super supreme, 1 slice	9	7	17.5	172	721
Veggie supreme, 1 slice	7	45	16.5	139	581
OTHER TAKE-AWAYS					
Cheesecake, 1 piece	6	22	30	342	1,430
Fish, battered, 1 piece	21	23	20	371	1,555
French fries, reg.	5	23	52	435	1,820
Hot potato chips	4	13	25	233	975
Meat pie	15	26	34	430	1,800
Meat pie, party size	3	7	8	107	450
Sausage roll, large	10	23	32	375	1,570
Sausage roll, party size	4	8	8	120	500
Wedges, reg.	4	20	50	396	1,660
CONFECTIONERY					
Boiled lollies, 1 av.	0	0	5	20	85
Chocolate, dark, 100 g	5	29	63	533	2,230
Chocolate, milk, 100 g	8	28	57	512	2,145
Cadbury Lite, 100 g	5	28	7	300	1,255
Chocolate, milk with nuts, 100 g	11	30	53	526	2,200
Caramello, 100 g	6	22	62	470	1,965
Jelly beans, 1	0	0	3	12	50
Jelly snakes, 1	0	0	4	16	67
Mars bar, 60 g	2	11	42	275	1,150
Mars bar lite, 45 g	2	5	29	169	705
Snickers bar, 60 g	6	13	36	285	1,195
Turkish Delight, 55 g	1	5	40	209	875

▶ *continued*

▶ continued

	Alcohol	Fat	Carbohydrate	Kilojoules	Calories
ALCOHOL					
Beer (per 375 mL)					
Beer, full strength	15	0	9	590	141
Beer, mid-strength	10	0	10	460	110
Beer, light, 2% alcohol	7	0	0	205	49
Spirits (per 30 mL)					
Spirits	10	0	0	295	70
Mixed drinks (per 375 mL)					
Bourbon and cola	15	0	30	940	225
Bundaberg rum and cola	18	0	40	1,195	286
Gin and tonic	15	0	32	975	233
Jim Beam and cola	18	0	37	1,145	274
Vodka, lime and lemon	15	0	35	1,025	245
Wine (per 120 mL glass)					
Champagne	10	0	3	345	82
Red wine	10	0	2	325	78
Sweet white wine	10	0	5	375	90
White wine	10	0	2	325	78
Fortified wine					
Port, 60 mL	10	0	7	410	98

Notes:1 standard drink = 10 g alcohol; 1 alcohol unit = 8 g alcohol (UK); No protein or fat is present in the alcoholic drinks in this table. Abbreviations: reg. = regular; tbsp = tablespoon; tsp = teaspoon; med. = medium; av. = average; choc. = chocolate; mL = millilitres; unproc. = unprocessed.

Data from: Food labels; Food company websites: Food Standards Australia and New Zealand. NUTTAB 2010 Online Version. www.foodstandards.gov.au/consumerinformation/nuttab2006/onlineversionintroduction/onlineversion.cfm.

Food Standards Agency. 2002. McCance and Widdowson's the composition of foods. 6th summary ed. Cambridge, UK: Royal Society of Chemistry. Pennington J.A.T., and J.S. Douglass. 2009. Bowes and Church's food values of portions commonly used. 19th ed. Baltimore: Lippincott Williams and Wilkins. U.S. Department of Agriculture National Nutrient Database.

Glossary

Adequate Intake (AI)—Indicates the amount of a nutrient required each day based on the best available data. It is not as precise as an RDA or an RDI (both in this glossary), which are based on more definitive data.

aerobic—An adjective to describe any activity that requires oxygen to be performed. In practical terms, this includes any activity that takes longer than 90 seconds. Aerobic activity improves fitness and endurance, and uses both glucose (via glycogen) and fat as a fuel.

amino acids—The building blocks of protein. Just as house bricks can be constructed into a house, so amino acids can be constructed into proteins. Amino acids are classified as either dispensable (previously known as nonessential) or indispensable (previously known as essential). The body can make dispensable amino acids, whereas indispensable amino acids must be provided by the diet.

anabolic—Meaning 'to build up'. Growing through childhood and repairing a wound are examples of anabolism. The term *anabolic* is most commonly heard when referring to anabolic steroids, drugs that promote muscle build-up. Unfortunately, anabolic steroids have serious side effects. (*Anabolic* is the opposite to *catabolic*, which means 'to break down'; during illness or insufficient food, the body becomes catabolic).

anaerobic—An adjective to describe any activity that doesn't require oxygen. In practical terms, this includes any activities that take less than 90 seconds, such as sprints and lifting weights. Most sports involve some anaerobic activity (e.g., a short sprint to catch a ball), but performing many sprints within a game requires aerobic fitness. Anaerobic activities use mainly glucose as a fuel.

antioxidant—An umbrella term for a range of compounds that may help to slow the aging process, protect against disease, and help the body to recover from exercise. Antioxidants are produced by the body and found in foods such as fruit, vegetables, mushrooms, nuts and grains.

ATP—Adenosine triphosphate. This molecule provides the energy for muscle contraction. ATP is manufactured from the metabolism of glucose.

beta-alanine—When combined with the amino acid histidine, beta-alanine creates carnosine, a natural buffer to the acid generated by sprint activity. Beta-alanine supplements may help the buffering effect.

bicarbonate—An acid buffer. Supplements of bicarbonate may help the body to buffer the acid produced by sprint activity.

caffeine—A stimulant naturally found in tea, coffee, the cocoa bean, the kola nut and the guarana plant. There is good evidence that caffeine can improve athletic endurance.

calcium—An essential mineral required for bone structure. Nearly all of the body's calcium is found in the bones and teeth. Only 1 per cent is found in blood, nerves and muscles for blood clotting and normal nerve and muscle function. Calcium requires vitamin D for absorption from food.

carbohydrate—A combination of carbon, hydrogen and oxygen to form either starches (bread, rice, potatoes) or sugars (glucose, fructose, sucrose). Often abbreviated to *carbs* or CHO (for carbon, hydrogen and oxygen).

carnitine—A supplement that was long promoted as helping reduce body fat and improving sports performance. Research could not back the claims. Not recommended.

carnosine—A compound in the body that helps to buffer acids generated by sprint activity. It is found in foods such as fish and chicken breast. Supplements of beta-alanine can increase carnosine levels in the body.

chondroitin—A compound found in joint cartilage. Supplements of chondroitin and glucosamine are taken to improve joint health and diminish osteoarthritis, although the balance of research has not shown a clear benefit to taking them.

chromium—A mineral that is part of the glucose tolerance factor that helps insulin work effectively. Often sold as chromium picolinate, it was thought to aid glycogen production and increase body fat loss, but research refuted the claims. Not recommended.

colostrum—The first milk produced by mammals after the birth of their young. It is high in immune factors needed by infants. Research continues as to whether supplements of cow colostrum assist the immune system of athletes.

creatine—A compound that helps the body to generate ATP quickly. Supplements of creatine can assist in sports that involved repeated sprints and repetitions (i.e., weight training).

Dietary Reference Intake (DRI)—A term used in the United States and Canada for the amount of each nutrient that will cover the health needs of virtually everyone. Because DRIs are set higher than the true needs of the body to give a margin of safety, they are not minimal requirements. The DRIs include the Recommended Dietary Allowances (RDAs) and Adequate Intakes (AIs). The RDA is based on many years of research; the AI is based on the best available data to date.

electrolyte drinks—Salts are electrolytes, and in commercial terms, electrolyte drinks are those that contain sodium and potassium. Most also contain carbohydrate in the form of sugars. Also known as sports drinks.

endurance—Usually, any continuous aerobic activity that takes longer than 60 minutes is a test of endurance fitness. The use of the term is subjective. Someone just starting a fitness program might consider 30 minutes an endurance test.

ergogenic—A term commonly used to imply performance enhancing. It's from the Greek words *ergon* ('work') and *genesis* ('create'). Most nutritional ergogenic aids don't live up to their claims.

fat—Also known as lipid. A concentrated source of kilojoules that is found in many foods including oils (100 per cent fat), butter and margarine (80 per cent fat), cheese, biscuits, cakes, pastries, fried and deep-fried foods, many take-aways, sausages, salami, devon, full-cream milk and yogurt.

glucosamine—A compound found in joint cartilage. It is thought that supplements of glucosamine and chondroitin may augment joint health in athletes, although the research has not yet established a benefit.

glutamine—An amino acid thought to increase muscle mass and boost immune function. The balance of the research does not support of this belief.

glycogen—A chain of glucose molecules stored in the liver and muscles to be used as an efficient fuel for muscle contraction. Glycogen is manufactured from the carbohydrate foods in our diet. When glycogen stores are low, fatigue sets in because the body has to rely on the less efficient fat as a major fuel.

HMB—Hydroxy methylbutyrate has been used as a bodybuilding aid for many years. Although thought to reduce muscle breakdown during training, there has been little scientific support for this supplement.

iron—An essential mineral important in the production of hemoglobin, a protein that transports oxygen to cells. Too little iron is a cause of anemia and tiredness.

maximum heart rate—The heart rate, or pulse, that you achieve at your highest exercise intensity. It is calculated at about 220 beats per minute, minus your age in years (it drops with age). It is commonly recommended that for fitness and good health you train at 60 to 80 per cent of your maximum heart rate, but this is a guide only and not a biological law.

If you are 30:
220 – 30 = 190
60 to 80% of 190 = 114 to 152

If you are 40:
220 – 40 = 180
60 to 80% of 180 = 108 to 144

If you are 50:
220 – 50 = 170
60 to 80% of 170 = 102 to 136

mitochondria—Very small (20,000 laid end to end would measure a millimetre) compartments in each cell of the body. They are the centre of energy production where ATP is transformed into energy. Larger numbers are found in muscle cells.

nitrate—Early research suggests that nitrate supplements (often taken as beetroot juice) make the body use oxygen more efficiently and improve endurance and time trial times.

Nutrient Reference Values (NRV)—A term used in the United States, the UK, Canada, Australia and New Zealand. It includes the estimated average requirement or the Adequate Intake of essential nutrients. From this the Dietary Reference Intakes (which include the Recommended Dietary Allowances in the United States and Canada), the Recommended Dietary Intakes (Australia and New Zealand) and the Reference Nutrient Intakes (UK) are determined. The NRV also includes an upper intake limit above which the intake of a nutrient, usually as a supplement, could be detrimental to health.

osteopenia—Reduced bone mass. It can occur in female athletes who stop menstruating. Further bone loss can lead to early osteoporosis.

osteoporosis—A condition in which bone mass drops and bones become brittle and more likely to break as a result of minor injury.

placebo effect—The perceived positive effect of an inactive substance purely because the user believes in its value. The term *placebo* comes from the Latin word meaning 'I shall please'.

potassium—An essential mineral found predominantly in plant foods and needed for normal fluid balance in cells. A diet with adequate potassium helps keep blood pressure normal.

probiotics—A general term for non-pathogenic bacteria present in foods (e.g., yogurt) and pass through the stomach and small intestine to live in the large bowel. Healthy bacteria in the large bowel assist both bowel and general health. Research on probiotics and athletes' immune function are ongoing.

protein—An essential nutrient made from chains of amino acids. Protein is found in large amounts in meat, fish, cheese, yogurt, milk (but not butter) and eggs. About 30 per cent of the protein in our diet comes from bread, breakfast cereals, rice, pasta and legumes.

Recommended Dietary Allowance (RDA)—A term used in the United States and Canada for the amount of each nutrient that will cover the health needs of virtually everyone. Because they are set higher than the true needs of the body to give a margin of safety, they are not minimal requirements.

Recommended Dietary Intake (RDI)—A term used in Australia and New Zealand for the amount of each nutrient that will cover the health needs of virtually everyone. Because they are set higher than the true needs of the body to give a margin of safety, they are not minimal requirements.

Reference Nutrient Intake (RNI)—A term used in the UK for the amount of each nutrient that will cover the health needs of virtually everyone. Because they are set higher than the true needs of the body to give a margin of safety, they are not minimal requirements.

sodium—A mineral that is a part of salt (sodium chloride) and other food additives such as monosodium glutamate. The sodium levels in foods can be found in the nutrition information panel on food labels.

ultra-endurance events—Events for the committed athlete prepared to do many hours of training. The ironman triathlon is a 3.8-kilometre (2.4-mile) swim, 180-kilometre (112-mile) bike ride, followed by a marathon (42 km, or 26 miles).

vitamins—Essential compounds that cannot be made by the body and therefore are required in the diet. The exception is vitamin D, which can be generated when the skin is exposed to sunlight. Vitamins are necessary for normal metabolic function. A diet low in vitamins over extended periods causes ill health. All the vitamins were discovered between 1912 and 1948.

zinc—An essential mineral widely distributed within the body. Too little in the diet impairs the immune function, possibly leading to frequent illness.

ZMA—Zinc magnesium aspartate was promoted with the view that athletes are low in zinc and magnesium. There is little evidence to support its use as a supplement.

References

Chapter 1 Nutrition and Fuel Systems for Sport

Australian Bureau of Statistics. 1998. *National nutrition survey: Nutrient intakes and physical measurements.* Canberra: Commonwealth of Australia.

Kirkendall, D.T. 1993. Effects of nutrition on performance in soccer. *Medicine & Science in Sports & Exercise* 25 (12): 1370-1374.

Mann, J., and A.S. Truswell. 2007. *Essentials of human nutrition.* Oxford: Oxford University Press.

Manore, M., and J. Thompson. 2000. *Sport nutrition for health and performance.* Champaign, IL: Human Kinetics.

Position of the American Dietetic Association, Dietitians of Canada and the American College of Sports Medicine: Nutrition and Athletic Performance. 2009. *Journal of the American Dietetic Association* 109 (3): 509-527.

Valtin, H. 2002. 'Drink at least eight glasses of water a day'. Really? Is there scientific evidence for '8 × 8'? *American Journal of Physiology* 283: R993-R1004.

Whitney, E.R., and S.R. Rolfes. 2005. *Understanding nutrition.* 10th ed. Belmont, CA: Wadsworth.

Chapter 2 Protein for Growth and Maintenance

Antonio, J., and J.R. Stout. 2002. *Supplements for strength-power athletes.* Champaign, IL: Human Kinetics.

Coultate, T. 2009. Food. The chemistry of its components. Cambridge: The Royal Society of Chemistry.

Fricker, P.A., S.K. Beasley and I.W. Copeland. 1988. Physiological growth hormone responses of throwers to amino acids, eating and exercise. *Australian Journal of Science and Medicine in Sport* March: 21-23.

Hayes, A. and P.J. Cribb. 2008. Effect of whey protein isolate on strength, body composition and muscle hypertrophy during resistance training. *Current Opinions in Clinical Nutrition and Metabolic Care* 11: 40-44

Lambert, M.I., J.A. Hefer, R.P. Millar and P.W. Macfarlane. 1993. Failure of commercial oral amino acid supplements to increase serum growth hormone concentrations in male bodybuilders. *International Journal of Sport Nutrition* 3: 298-305.

Manninen, A.H. 2004. Protein hydrolysates in sports and exercise: A brief review. *Journal of Sports Science and Medicine* 3: 60-63.

Paul, G.L. The rationale for consuming protein blends in sports nutrition. 2009. *Journal of the American College of Nutrition* 28 (4): 464S-472S

Position of the American Dietetic Association, Dietitians of Canada and the American College of Sports Medicine: Nutrition and Athletic Performance. 2009. *Journal of the American Dietetic Association* 109 (3): 509-527.

Saunders, M.J., M.D. Kane and M.K. Todd. 2004. Effects of a carbohydrate-protein beverage on cycling endurance and muscle damage. *Medicine & Science in Sports & Exercise* 36: 1233-1238.

Silk, D.B.A. 1980. Use of a peptide rather than free amino acid nitrogen source in chemically defined 'elemental' diets. *Journal of Parenteral and Enteral Nutrition* 4 (6): 548-553.

Tarnopolsky, M. 2010. Protein and amino acid needs for training and bulking up. In L. Burke and V. Deakin, eds., *Clinical Sports Nutrition.* North Ryde: McGraw-Hill Australia.

Tipton, K.D., and R.R. Wolfe. 2001. Exercise, protein metabolism, and muscle growth. *International Journal of Sport Nutrition and Exercise Metabolism* 11: 109-132.

Chapter 3 Carbohydrate for Energy

Atkinson, F.S., K. Foster-Powell and J.C. Brand-Miller. 2008. International tables of glycemic index and glycemic load values: 2008. *Diabetes Care* 31 (12). http://care.diabetesjournals.org/content/31/12/2281/suppl/DC1.

Bergström J., and E. Hultman. 1966. Muscle glycogen synthesis after exercise: An enhancing factor localised to the muscle cells in man. *Nature* 210: 309-310.

Brand-Miller, J., T.M.S. Wolever, K. Foster-Powell and S. Colagiuri. 2007. *The new glucose revolution*. 3rd ed. New York: Marlowe & Company.

DeMarco, H.M., K.P. Sucher, C.J Cisar and G.E. Butterfield. 1999. Pre-exercise carbohydrate meals: Application of the glycemic index. *Medicine & Science in Sports & Exercise* 31: 164-170.

Donaldson, C.M., T.L. Perry and M.C. Rose. 2010. Glycemic Index and endurance performance. *International Journal of Sport Nutrition and Exercise Metabolism* 20: 154-165.

Flatt, J.-P. 1995. Use and storage of carbohydrate and fat. *American Journal of Clinical Nutrition* 61 (Suppl): 952S-959S.

Hawley, J.A., and L.M. Burke. 1997. Effect of meal frequency and timing on physical performance. *British Journal of Nutrition* 77 (Suppl): S91-S103.

McWhirter, N. (Ed). 1980. *Guinness book of records*. 27th ed. Middlesex: Guinness Superlatives.

Position of the American Dietetic Association, Dietitians of Canada and the American College of Sports Medicine: Nutrition and Athletic Performance. 2009. *Journal of the American Dietetic Association* 109 (3): 509-527.

Sherwood, S. 2001. *Human physiology*. 4th ed. Pacific Grove, CA: Brooks/Cole.

Chapter 4 Calcium, Iron and Vitamins for Health and Performance

AIS Sports Supplement Program Website Fact Sheet August 2011 http://www.ausport.gov.au/__data/assets/pdf_file/0008/446723/Multivitamins11_-_Website_fact_sheet.pdf.

Beard, J. 2002. Iron status and exercise. *American Journal of Clinical Nutrition* 72 (Suppl): 594S-597S.

Clarkson, P. 1995. Antioxidants and physical performance. *Critical Reviews in Food Science and Nutrition* 35 (1 and 2): 131-141.

Cobiac, L., and K. Baghurst. 1993. Iron status and dietary iron intakes of Australians. *Food Australia* (Suppl) April.

Constantini, N.W., R. Arieli, G. Chodick and G. Dubnov-Raz. 2010. High prevalence of vitamin D insufficiency in athletes and dancers. *Clinical Journal of Sport Medicine* 20: 368-371.

Fogelholm, M. 1994. Vitamins, minerals and supplementation in soccer. *Journal of Sports Sciences* 12: S23-S27.

Hallberg, L., and L. Hulthén. 2000. Prediction of dietary iron absorption: An algorithm for calculating absorption and bioavailability of dietary iron.

American Journal of Clinical Nutrition 71: 1147-1160.

Institute of Medicine. 2010. Dietary reference intakes for calcium and vitamin D (http://www.iom.edu/Reports/2010/Dietary-Reference-Intakes-for-Calcium-and-Vitamin-D.aspx).

Lönnerdal, B. 2010. Calcium and iron absorption: Mechanisms and public health relevance. *International Journal for Vitamin and Nutrition Research* 80 (4-5): 293-299.

Multivitamins and Minerals. AIS Sports Supplement Website Fact Sheet. Australian Institute of Sport. August 2011. http://www.ausport.gov.au/__data/assets/pdf_file/0008/446723/Multivitamins11_-_Website_fact_sheet.pdf.

Nielsen, P., and D. Nachtigall. 1998. Iron supplementation in athletes. *Sports Medicine* 26: 207-216.

Nutrient reference values for Australia and New Zealand. Executive summary. Commonwealth of Australia 2006. Canberra.

Peake, J.M. 2003. Vitamin C: Effects of exercise and requirements with training. *International Journal of Sport Nutrition and Exercise Metabolism* 13: 125-151.

Piantadosi, C.A. 2006. 'Oxygenated' water and athletic performance. *British Journal of Sports Medicine*. 40: 740.

Position of the American Dietetic Association, Dietitians of Canada and the American College of Sports Medicine: Nutrition and Athletic Performance. 2009. *Journal of the American Dietetic Association* 109 (3): 509-527.

Report of the Panel on Dietary Reference Values of the Committee on Medical Aspects of Food Policy. 1991. London: Her Majesty's Stationery Office.

Sports Dietitians Australia. 2010. Fact sheet: Bone health. Melbourne: Sports Dietitians Australia. www.sportsdietitians.com.au/content/2540/BoneHealth.

Sports Dietitians Australia. 2009. Fact sheet: Iron depletion in athletes. Melbourne: Sports Dietitians Australia. www.sportsdietitians.com.au/resources/upload/Iron_depletion_in_athletes.pdf.

Chapter 5 Liquids for Hydration, Cooling and Energy

American College of Sports Medicine Position Stand. 2007. Exercise and fluid replacement. *Medicine & Science in Sports & Exercise* 39 (2): 377-390.

Armstrong, L.E., D.L. Costill and W.J. Fink. 1985. Influence of diuretic-induced dehydration on competitive running performance. *Medicine & Science in Sports & Exercise* 14: 456-461.

Australian Institute of Health and Welfare. 2010. *Australia's health 2010*. Canberra: Australian Institute of Health and Welfare.

Australian Institute of Sport. 2009. Fact sheet: Fluid—

who needs it? www.ausport.gov.au/ais/nutrition/factsheets/hydration2/fluid_-_who_needs_it.

Bar-Or, O. 1994. Children's responses to exercise in hot climates: Implications for performance and health. *Sports Science Exchange* 77 (2).

Brouns, F., J. Senden, E.J. Beckers and W.H.M. Saris. 1995. Osmolarity does not affect the gastric emptying rate of oral rehydration solutions. *Journal of Parenteral and Enteral Nutrition* 19 (5): 403-406.

Burdon, C.A., H.T. O'Connor, J.A. Gifford and S.M. Shirreffs. 2010. Influence of beverage temperature on exercise performance in the heat: A systematic review. *International Journal of Sports Nutrition and Exercise Metabolism.* 20 (2): 166-174.

Cox, G.R., E.M. Broad, M.D. Riley and L.M. Burke. 2002. Body mass changes and voluntary fluid intakes of elite level water polo players and swimmers. *Journal of Science and Medicine in Sport* 5 (3): 183-193.

Davis, M.J., D.A. Jackson, M.S. Broadwell, J.L. Queary and C.L. Lambert. 1997. Carbohydrate drinks delay fatigue during intermittent, high-intensity cycling in active men and women. *International Journal of Sport Nutrition* 7: 261-273.

Epstein, Y., and L.E. Armstrong. 1999. Fluid-electrolyte balance during labor and exercise: Concepts and misconceptions. *International Journal of Sport Nutrition* 9: 1-12.

Fixx J. 1978. *Jim Fixx's second book of running.* New York: Random House.

Gardner, J.W. 2002. Death by water intoxication. *Military Medicine* 167 (5): 432-434.

Gisolfi, C.V. 1995. Effect of sodium concentration in a carbohydrate-electrolyte solution on intestinal absorption. *Medicine & Science in Sports & Exercise* 27: 1414-1420.

Gore, C.J., P.C. Bourdon, S.M. Woolford and D.G. Pederson. 1993. Involuntary dehydration during cricket. *International Journal of Sports Medicine* 14: 387-395.

Hargreaves, M. 1996. Physiological benefits of fluid and energy replacement during exercise. *Australian Journal of Nutrition and Dietetics* 53 (4 Suppl): S3-S7.

Hew-Butler T., J.C. Ayus, C. Kripps, R.J. Maughan, S. Mettler, W.H. Meeuwisse, A.J. Page, S.A. Reid, N.A. Rehrer, W.O. Roberts, I.R. Rogers, M.H. Rosner, A.J. Siegal, D.B. Speedy, K.J. Stuempfle, J.G. Verbalis, L.B. Weschler and P. Wharam. 2008. Statement of the 2nd International Exercise-Associated Hyponatremia Consensus Development Conference, New Zealand, 2007. *Clinical Journal of Sports Medicine* 18: 111-121.

Institute of Medicine, Food and Nutrition Board. 2004 Press release. www8.nationalacademies.org/onpinews/newsitem.aspx?RecordID=10925.

International Olympic Committee Consensus Statement on Sports Nutrition 2010 http://www.olympic.org/Documents/Reports/EN/CONSENSUS-FINAL-v8-en.pdf.

Jeukendrup, A.E. 2010. Carbohydrate and exercise performance: The role of multiple transport carbohydrates. *Current Opinion in Clinical Nutrition and Metabolic Care* 13: 452-457.

Luetkemeier, M.J., M.G. Coles and E.W. Askew. 1997. Dietary sodium and plasma volume levels with exercise. *Sports Medicine* 23: 279-286.

Lyle, D.M., P.R. Lewis, D.A.B. Richards, R. Richards, A.E. Bauman, J.R. Sutton and I.D. Cameron. 1994. Heat exhaustion in the Sun-Herald City to Surf fun run. *Medical Journal of Australia* 161: 361-365.

Maughan, R.J., and J.B. Leiper. 1995. Sodium intake and post-exercise rehydration in man. *European Journal of Applied Physiology and Occupational Physiology* 71 (4): 311-319.

Maughan, R.J., and J. Griffin. 2003. Caffeine ingestion and fluid balance: A review. *Journal of Human Nutrition and Dietetics.* 16: 411-420.

Meyer, F., O. Bar-Or, A. Salsberg, D. Passe. 1994. Hypohydration during exercise in children: effect on thirst, drink preferences, and hydration. *International Journal of Sport Nutrition* 4 (1): 22-35.

Millward A., L. Shaw, E. Harrington and A.J. Smith. 1997. Continuous monitoring of salivary flow rate and pH at the surface of the dentition following consumption of acidic beverages. *Caries Research* 31: 44-49.

Milosevic A. 1997. Sports drinks hazard to teeth. *British Journal of Sports Medicine* 31: 28-30 (see also responses: Brouns F., and L. Muntjewerf. 1997 Sports drinks and teeth. *British Journal of Sports Medicine* 31: 258; and Murray R. 1997. Sports drinks and teeth. *British Journal of Sports Medicine* 31: 352.

Morton, D.P., and R. Callister. 2000. Characteristics and etiology of exercise-related transient abdominal pain. *Medicine & Science in Sports & Exercise* 32: 432-438.

Morton, D.P., and R. Callister. 2002. Factors influencing exercise-related transient abdominal pain. *Medicine & Science in Sports & Exercise* 34: 745-749.

Moss, S.J. 1998. Dental erosion. *International Dental Journal* 48: 529-539.

National Health and Medical Research Council. 2009. Australian guidelines to reduce health risks from drinking alcohol. Canberra: Commonwealth of Australia.

National Health and Medical Research Council. 2003. Dietary guidelines for Australian adults. A guide to healthy eating. Canberra: Commonwealth of Australia.

Passe, D.H., M. Horn and R. Murray. 1997. The effects of beverage carbonation on sensory responses and voluntary fluid intake following exercise. *International Journal of Sport Nutrition* 7: 286-297.

Ploutz-Snyder, L., J. Foley, R. Ploutz-Snyder, J. Kanaley, K. Sagendorf and R. Meyer. 1999. Gastric gas and fluid emptying assessed by magnetic resonance imaging. *European Journal of Applied Physiology and Occupational Physiology* 79: 212-220.

Plunkett, B.T. and W.G. Hopkins. 1999. Investigation of the side pain 'stitch' induced by running after fluid ingestion. *Medicine & Science in Sports & Exercise* 31: 1169-1175.

Position of the American Dietetic Association, Dietitians of Canada and the American College of Sports Medicine: Nutrition and Athletic Performance. 2009. *Journal of the American Dietetic Association* 109 (3): 509-527.

Rehrer, N.J. 1996. Factors influencing fluid bioavailability. *Australian Journal of Nutrition and Dietetics* 53 (4 Suppl): S8-S12.

Rehrer, N.J., and L.M. Burke. 1996. Sweat losses during various sports. *Australian Journal of Nutrition and Dietetics* 53 (4 Suppl): S13-S16.

Saunders, M.J., M.D. Kane and M.K. Todd. 2004. Effects of a carbohydrate-protein beverage on cycling endurance and muscle damage. *Medicine & Science in Sports & Exercise* 36 (7): 1233-1238.

Schwellnus, M.P. 2009. Cause of Exercise Associated Muscle Cramps (EAMC) —Altered neuromuscular control, dehydration or electrolyte depletion? *British Journal of Sports Medicine* 43: 401-408.

Shi, X., and D.H. Passe. 2010. Water and solute absorption from carbohydrate-electrolyte solutions in the human proximal small intestine: A review and statistical analysis. *International Journal of Sport Nutrition and Exercise Metabolism* 20: 427-442.

Shi, X., R.W. Summers, H.P. Schedl, S.W Flanagan, R. Chang and C.V. Gisolfi. 1995. Effects of carbohydrate type and concentration and solution osmolality on water absorption. *Medicine & Science in Sports & Exercise* 27: 1607-1615.

Shirreffs, S.M., A.J. Taylor, J.B. Leiper and R.J. Maughan. 1996. Post-exercise rehydration in man—Effects of volume consumed and drink sodium content. *Medicine & Science in Sports & Exercise* 28 (10): 1260-1271.

Skillen, R.A., M. Testa, E.A. Applegate, E.A. Heiden, A.J. Fascetti and G.A. Casazza. 2008. Effects of an amino acid-carbohydrate drink on exercise performance after consecutive-day exercise bouts. *International Journal of Sport Nutrition and Exercise Metabolism* 18: 473-492.

Stearns, R.L., H. Emmanuel, J.S. Volek and D.J. Casa. 2010. Effects of ingesting protein in combination with carbohydrate during exercise on endurance performance: A systematic review with meta-analysis. *Journal of Strength & Conditioning Research* 24 (8): 2192-2202.

Vist, G.E., and R.J. Maughan. 1995. The effect of osmolality and carbohydrate content on the rate of gastric emptying of liquids in man. *Journal of Physiology* 486: 523-531.

Walsh, R.M., T.D. Noakes, J.A Hawley and S.C. Dennis. 1994. Impaired high-intensity cycling performance time at low levels of dehydration. *International Journal Sports Medicine* 15: 392-398.

Wongkhantee, S., V. Patanapiradej, C. Maneenut and D. Tantbirojn. 2005. Effect of acidic food and drinks on surface hardness of enamel, dentine, and tooth-coloured filling materials. *Journal of Dentistry* 34 (3): 214-220.

Chapter 7 Digestion and Timing of Meals

Bergeron, M.F. 1996. Heat cramps during tennis: A case report. *International Journal of Sport Nutrition* 6: 62-68.

Maughan, R. 2010. Fluid and carbohydrate intake during exercise. In L. Burke and V. Deakin, eds., *Clinical sports nutrition.* North Ryde: McGraw-Hill Australia.

Morton, D.P., D. Richards and R. Callister. 2005. Epidemiology of exercise-related transient abdominal pain at the Sydney City to Surf community run. *Journal of Science & Medicine in Sport* 8 (2): 152-162.

Sherwood, L. 2001. *Human physiology.* 4th ed. Pacific Grove, CA: Brooks/Cole.

Whitney, E.R., and S. R. Rolfes. 2005. *Understanding nutrition.* 10th ed. Belmont, CA: Wadsworth.

Stofan, J.R., J.J. Zachwieja, C.A. Horswill, R. Murray, S.A. Anderson and E.R. Eichner. 2005. Sweat and sodium losses in NCAA football players: A precursor to heat cramps? *International Journal of Sport Nutrition and Exercise Metabolism* 15: 641-652.

Chapter 8 What to Eat and Drink Before, During and After Exercise

Burke, L.M., G.R. Collier and S.K. Beasley. 1995. Effect of co-ingestion of fat and protein with CHO feedings on muscle glycogen storage. *Journal of Applied Physiology* 78: 2187-2192.

Burke, L., and V. Deakin, eds. 2010. *Clinical sports nutrition.* 4th ed. North Ryde: McGraw-Hill Australia.

Fallon, K.E., E. Broad, M.W. Thompson and P.A. Reull. 1998. Nutritional and fluid intake in a 100 km ultramarathon. *International Journal of Sport Nutrition* 8: 24-35.

Hawley, J.A., and L.M. Burke. 1997. Effect of meal frequency and timing on physical performance. *British Journal of Nutrition* 77 (Suppl): S91-S103.

Ivy, J.L., H.W. Goforth, B.M. Damon, T.R. McCauley, E.C. Parsons and T.B. Price. 2002. Early postexercise muscle glycogen recovery is enhanced with a carbohydrate-protein supplement. *Journal of Applied Physiology* 93: 1337-1344.

Kang, J., R.J Robertson, B.G. Denys, S.G. DaSilva, P. Visich, R.R. Suminski, A.C. Utter, F.L. Goss and K.F. Metz. 1995. Effect of carbohydrate ingestion subsequent to carbohydrate supercompensation on endurance performance. *International Journal of Sport Nutrition* 5: 329-343.

Lucia, A., C. Earnest and C. Arribas. 2003. The Tour de France: A physiological review. *Scandinavian Journal of Medicine and Science in Sports* 13: 275-283.

Position of the American Dietetic Association, Dietitians of Canada and the American College of Sports Medicine: Nutrition and Athletic Performance. 2009. *Journal of the American Dietetic Association* 109 (3): 509-527.

Saris, W.H. 1990. The Tour de France: Food intake and energy expenditure during extreme sustained exercise. *Cycling Science* 2 (4): 17-21.

Stroud, M.A., P. Ritz, W.A. Coward, M.B. Sawyer, D. Constantin-Teodosiu, P.L. Greenhaff and I.A. Macdonald. 1997. Energy expenditure using isotope-labelled water ($^2H_2$ ^{18}O), exercise performance, skeletal muscle enzyme activities and plasma biochemical parameters in humans during 95 days of endurance exercise with inadequate energy intake. *European Journal of Applied Physiology* 76: 243-252.

Zawadski, K.M., B.B. Yaspelkis and J.L. Ivy. 1992. Carbohydrate-protein complex increases the rate of muscle glycogen storage after exercise. *Journal of Applied Physiology* 72 (5): 1854-1859.

Chapter 9 Nutritional Supplements

American Dietetic Association. n.d. Supplements and ergogenic aids for athletes. www.eatright.org/Public/content.aspx?id=7088.

Antonio, J., and J.R. Stout. 2002. *Supplements for endurance athletes*. Champaign, IL: Human Kinetics.

Antonio, J., and J.R. Stout. 2002. *Supplements for strength-power athletes*. Champaign, IL: Human Kinetics.

Armstrong, L.E. 2002. Caffeine, body fluid-electrolyte balance, and exercise performance. *International Journal of Sport Nutrition and Exercise Metabolism* 12: 189-206.

Artioli, G.G., B. Gualano, A. Smith, J. Stout and A.H. Lancha. 2010. Role of β-alanine supplementation on muscle carnosine and exercise performance. *Medicine & Science in Sports & Exercise* 42 (6): 1162-1173.

Australian Institute of Sport. 2011. AIS Sports Supplement Program 2011. http://www.ausport.gov.au/ais/nutrition/supplements/overview2.

Bahrke, M.S, W.P. Morgan and A. Stegner. 2009. Is ginseng an ergogenic aid? *International Journal of Sports Nutrition and Exercise Metabolism* 19: 298-322.

Bailey, S.J., P. Winyard, A. Vanhatalo, J.R. Blackwell, F.J. DiMenna, D.P. Wilkerson, J. Tarr, N. Benjamin and A.M. Jones. 2009. Dietary nitrate supplementation reduces the O2 cost of low-intensity exercise and enhances tolerance to high-intensity exercise in humans. *Journal of Applied Physiology* 107: 1144-1155.

Beedie, C.J., and A.J. Foad. 2009. The placebo effect in sports performance. *Sports Medicine* 39 (4): 313-329.

Brilla, L.R., and V. Conte. 2000. Effects of a novel zinc-magnesium formulation on hormones and strength. *Journal of Exercise Physiology* 3: 26-36.

British Dietetic Association. n.d. Food fact sheets. www.bda.uk.com/foodfacts/index.html#supplements.

Broad, E.M., R.J. Maughan and S.D.R. Galloway. 2008. Carbohydrate, protein, and fat metabolism during exercise after oral carnitine supplementation in humans. *International Journal of Sport Nutrition and Exercise Metabolism* 18: 567-584.

Brouns, F., and G.J. van der Vusse. 1998. Utilisation of lipids during exercise in human subjects: Metabolic and dietary constraints. *British Journal of Nutrition* 79: 117-128.

Buckley, J.D., M.J. Abbott, G.D. Brinkworth, P.B. White. 2002. Bovine colostrum supplementation during endurance running training improves recovery, but not performance. *Journal of Science and Medicine in Sport* 5 (2): 65-79.

Buford, T.W., R.B. Kreider, J.R. Stout, M. Greenwood, B. Campbell, M. Spano, T. Ziegenfuss, H. Lopez, J. Landis and J. Antonio. 2007. International Society of Sports Nutrition position stand: Creatine supplementation and exercise. *Journal of the International Society of Sports Nutrition* 4: 6 www.jissn.com/content/4/1/6.

Burke, L. 1995. The complete guide to food for sports performance. Allen & Unwin, St. Leonards. Australia.

Burke, L. 2008. Caffeine and sports performance. *Applied Physiology, Nutrition, and Metabolism* 33: 1319-1334.

Burke, L., and V. Deakin, eds. 2010. *Clinical sports nutrition*. 4th ed. North Ryde: McGraw-Hill Australia.

Candow, D.G., P.D. Chilibeck, D.G. Burke, K.S. Davison and T. Smith-Palmer. 2001. Effect of glutamine supplementation combined with resistance training in young adults. *European Journal of Applied Physiology* 86: 142-149.

Clancy, S.P., P.M. Clarkson, M.E. De Cheke, K. Nosaaka, P.S. Freedson, J.J. Cunningham and B. Valentine. 1994. Effects of chromium picolinate supplementation on body composition, strength, and urinary chromium loss in football players. *International Journal of Sport Nutrition* 4: 142-153.

Clark, K.L, W. Sebastianelli, K.R. Flechsenhar, D.F. Aukermann, R.L. Millard, J.R. Deitch, P.S. Sherbondy and A. Albert. 2008. 24-week study on the use of collagen hydrolysate as a dietary supplement in athletes with activity-related joint pain. *Current Medical Research Opinion* 24 (5): 1485-1496.

Clarkson, P.M. 1997. Effects of exercise on chromium levels. *Sports Medicine* 23: 341-349.

Clarkson, P.M. 1996. Nutrition for improved sports performance. *Sports Medicine* 21: 393-401.

Cox, A.J., D.B. Pyne, P.U. Saunders and P.A. Fricker. 2010. Oral administration of the probiotic Lactobacillus fermentum VRI-003 and mucosal immunity in endurance athletes. *British Journal of Sports Medicine* 44 (4): 222-226.

Dalbo, V.J., M.D. Roberts, R.J Stout and C.M. Kerksick. 2010. Putting to rest the myth of creatine supplementation leading to muscle cramps and dehydration. *British Journal of Sports Medicine.* 42: 567-573.

Davidson, G., and B.C. Diment. 2010. Bovine colostrum supplementation attenuates the decrease of salivary lysozyme and enhances the recovery of neutrophil function after prolonged exercise. *British Journal of Nutrition* 103: 1425-1432.

Derave, W., I. Everaert, S. Beeckman and A. Baguet. 2010. Muscle carnosine metabolism and β-alanine supplementation in relation to exercise and training. *Sports Medicine* 40 (3): 247-263.

Desbrow, B., R. Hughes, M. Leveritt and P. Scheelings. 2007. An examination of consumer exposure to caffeine from retail coffee outlets. *Food and Chemical Toxicology* 45: 1588-1592.

Diaz, M.L., B.A. Watkins, Y. Li, R.A. Anderson and W.W. Campbell. 2008. Chromium picolinate and conjugated linoleic acid do not synergistically influence diet- and exercise-induced changes in body composition and health indexes in overweight women. *Journal of Nutritional Biochemistry* 19: 61-68.

Dietitians Association of Australia. n.d. Nutrition A-Z. www.daa.asn.au/index.asp?pageID=2145842141.

Fiala, K.A., D.J. Casa and M.W. Roti. 2004. Rehydration with a caffeinated beverage during the non-exercise periods of 3 consecutive days of 2-a-day practices. *International Journal of Sport Nutrition and Exercise Metabolism* 14: 419-429.

Gleeson, M. 2008 Dosing and efficacy of glutamine supplementation in human exercise and sport training. *The Journal of Nutrition* 138: 2045S-2049S.

Gleeson, M., N.C. Bishop, M. Oliveira and P. Tauler. 2011. Daily probiotic's (Lactobacillus casei Shirota) reduction of infection incidence in athletes. *International Journal of Sports Nutrition and Exercise Metabolism* 21 (1): 55-64.

Greenhaff, P.L. 1995. Creatine and its application as an ergogenic aid. *International Journal of Sport Nutrition* 5: S100-S110.

Heckman, M.A., J. Weil and E.G. de Mejia. 2010. Caffeine (1,3,7-trimethylxanthine) in foods: A comprehensive review on consumption, functionality, safety, and regulatory matters. *Journal of Food Science* 75 (3): R77-R87.

Horswill, C.A. 1995. Effects of bicarbonate, citrate, and phosphate loading on performance. *International Journal of Sport Nutrition* 5: S111-S119.

International Olympic Committee Consensus Statement on Sports Nutrition 2010 http://www.olympic.org/Documents/Reports/EN/CONSENSUS-FINAL-v8-en.pdf.

Kanter, M. 1998. Free radicals, exercise and antioxidant supplementation. *Proceedings of the Nutrition Society* 57: 9-13.

Lansley, K.E., P.G. Winyard, S.J. Bailey, A. Vanhatalo, D.P. Wilkerson, J.R. Blackwell, M. Gilchrist, N. Benjamin and A.M. Jones. 2011. Acute dietary nitrate supplementation improves cycling time trial performance. *Medicine & Science in Sports & Exercise* 43 (6): 1125-1131.

Lee, Y.H., J.H. Woo, S.J. Choi, J.D. Ji and G.G. Song. 2010. Effect of glucosamine or chondroitin sulfate on the osteoarthritis progression: a meta-analysis. *Rheumatology International* 30: 357-363.

Maughan, R.J., and J. Griffin. 2003. Caffeine ingestion and fluid balance: A review. *Journal of Human Nutrition and Dietetics.* 16: 411-420.

McCusker, R.R., B.A. Goldberger and E.J.Cone. 2003. Caffeine content of specialty coffees. *Journal of Analytical Toxicology* 27: 520-522.

McGinley, C., A. Shafat and A. E. Donnelly. 2009. Does antioxidant vitamin supplementation protect against muscle damage? *Sports Medicine* 39 (12): 1011-1032.

McNaughton, L.R., J. Siegler and A. Midgeley. 2008. Ergogenic effects of sodium bicarbonate. *Current Sports Medicine Reports* 7 (4): 230-236.

Nissen, S.L. 2004 Beta-hydroxy-beta-methylbutyrate. In I. Wolinsky and J.A. Driskell, eds, *Nutritional ergogenic aids.* Boca Raton, FL: CRC Press.

Phillips, G.C. 2007. Glutamine: The nonessential amino acid for performance enhancement. *Current Sports Medicine Reports* 6: 265-268.

Piantadosi, C.A. 2006. 'Oxygenated' water and athletic performance. *British Journal of Sports Medicine.* 40: 740.

Position of the American Dietetic Association, Dietitians of Canada and the American College of Sports Medicine: Nutrition and Athletic Performance. 2009. *Journal of the American Dietetic Association* 109 (3): 509-527.

Powers, S.K., and K. Hamilton. 1999. Antioxidants and exercise. *Clinics in Sports Medicine* 18: 525-536.

Rowlands, D.S., and J.S. Thompson. 2009. Effects of beta-hydroxy-beta-methylbutyrate supplementation during resistance training on strength, body composition, and muscle damage in trained and untrained young men: A meta-analysis. *Journal of Strength and Conditioning Research* 23 (3): 836-846.

Sale, C., B. Saunders, R.C. Harris. 2010. Effect of beta-alanine supplementation on muscle carnosine concentrations and exercise performance. *Amino Acids* 39: 321-333.

Shing, C.M., D.C. Hunter and L.M. Stevenson. 2009. Bovine colostrum supplementation and exercise performance. *Sports Medicine* 39 (12): 1033-1054.

Smith, W.A., A.C. Fry, L.C. Tschume and R.J. Bloomer. 2008. Effect of glycine propionyl-l-carnitine on aerobic and anaerobic exercise performance. *International Journal of Sport Nutrition and Exercise Metabolism* 18: 19-36.

Sports Dietitians Australia. n.d. Supplements. www.sportsdietitians.com.au/content/498/Supplements.

U.S. Food and Drug Administration. n.d. Consumer education and general information on dietary supplements. www.fda.gov/food/dietarysupplements/consumerinformation/ucm110417.htm.

Volek, J.S., R. Silvestre, J.P. Kirwan, M.J. Sharman, D.A. Judelson, B.A. Spiering, J.L. Vingren, C.M. Maresh, J.L. Vanheest and W.J. Kraemer. 2006. Effects of chromium supplementation on glycogen synthesis after high-intensity exercise. *Medicine and Science in Sports and Exercise* 38 (12): 2102-2109.

Wandell, S., P. Juni, B. Tendal, E. Nüesch, P.M. Villiger, N.J. Welton, S. Reichenbach and S. Trelle. 2010. Effects of glucosamine, chondroitin, or placebo in patients with osteoarthritis of hip or knee: Network meta-analysis. *British Medical Journal* 341: c4675. doi: 10.1136/bmj.c4675.

Warren, J., and A. Dettre. 1974. Soccer in Australia. Paul Hamlyn Pty Ltd, Dee Why West. Australia.

Webb, A.J., N. Patel, S. Loukogeorgakis, M. Okorie, Z. Aboud, S. Misra, R. Rashis, P. Miall, J. Deanfield, N. Benjamin, R. MacAllister, A.J. Hobbs and A. Ahluwalia. 2008. Acute blood pressure lowering, vasoprotective, and antiplatelet properties of dietary nitrate via bioconversion to nitrite. *Hypertension* 51: 784-790.

Wemple, R.D, D.R. Lamb and K.H. McKeever. 1997. Caffeine vs caffeine-free sports drinks: Effects on urine production at rest and during prolonged exercise. *International Journal of Sports Medicine* 18: 40-46.

West, N.P., D.B. Pyne, J.M. Peake and A.W. Cripps. 2009. Probiotics, immunity and exercise: A review. *Exercise Immunology Reviews* 15: 107-126.

West, N.P., D.B. Pyne, A.W. Cripps, W.G. Hopkins, D.C. Eskesen, A. Jairath, C.T. Christophersen, M.A. Conlon, P.A. Fricker. 2011. Lactobacillus fermentum (PCC®) supplementation and gastrointestinal and respiratory-tract illness symptoms: a randomised control trial in athletes. *Nutrition Journal* 10: 30.

Wilborn, C.D., C.M. Kersick, B.I. Campbell, L.W. Taylor, B.M. Marcello, C.J. Rasmussen, M.C. Greenwood, A. Almada and R.B. Kreider. 2004. Effects of Zinc Magnesium Aspartate (ZMA) supplementation on training adaptations and markers of anabolism and catabolism. *Journal of the International Society of Sports Nutrition* 1 (2): 12-20.

Williams, M.H. 1998. *The ergogenics edge*. Champaign, IL: Human Kinetics.

Wolinsky, I., and J.A. Driskell. 2004. *Nutritional ergogenic aids*. Boca Raton, FL: CRC Press.

World Anti-Doping Agency 2004 http://www.wada-ama.org/rtecontent/document/ds_english.pdf.

Yoshimura, M., K. Sakamoto, A. Tsuruta, T. Yamamoto, K. Ishida, H. Yamaguchi and I. Nagaoka. 2009. Evaluation of the effect of glucosamine administration on biomarkers for cartilage and bone metabolism in soccer players. *International Journal of Molecular Medicine* 24: 487-494.

Chapter 10 Nutrition for Vegetarian Athletes

Burke, L., and V. Deakin, eds. 2010. *Clinical sports nutrition*. 4th ed. North Ryde: McGraw-Hill Australia, pp. 602-616.

Food Standards Agency (2002) McCance and Widdowson's The Composition of Food, Sixth summary edition. Cambridge: Royal Society of Chemistry.

National Health and Medical Research Council. 2006. Nutrient Reference Values for Australia and New Zealand. Canberra: Commonwealth of Australia.

National Heart Foundation of Australia. 2009. Position statement: Dietary fats and dietary sterols for cardiovascular health. National Heart Foundation of Australia. Sydney, New South Wales.

NUTTAB 2010 Online Searchable Database; Food Standards Australia New Zealand. http://www.foodstandards.gov.au/consumerinformation/nuttab2010/nuttab2010onlinesearchabledatabase/onlineversion.cfm.

Position of the American Dietetic Association: Vegetarian diets 2009. *Journal of the American Dietetic Association* 109: 1266-1282.

Position of the American Dietetic Association, Dietitians of Canada and the American College of Sports Medicine: Nutrition and Athletic Performance. 2009. *Journal of the American Dietetic Association* 109 (3): 509-527.

Venderley, A.M., and W.W. Campbell. 2006. Vegetarian diets. Nutrition considerations for athletes. *Sports Medicine.* 36 (4): 293-305.

Chapter 11 Meal Tips for Restaurants and Road Trips

Australian Institute of Sport. 2009. AIS Sports Nutrition: Tips for surviving travel challenges. www.ausport.gov.au/ais/nutrition/factsheets/travel2/tips_for_surviving_travel_challenges.

Eastman, C.I., and H.J. Burgess. 2009. How to travel the world without jet lag. *Sleep Medicine Clinics*. 4: 241-255.

Manfredini, R., F. Manfredini, C. Fersini and F. Conconi. 1998. Circadium rhythms, athletic performance, and jet lag. *British Journal Sports Medicine* 32: 101-106.

Reilly, T., J. Waterhouse, L.M. Burke and J.M. Alonso. 2007. Nutrition for travel. *Journal of Sports Sciences*. 25 (S1): S125-S134.

Sack, R.L. 2010. Jet lag. *New England Journal of Medicine* February 4: 440-447.

Sports Dietitians Australia. 2009. Nutrition & the travelling athlete. Fact sheet. Melbourne: Sports Dietitians Australia. www.sportsdietitians.com.au/resources/upload/file/The%20Travelling%20Athlete.pdf.

Waterhouse, J., B. Edwards, A. Nevill, S. Carvalho, G. Atkinson, P. Buckley, T. Reilly, R. Godfrey and R. Ramsay R. 2002. Identifying some determinants of 'jet lag' and its symptoms: A study of athletes and other travellers. *British Journal Sports Medicine* 36: 54-60.

Chapter 12 Muscle Building and Weight Gain Strategies

Antonio, J., and J.R. Stout. 2002. *Supplements for strength-power athletes*. Champaign, IL: Human Kinetics.

Balon, T.W., J.F. Horowitz and K.M. Fitzsimmons. 1992. Effects of carbohydrate loading and weight lifting on muscle girth. *International Journal of Sport Nutrition* 2: 328-334.

Børsheim, E., A. Aarsland and R.R. Wolfe. 2004. Effect of an amino acid, protein, and carbohydrate mixture on net muscle protein balance after resistance exercise. *International Journal of Sport Nutrition and Exercise Metabolism* 14: 255-271.

Fussell, S. 1991. *Muscle: Confessions of an unlikely bodybuilder*. London: Cardinal.

International Olympic Committee Consensus Statement on Sports Nutrition 2010 http://www.olympic.org/Documents/Reports/EN/CONSENSUS-FINAL-v8-en.pdf.

Koopman, R., W.H.M. Saris, A.J.M. Wagenmakers and L.J.C. van Loon. 2007. Nutritional interventions to promote post-exercise muscle protein synthesis. *Sports Medicine*. 37 (10): 895-906.

Lambert, C.P., L.L. Frank and W.J. Evans. 2004. Macronutrient considerations for the sport of bodybuilding. *Sports Medicine* 34: 317-327.

Lukin, D. 1993, *The Dean Lukin Diet*. Margaret Gee Publishing, McMahons Point, New South Wales.

Seid, R.P. 1989. *Never Too Thin*. Prentice Hall Press, New York.

Volek, J.S., C.E. Forsythe and W.J. Kraemer. 2006. Nutritional aspects of women strength athletes. *British Journal of Sports Medicine* 40: 742-748.

Wolinsky, I., and J.A. Driskell. 2004. *Nutritional ergogenic aids*. Boca Raton, FL: CRC Press.

Chapter 13 Fat Burning and Weight Loss Strategies

Astrup, A., M.T. Larsen and A. Harper. 2004. Atkins and other low-carbohydrate diets: Hoax or an effective tool for weight loss? *Lancet* 364: 897-899.

Beals, K.A., and M.M. Manore. 1994. The prevalence and consequences of subclinical eating disorders in female athletes. *International Journal of Sport Nutrition* 4: 175-195.

Bravata, D.M., L. Sanders, J. Huang, H.M. Krumholz, I. Olkin, C.D. Gardner and D.M. Bravata. 2003. Efficacy and safety of low-carbohydrate diets. *Journal of the American Medical Association* 289: 1837-1850.

Bray, G.A., and B.M. Popkin. 1998. Dietary fat intake does affect obesity! *American Journal of Clinical Nutrition* 68: 1157-1173.

Cellulite. 2009. *Taber's Cyclopedic Medical Dictionary*. 21st edition online. www.tabers.com/tabersonline/ub/index/Tabers/Entries/. Philadelphia: F.A. Davis.

Centre for Nutrition Policy and Promotion, U.S. Department of Agriculture. 2010. Dietary Guidelines for Americans. www.cnpp.usda.gov/dietaryguidelines.htm.

Crutcher, M. 2002, February 24. Warne diets to become second leading wicket-taker. ESPN Cricinfo. www.espncricinfo.com/wctimeline/content/story/114575.html.

Fogelholm, M. 1994. Effects of bodyweight reduction on sports performance. *Sports Medicine* 18 (4): 248-267.

Food and Agriculture Organisation of the United Nations. 1998. Report of a joint FAO/WHO expert Consultation. Carbohydrates in human nutrition. FAO food and nutrition paper. Rome: Food and Agriculture Organisation.

Gades, D.M., and J.S. Stern. 2003. Chitosan supplementation and fecal fat excretion in men. *Obesity Research* 11: 683-688.

Holt, S.H.A., J.C. Brand-Miller, P. Petocz and E. Farmakalidis. 1995. A satiety index of common foods. *European Journal of Clinical Nutrition* 49: 675-690.

Jeukendrup, A., and M. Gleeson. 2010. *Sport nutrition*. Champaign, IL: Human Kinetics.

Khan, M.H., F. Victor, B. Rao and N.S. Saddick. 2010a. Treatment of cellulite. Part 1. Pathophysiology. *Journal of the American Academy of Dermatology* 62 (3): 361-370.

Khan, M.H., F. Victor, B. Rao and N.S. Saddick. 2010b. Treatment of cellulite. Part 2. Advances and controversies. *Journal of the American Academy of Dermatology* 62 (3): 373-384.

Manore, M., and J. Thompson. 2000. *Sport nutrition for health and performance*. Champaign, IL: Human Kinetics.

Movahedi, A. 1999. Simple formula for calculating basal energy expenditure. *Nutrition Research* 19: 989-995.

Ni Mhurchu, C., S.D. Poppitt, A.-T. McGill, F.E. Leahy, D.A. Bennett, B.B. Lin, D. Ormrod, I. Ward, C. Strik and A. Rodgers. 2004. The effect of the dietary supplement, Chitosan, on body weight: A randomized controlled trial in 250 overweight and obese adults. *International Journal of Obesity* 28: 1149-1156.

Phelan, S., T. Liu, A. Gorin, M. Lowe, J. Hogan, J. Fava and R.R. Wing. 2009. What distinguishes weight-loss maintainers from the treatment-seeking obese? Analysis of environmental, behavioral, and psychosocial variables in diverse populations. *Annals of Behavioral Medicine* 38: 94-104.

Position of the American Dietetic Association, Dietitians of Canada and the American College of Sports Medicine: Nutrition and Athletic Performance. 2009. *Journal of the American Dietetic Association* 109 (3): 509-527.

Rolls, B.J., and E.A. Bell. 1999. Intake of fat and carbohydrate: Role of energy density. *European Journal of Clinical Nutrition* 53: S166-S173.

Rosenbaum, M., V. Prieto, J. Hellmer, M. Boschmann, J. Krueger, R. Leibel and A. Ship. 1998. An exploratory investigation of the morphology and biochemistry of cellulite. *Plastic and Reconstructive Surgery* 101: 1934-1939.

Rossi, A.B.R., and A.L. Vergnanini. 2000. Cellulite: A review. *Journal of the European Academy of Dermatology and Venerology* 14: 251-262.

Seid, R.P. 1989. *Never Too Thin*. Prentice Hall Press, New York.

Sherwood, L. 2001. *Human physiology*. 4th ed. Pacific Grove, CA: Brooks/Cole.

Sundgot-Borgen, J. 1994. Eating disorders in female athletes. *Sports Medicine* 17 (3): 176-188.

U.S. Department of Agriculture, Center for Nutrition Policy and Promotion. 2010. Dietary Guidelines for Americans. www.cnpp.usda.gov.

Wing, R.R., and J.O. Hill. 2001. Successful weight loss maintenance. *Annual Reviews of Nutrition* 21: 323-341.

World Health Organisation. 2003. Technical Report Series 916. Joint WHO/FAO expert consultation on diet, nutrition and the prevention of chronic diseases. Geneva, Switzerland: World Health Organisation. www.who.int/hpr/NPH/docs/who_fao_expert_report.pdf.

Chapter 14 Nutrition for Selected Sports

Australian Institute of Sport. 2009. Fact Sheet Swimming http://www.ausport.gov.au/ais/nutrition/factsheets/sports/swimming.

Currell, K., S. Conway and A.E. Jeukendrup. 2009. Carbohydrate ingestion improves performance of a new reliable test of soccer performance. *International Journal of Sport Nutrition and Exercise Metabolism* 19 (1): 34-36.

International Olympic Committee Consensus Statement on Sports Nutrition 2010 http://www.olympic.org/Documents/Reports/EN/CONSENSUS-FINAL-v8-en.pdf.

Kirkendall, D.T. 1993. Effects of nutrition on performance in soccer. *Medicine & Science in Sports & Exercise* 25 (12): 1370-1374.

Maughan, R.J., L.A. Dargavel, R. Hares and S.M. Shirreffs. 2009. Water and salt balance of well-trained swimmers in training. *International Journal of Sport Nutrition and Exercise Metabolism* 19: 598-606.

Shirreffs, S.M. 2010. Hydration: Special issues for playing football in warm and hot environments. *Scandinavian Journal of Medicine and Science in Sports* 20 (Suppl 3): 90-94.

Resources

Recommended Reading

Antonio, J., and J.R. Stout. 2002. *Supplements for endurance athletes*. Champaign IL: Human Kinetics.

Antonio, J., and J.R. Stout. 2002. *Supplements for strength-power athletes*. Champaign, IL: Human Kinetics.

Brand-Miller, J., K. Foster-Powell and S. Colaguiri. 2008. *The low GI handbook*. Sydney: Hachette Australia.

Burke, L. 2007. *Practical sports nutrition*. Champaign, IL: Human Kinetics.

Burke, L., and V. Deakin, eds. 2010. *Clinical sports nutrition*. New York: McGraw-Hill.

Jeukendrup, A., and M. Gleeson. 2010. *Sport nutrition*. Champaign, IL: Human Kinetics.

Manore, M., and J. Thompson. 2000. *Sport nutrition for health and performance*. Champaign, IL: Human Kinetics.

Rolls, B., and R.A. Barnett. 2000. *Volumetrics weight control plan*. New York: Quill.

Saxelby, C. 2006. *Nutrition for life*. South Yarra: Hardie Grant Books.

For books on all aspects of sports science, including sports nutrition, contact Human Kinetics in your country for a catalogue, or go to www.humankinetics.com.

Sports Nutrition and General Nutrition Websites

American Dietetic Association

www.eatright.org

Go to the 'Food and Nutrition Information' section for good-quality resources.

Australian Institute of Sport, Department of Sports Nutrition

www.ausport.gov.au/ais/nutrition

This site has everything—stuff on supplements, recipes, resources and, of course, sports nutrition.

British Dietetic Association

www.bda.uk.com

The home of dietitians in the UK. Check out their 'Food Facts' section.

Dietitians Association of Australia

www.daa.asn.au

This site has lots of useful general nutrition information for the public.

Freelance Dietitians Group of the British Dietetic Association

www.dietitiansunlimited.co.uk

Use this site to find a sports dietitian in the UK.

Gatorade Sports Science Institute

www.gssiweb.com

A good-quality site for sports nutrition issues with a bent toward sports drinks.

Glenn Cardwell

www.glenncardwell.com

The author's own website from which you can get a free nutrition newsletter.

International Society of Sports Nutrition

www.sportsnutritionsociety.org

Lucozade Sports Science

www.lucozadesport.com

This site has lots of information on sports drinks and sports nutrition.

National Sports Medicine Institute (UK)

www.nsmi.org.uk

This site explains the causes and possible treatments for most injuries you may sustain during sport.

Nutrition Australia

www.nutritionaustralia.org

Information produced by nutrition professionals. Subscribe to their free online newsletter and check their FAQs on nutrition.

Sports, Cardiovascular, and Wellness Nutrition (USA)

www.scandpg.org

This is the website of sports dietitians in the United States. It provides nutrition advice, fact sheets and manuals.

Sports Dietitians Australia

www.sportsdietitians.com

Click on 'Fact Sheets' for free sports nutrition pdf files. This site also has information on nutrition for various sports. It is produced for the general public by sports dietitians.

Sports Dietitians UK

www.sportsdietitians.org.uk

This site has the basics of sports nutrition and tips on popular sports.

Websites About Food Labelling

Australia and New Zealand

http://www.foodstandards.gov.au/consumer-information/labellingoffood/

www.foodstandards.gov.au/consumerinformation/labellingoffood/

United Kingdom

http://food.gov.uk:80/foodlabelling/ull/

www.food.gov.uk/foodlabelling/

www.nutrition.org.uk/nutritionscience/foodfacts

www.eatwell.gov.uk/foodlabels/understand-labels/

In 2010, the responsibility for food labelling moved from the Food Standards Agency to the Department for Environment, Food and Rural Affairs, which means that website URLs could change.

United States

www.fda.gov/Food/ResourcesForYou/Consumers/ucm079449.htm

www.fda.gov/Food/LabelingNutrition/Label-Claims/default.htm

www.mayoclinic.com/health/nutrition-facts/NU00293/METHOD=print

Canada

http://www.inspection.gc.ca/english/fssa/labeti/guide/toce.shtml

www.fcpmc.com/issues/labelling/index.html

Agency Websites

European Food Information Council

www.eufic.org

Has lots of useful information on nutrition, food safety and consumer information.

Food and Drug Administration (USA)

www.fda.gov

Offers information on food additives such as sweeteners.

Food Standards Australia New Zealand

www.foodstandards.gov.au

Offers information on labelling, consumer information and food additives such as sweeteners.

Index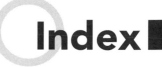

Note: The italicized *f* and *t* following page numbers refer to figures and tables, respectively.

About the Author

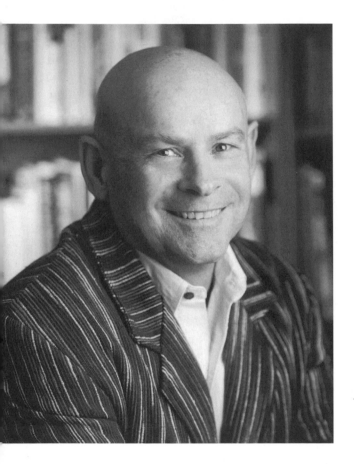

Glenn Cardwell is a qualified sports dietitian and an Accredited Practising Dietitian with more than 30 years of experience. He has advised athletes from junior ranks through elite levels, and he has run sports nutrition courses for fitness leaders, personal trainers and university students since 1986.

Cardwell was one of the first sports dietitians in Australia and helped to establish the professional organisation Sports Dietitians Australia; he served as its magazine editor for 10 years. He was the sports nutrition adviser to the West Coast Eagles (Australian Football League) for 14 seasons and the Western Force (Super 14 Rugby Union) for their first two seasons.

Cardwell has written many articles on sports nutrition for magazines and professional newsletters. In 2002 he was privileged to accompany Australian fast bowler Brett Lee to Chicago to study his sweat composition and losses. In 2003 he was made life member of Nutrition Australia for services to nutrition education. In 2011 he was given the honour of life membership of Sports Dietitians Australia for more than 25 years of service in promoting sports nutrition. He runs his own nutrition consultancy, advising international and national companies, as well as fresh produce companies.